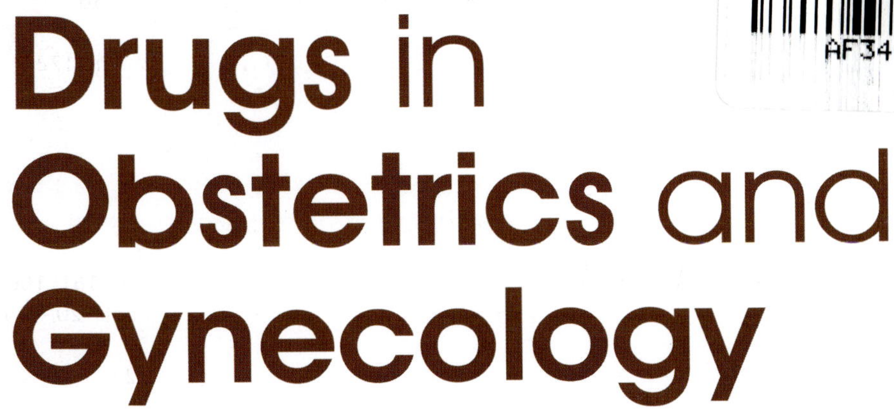

Drugs in Obstetrics and Gynecology

A Practical Approach

Part I Obstetrics

Drugs in Obstetrics and Gynecology
A Practical Approach

Part I Obstetrics

Ruchika Garg
Fellow Indian Menopause Society FIMS
Professor, Department of Gynecology
SN Medical College, Agra, India
Editor-in-Chief Journal of Midlife Health
Executive Editor Journal of SAFOG

Priya Vora Thakur
DNB, FICOG, FCPS, DFP, DGO, MBBS
Consultant, Department of Gynecology, Saint Elizabeth
Bhatia, Ruxmani and Dr Vora's Hospitals
Mumbai, India

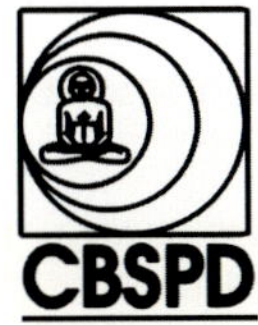

CBS Publishers & Distributors Pvt Ltd

New Delhi • Bengaluru • Chennai • Kochi • Kolkata • Lucknow • Mumbai
Hyderabad • Jharkhand • Nagpur • Patna • Pune • Uttarakhand

Drugs in Obstetrics and Gynecology
A Practical Approach

Part I Obstetrics

ISBN: 978-93-5466-855-5

Published by Satish Kumar Jain and produced by Varun Jain for

CBS Publishers & Distributors Pvt Ltd

4819/XI Prahlad Street, 24 Ansari Road, Daryaganj, New Delhi 110 002, India

Ph: 011-23289259, 23266838
Website: www.cbspd.com
Fax: 011-23243014
e-mail: delhi@cbspd.com

Corporate Office: 204 FIE, Industrial Area, Patparganj, Delhi 110 092, India
Ph: 011-49344934
Fax: 011-49344935
e-mail: publishing@cbspd.com; publicity@cbspd.com

Branches

- Bengaluru: Seema House 2975, 17th Cross, KR Road, Banasankari 2nd Stage, Bengaluru 560 070, Karnataka, India
  Ph: +91-80-26771678/79 Fax: +91-80-26771680 e-mail: bangalore@cbspd.com
- Chennai: 18/8B, Subbarayan Street, Shenoy Nagar, Chennai 600 030, Tamil Nadu, India
  Ph: +91-44-42032115, 26681266 e-mail: chennai@cbspd.com
- Kochi: 42/1325, 1326, Power House Road, Opposite KSEB, Power House, Ernakulum 682018, Kochi, Kerala, India
  Ph: +91-484-4059061–67 Fax: +91-484-4059065 e-mail: kochi@cbspd.com
- Kolkata: 147, Hind Ceramics Compound, 1st Floor, Nilgunj Road, Belghoria, Kolkata 700 056, West Bengal, India
  Ph: +91-33-25330055/56 e-mail: kolkata@cbspd.com
- Lucknow: Basement, Khushuma Complex, 7 Meerabai Marg (behind Jawahar Bhawan), Lucknow 226 001, UP, India
  Ph: +91-522-4000032 e-mail: tiwari.lucknow@cbspd.com
- Mumbai: PWD Shed, Gala No. 25/26, Ramchandra Bhatt Marg, Next JJ Hospital Gate No. 2, Opp. Union Bank of India, Noorbaug, Mumbai 400 009, Maharashtra, India
  Ph: +91-22-66661880/89 e-mail: mumbai@cbspd.com

Representatives

- **Hyderabad** 0-9885175004
- **Jharkhand** 0-9811541605
- **Nagpur** 0-8692091830
- **Patna** 0-9334159340
- **Pune** 0-9664372571
- **Uttarakhand** 0-9716462459

Printed at HT Media Ltd, Greater Noida, UP, India

Contributors

Aaishwarya R MBBS MS DNB
Assistant Professor
Department of Obstetrics and Gynecology
Seth GS Medical College and
Wadia Maternity Hospital, Mumbai

Amarjeet Kaur Bava DGO MD
Associate Professor
Department of Obstetrics and Gynecology
LTMMC and LTMGH Sion Hospital, Mumbai

Ameya Medhekar MD DTM and H CTropMed
Consultant Physician
Department of Medicine
Specialist in Tropical Medicine
Lilavati Hospital and Resem arch Centre, Mumbai

Ameya Purandare MBBS DGO FICOG DNB MD
Consultant
Department of Obstetrics and Gynecology, Bhatia
Hospital, HN Reliance, Purandare Hospitals
Naigaon Maternity Hospital, Mumbai

Anahita Chauhan MD DGO MBBS
Consultant
Department of Obstetrics and Gynecology
Saifee and St. Elizabeth Hospitals Mumbai

Arundhati Tilve DNB DGO
Assistant Professor
Department of Obstetrics and Gynecology
TNMC and BYL Nair Hospital, Mumbai

Anjaly Raj MBBS MD
Consultant, Department of Gynecology
All India Institute of Medical Sciences
New Delhi

Anusha Devalla MBBS MS DNB
Assistant Professor
Department of Obstetrics and Gynecology
All India Institute of Medical Sciences, Bibinagar
Private Practitioner
Gayatri Hospital, Ramanthapur, Hyderabad

Archana Bhosale MS DGO FCPS FICOG
Associate Professor
Department of Obstetrics and Gynecology
LTMMC and LTMGH, Sion Hospital, Mumbai

Asha Dalal MD DGO MBBS
Head, Department Obstetrics and Gynecology
Sir HN Reliance Foundation and Research Centre
Mumbai

Ashwin Shetty MD DFFP MRCOG CCST FRCOG
Consultant, Department of Obstetrics and Gynecology
Sir HN Reliance Foundation Hospital and Research
Centre, Mumbai

Ashwini Hotkar MS DNB ADART FII (Fellowship in infertility
Senior Resident
Department of Obstetrics and Gynecology
LTMMC and GH, Sion Hospital, Mumbai

Asmita Patil MS
Associate Professor and Unit In-charge
Department of Obstetrics and Gynecology
HBT Medical College and Dr RN Cooper Hospital
Mumbai

Amrita Tandon MS DNB FMAS MRM (London)
Consultant, Department of Obstetrics and
Gynecology, IVF and Endoscopic Surgeon
Dr Sudha Tandon IVF Maternity and
Gyn Endoscopy Hospital Chembur and Vashi

Avir Sarkar MBBS MD
Senior Resident
ESIC Medical College and Hospital NIIT
Faridabad

Bhavini Shah DGO DNB
Consultant
Department of Obstetrics and Gynecology
Saifee Hospital and Medical Research Centre and
Masina Hospital, Mumbai

Bhumika Kotecha Mundhe DGO DNB MNAMs FICOG
Consultant
Department of Obstetrics and Gynecology
Masina, Saifee, Ruxmani, Wockhardt,
St. Elizabeth and NH-SRCC Hospitals, Mumbai

Charumati V Pekhale MBBS DGO DNB
Infertility Specialist
Consultant, Department of Obstetrics and
Gynecology, NOVA IVF, Nasik

Devika Chopra MBBS DNB MSC (Oxford UK)
Department of Obstetrics and Gynecology
Bhatia, Elizabeth, Wockhardt
SRCC Hospitals, Mumbai

Danny Laliwala MD FCPS DGO DFP
Consultant
Department of Obstetrics and Gynecology
Jaslok Breach Candy, Saifee, Masina, Wockardt,
SRCC Hospitals, Mumbai

Ganpat Sawant
DNB DICOG DFP FCPS DGO MD
Ex-Professor and Head
Department of Obstetrics and Gynecology
DY Patil Medical College, Navi Mumbai

Geetha Agarwal CIMP FAMS MD
Consultant, Department of Obstetrics and
Gynecology, Heritage Hospital, Raipur

Geetha Balsarkar MD
Professor and Head
Department of Obstetrics and Gynecology
Seth GS Medical College, Nowrosjee Wadia
Maternity Hospital, Parel, Mumbai

Isha Wadhawan
MBBS MD MRCOG Diplomate ABOG
Consultant
Department of Obstetrics and Gynecology
Fortis Escorts Hospital, NIT, Faridabad

Indra Prasad MBBS MS
Associate Professor
Department of Obstetrics and Gynecology
All India Institute of Medical Sciences, Patna

Jagruti Ghosh MBBS DNB OBGY
Consultant
Department of Obstetrics and Gynecology
JUANA Mother and Child Care Hospital LLP
Wockhardt and Family Care Hospital, Mumbai

Jiteeka Thakkar
MBBS DGO DFP BDRME (Germany) ADRM (Germany)
Consultant
Department of Gynecology
Bloom IVF Lilavati Hospital
PPNH Opera House

Kairavi H Gokani MBBS DNB MRCOG ICOG
Consultant
Department of Gynecology
Ankur Fertility Clinic
Fellowship in Reproductive Medicine Diploma in
Reproductive Medicine and IVF (Kiel, Germany)
Fellowship in Minimal Access Surgery, Mumbai

Kedar N Ganla MBBS MD DNB FCPS DGO DFP
Consultant
Department of Obstetrics and Gynecology
Family Physician, Ankoor Fertility Clinic, Mahim,
Mumbai

Kinjal Shah MBBS DGO DNB
Consultant
Department of Obstetrics and Gynecology
Bhatia Ruxmani Hospital, Mumbai

Kiran Guleria MBBS MS
Professor and Director
Department of Obstetrics and Gynecology
UCMS and GTB Hospital, Delhi

Komal Chavan
MD DNB MNAMS FCPS DGO FICOG
Diploma in Reproductive Medicine (UK-SH)
Chairperson FOGSI Medical Disorders in Pregnancy
Committee (2019-2022)
Senior Consultant
Department of Obstetrics and Gynecology
DNB Teacher, V N Desai Hospital Mumbai

Madhuri Patel MD DGO FICOG
Secretary General, FOGSI
Hon. Consultant, Police Hospital
Visiting Consultant, St. Elizabeth Hospital, Mumbai

Madhuri Mehendale DNB FCPS DGO
Diploma in Advance Laparoscopy and Infertility
Assistant Professor
Department of Obstetrics and Gynecology
LTMMC and LTMGH Sion Hospital
Consultant, Department of Obstetrics and
Gynecology
ZYNOVA Multispeciality Hospital, Mumbai

Malavika JC MBBS MS
Associate Professor
Department of Gynecology
SS Institute of Medical Sciences and Research
Centre, Davangere, Karnataka

Manan Boob MBBS MS (ObGy)
Consultant
Department of Obstetrics and Gynecology
Subham Hi Tech Hospital, Amravati

Mandakini Megh MD DGO FICMCH FICMU FICOG
Chairperson, ICOG-FOGSI
International Vice President, MWIA Central Asia
Consultant, Department of Obstetrics and
Gynecology, Gynae-O-Care Clinic, Mumbai

Mansi Medhekar MBBS MS DNB FICOG
Consultant
Department of Obstetrics and Gynecology
Lilavati Hospital and Research Centre
SL Raheja, Fortis Hospital, Surya Hospital
Mumbai

Mamta Gupta MD (Obs. Gynae)
Consultant Gynecologist and Former Head
Department of Obstetrics and Gynecology
Hindu Rao Hospital and associated NDMC Medical
College, Delhi, India

Mala Arora FRCOG (UK) FICOG DA (UK) D OBST (Ire)
Director
Department of Obstetrics and Gynecology
Noble IVF Centre, Faridabad
Senior Consultant
Department of Obstetrics and Gynecology
Fortis La Femme GK2, New Delhi

Meenal Sarmalkar MD DGO MBBS
Associate Professor
Department of Obstetrics and Gynecology
LTMMC and LTMGH, Sion Hospital, Mumbai

Milan Balakrishnan MBBS MD
Consultant, Department of Psychiatry
Bombay Hospital and Medical Research Centre,
Mumbai

Moushmi Parpillewar Tadrs
MBBS DGO DNB FICOG FMAS
Associate Professor
Department of Obstetrics and Gynaecology
Government Medical College, Nagpur

Mukta Agarwal MBBS MD FICOG
Additional Professor
Department of Obstetrics and Gynecology
AIIMS, Patna

Neha Kamath MD DNB
Assistant Professor
Department of Obstetrics and Gynecology,
LTMMC and LTMGH Sion Hospital, Mumbai

Neha Rajji Matthews MBBS DGO DNB
Consultant
Department of Obstetrics and Gynecology
Mulund Fortis Hospital, Mumbai

Niraj Mahajan MBBS MS
Head of Unit
Department of Obstetrics and Gynecology TNMC
and BYL Nair Hospital, Mumbai

Nishita Shah MBBS DGO MD
Consultant
Department of Obstetrics and Gynecology
St. Elizabeth and Saifee Hosptials, Mumbai

Nidhi Shah DNB DGO IFCPC-IARC Colposcopy
Consultant
Department of Gynecology
Jaslok Hospital and Dr Vora's Hospitals, Mumbai

Niharika Sethi
Senior Resident
Department Obstetrics and Gynecology
VMMC and SJ Hospital, New Delhi

Pariskshit Tank
MD DNB FCPS DGO DFP MNAMS FICOG FRCOG
Consultant, Department of Obstetrics and
Gynecology, Ashwini Maternity and Surgical Hospital
and Jupiter Hospital, Mumbai

Pradnya Changede MS FICOG FCPS DGO IBCLC
Associate Professor
Department Obstetrics and Gynecology
LTMMC and LTMGH, Sion Hospital, Mumbai

Priyanka Vora MBBS DGO FCPS DFP (GOLD) BIMIE
Masters In Reproductive Medicine and IVF (UK)
Diploma in Reproductive Medicine and IVF (Kiel,
Germany)
Associate Consultant
Department of Gynecology
Ankoor Fertility Clinic, Mahim, Mumbai

Priyanka Mathe MBBS MS
Assistant Professor
Department of Obs and Gyn
UCMS and GTB Hospital, Delhi

Punit Bhojani MS DNB FICOG FCPS
Consultant
Department of Obstetrics and Gynecology
Bhojani Clinic, Consultant at Surya, SRCC, Somaiya
and Masina Hospitals, Mumbai

Purnima Satoskar MD DNB FRCOG
Consultant
Department Obstetrics and Gynecology
Jaslok Hospital
Wadia Hospital, Mumbai

Pradnya Supe MS Obs and Gyn, IBCLS
Fellowship in Laparoscopy, *Ex*-Assistant Professor
Department of Gynecology
LTMMC and LTMGH, Sion, Zen and SRV Hospitals
Mumbai

Preeti Frank Lewis MD
Associate Professor
Department Obstetrics and Gynecology
GGMC and Sir JJ Group of Hospital, Mumbai

Priti Vyas MD DGO FCPS FICOG MSC
Consultant, Department Obstetrics and Gynecology
Sangita Maternity Surgical and Diagnostic Centre
Hinduja Hospital, Surya Mother and Child Care Centre
KLS Memorial Hospital, Mumbai

Priya Vora MBBS DNB FCPS FICOG DGO DFP
Senior Consultant
Department of Obstetrics and Gynecology
Dr Vora's hospital, Saint Elizabeth, Ruxmani, Bhatia,
Wockhardt Hospitals, Mumbai

Prabhat Kumar Agrawal
Professor, Department of Medicine
SN Medical College, Agra

Pratima Verma MBBS MS
Associate Professor
Department of Gynecology
GSVM Medical College, Kanpur

Pooja Mishra MS
Senior Resident
Department of Obstetrics and Gynecology
KG Medical College, Lucknow

Rahul Mayekar MD DGO
Associate Professor and Head of Unit
Department Obstetrics and Gynecology
LTMMC and LTMGH Sion Hospital, Mumbai

Rajendra Nagarkatti MD FICOG FCPS DGO DFP
Consultant
Department of Obstetrics and Gynecology and IVF
Specialist Ashirwad Maternity and General Hospital
Mira Bhayander, Mumbai

Rajeshwari L Khyade MBBS DGO DNB FMAS
Senior Consultant and DNB Teacher
Department of Gynecology
KB Bhabha Hospital, Mumbai

Rajshree D Katke MD OBGY FICOG FMAS
Professor
Department of Obstetrics and Gynecology
Grant Government Medical College, Mumbai

Rana Choudhary
MBBS DNB DGO DFP DCR FCPS FICOG FICMCH MNAMS
Masters in Reproductive Medicine and IVF (UK)
Senior Consultant
Department of Obstetrics and Gynecology
Wockhardt Hospital, Mumbai

Rashmi Jalvee MS DGO DNB MRCOG
Assistant Professor
Department Obstetrics and Gynecology
HBT Medical College and Dr RN Cooper Hospital,
Mumbai

Rashmi Kahar MBBS DGO FICOG FICMCH
Consultant, Department of Gynecology
Kharodkar Hospital, Sai Nagar, Amaravti

Rashmi Upadhyay MBBS MS
Senior Resident, Department of Gynecology
GSVM Medical College, Kanpur
414/2 Adarsh Nagar, Manduadih, Varanasi

Reena Wani
MD FRCOG FICOG DNBE DGO DFP FCPS
Additonal Professor and Head
Department of OBGY, HBT Medical College and Dr
RN Cooper Hospital, Mumbai

Reeta Bansiwal
Professor, Department of Obstetrics and Gynecology
VMMC and Safdarjung Hospital, New Delhi

Reshma Palep MS DNB MRCS(Ed)
Consultant
Department of Gynecology
Breast Surgeon, Sir HN Reliance Saifee, Dr Palep's
Nursing Home, Mumbai

Ritu Bharadwaj MBBS MS
Junior Resident, Department Gynecology
SN Medical College, Agra

Rohan Palshetkar MS FRM IVF Specialist ADRM
(Germany) DRME (Gemany)
Consultant, Department Obstetrics and
Gynecology, Palshetkar-Patil Nursing Home Breach
Candy Hospital, Surya Hospital, Mumbai

Roopali Sehgal MBBS MS
Resident, Department of Obstetrics and Gynecology
GGMC and Sir JJ Group of Hospital, Mumbai

Ruchika Garg
Fellow Indian Menopause Society FIMS
Professor, Department of Gynecology
SN Medical College, Agra, India
Editor-in-Chief Journal of Midlife Health
Executive Editor Journal of SAFOG

Sangeeta Agrawal MD DNB DGO FRCOG
Consultant
Department of Obstetrics and Gynecology
Bhatia and Breach Candy hospital, Mumbai

Sarita Bhalerao MD DNB FRCOG
Senior Consultant
Obstetrics and Gynecology, Reliance HNH, Bhatia,
Saifee, Breach Candy Hospital St. Elizabeth, Wadia
Maternity Hospital, Mumbai

Seema Mehrotra MS
Professor, Department of Obstetrics and
Gynecology, KGMC, Lucknow

Shailesh Kore
MD DNB MNAMS FCPS DGO DFP DICOG
Head, Department Obstetrics and Gynecology
Nair Hospital and TN Medical College, Mumbai

Shaily Agarwal MBBS MS
Professor, Department of Gynecology
GSVM Medical College, Kanpur

Shraddha Mevada MS
Assistant Professor
Department of Obstetrics and Gynecology
HBT Medical College and
Dr RN Cooper Hospital, Mumbai

Shweta Khade DNB (OBGY) DGO Dip. ART
Assistant Professor
Department Obstetrics and Gynecology
LTMMC and LTMGH, Sion Hospital, Mumbai

Shilpa Agrawal DGO FCPS DNB FNB
Consultant
Department Obstetrics and Gynecology
High Risk Pregnancy and Fetal Medicine Specialist.
Jaslok Hospital and Research Centre
Dr G Deshmukh Road, Mumbai

Shreedevi Tanksale
DNB DGO DFP Diploma in Reprod. Med.
Little Miracles Fertility Clinic
Consultant, Department of Obstetrics and Gynecology
Surya Mother and Child Care, Criticare Asia Hospital,
Apollo Spectra, Mumbai

Shreya Prabhoo MBBS DNB DGO MNAMS FICOG
Consultant
Department of Obstetrics and Gynecology
Mukund Hospital, L&T Healthcare Centre
Visiting Consultant, Surya Hospital, Mumbai

Siddesh Iyer MBBS DGO DNB MRCOG (London)
Consultant
Department Obstetrics and Gynecology
Laparoscopic Surgeon, Director, Saukhyam
Hospital
Ex-Assistant Professor, Cooper and JJ Hospital DNB
Consultant BDBA, Mumbai

Suchitra N Pandit MBBS FRCOG MD
Senior Consultant
Department of Obstetrics and Gynecology
Surya Hospital, Mumbai

Sudha Tandon MD DGO
Director, Dr Sudha Tandon IVF
Maternity and Gyn Endoscopy Hospital
Chembur and Vashi

Sana Ismail MS
Senior Resident
Department of Gynecology
SN Medical College, Agra

Sujata Dalvi MD DGO FCPS FICOG
Consultant
Department of Obstetrics and Gynecologist
Global Saifee, Bhatia, St. Elizabeth Hospitals
Hon Clinical Associate–Nowrosjee Wadia
Jagjivan Ram Hospital, Mumbai

Sunil Tambvekar
MBBS DNB MNAMS DFB FMAS PGDMLS
Consultant
Department of Obstetrics and Gynecology
Assistant Professor, Department of Obstetrics and
Gynecology, Nowrosjee Wadia Maternity Hospital
Seth GS Medical College, Mumbai

Shalini Bhatija MBBS DNB MS
Clinical Associate
Department of Obstetrics and Gynecology Jaslok
Hospital, Mumbai

Tejal Poddar MS DFP
Consultant
Department in Reproductive Medicine
Little Miracles Fertility Clinic, Saifee, Bhatia
Elizabeth, Apollo Spectra, SRCC, Ruxmani
Hospitals, Mumbai

Usha Saraiya MD DGO FIAC FRCOG (UK)
Consultant, Department Obstetrics and Gynecology
Saifee, Breach Candy and St. Elizabeth Hospitals
Mumbai

Vandana Walvekar MD DGO DPF FAMS
Consultant, Department Obstetrics and Gynecology
Wadia Hospital and Bhatia Breach Candy Hospital
Mumbai

Vidya Thobi MD MS FICOG
Professor, Department Obstetrics and Gynecology
AL-Ameen Medical College, Bijapur

Vijaya Babre2
MS DNB FCPS DGO DFP FICOG MNAMS DHA
Senior Consultant
Department Obstetrics and Gynecology
DNB Teacher, Khan Bahadur Bhabha Municipal
Hospital, Kurla, Mumbai

Foreword

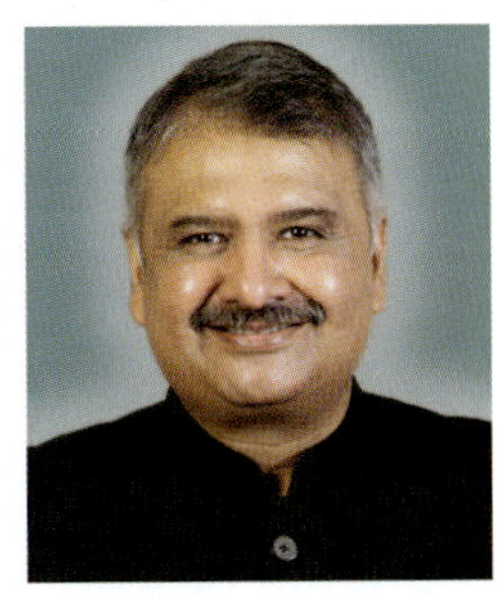

As the field of obstetrics and gynaecology continues to advance, it is essential for healthcare professionals to remain up-to-date and well-informed. The book *Drugs in Obstetrics and Gynecology: A Practical Approach* covers a wide range of topics, from the use of drugs during pregnancy and lactation to the management of common gynecological conditions, such as endometriosis, polycystic ovary syndrome (PCOS), and menopause. The discussion on the use of hormonal therapies, including oral contraceptives and hormone replacement therapy, is particularly informative and highlights the potential risks and benefits associated with these drugs.

The book also provides detailed information on the use of drugs in the management of infertility and assisted reproductive technologies, as well as the management of obstetric complications, such as pre-eclampsia, gestational diabetes, and postpartum hemorrhage. Additionally, the book provides information on the use of drugs for the management of gynecological cancer, such as ovarian, endometrial, and cervical cancer.

One of the unique features of this book is the practical approach in which it is written. The book provides breadth, depth and expansive research from many medical experts in the field of reproductive and sexual health. The book honours fact-based information and provides cutting-edge interpretation of various obstetrics and gynaecology in its both parts. The book provides up-to-date resources and approach to obstetrics and gynaecology.

Jaydeep Tank
President FOGSI 2024-2025
Mumbai, India

Foreword

The book *Drugs in Obstetrics and Gynecology: A Practical Approach* provides clear and concise information on the indications, dosages, side effects, and contraindications of commonly used drugs in obstetrics and gynecology. It also includes case studies, algorithms, and tables to help readers understand and apply the information presented in the book.

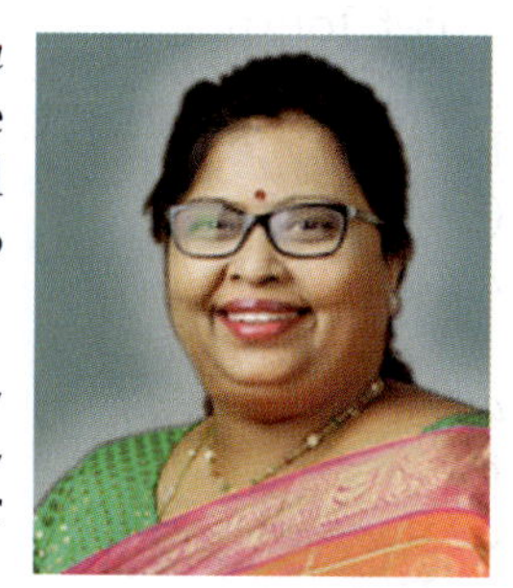

This book is an invaluable resource for healthcare professionals, including obstetricians, gynecologists, and primary care physicians, who are involved in the care of women. It is also a useful resource for medical students and residents who are training in this field.

Prof Ruchika and Dr Priya, the authors, have done an excellent job of providing a comprehensive and up-to-date guide to the safe and effective use of drugs in obstetrics and gynecology in a practical approach. I highly recommend this book to anyone involved in the care of women.

S Shantha Kumari
MD, FRCOG (UK) FRCPI (Ireland)
Hyderabad
President FOGSI 2021–2023
Honorary Treasurer FIGO 2021–2023

Foreword

Dr Ruchika Garg is a Professor in the Department of Obstetrics and Gynaecology in SN Medical College, Agra, India. She is Editor-in-Chief, Journal of South Asian Federation of Obstetrics and Gynecology (SAFOG), and Associate Editor in Journal Midlife Health and Joint Editor of Journal of South Asian Federation of Menopause Societies (SAFOMS). She is President, Agra Chapter of Indian Menopause Society Agra Society 2023-25.

I am honoured to write the foreword for the book, *Drugs in Obstetrics and Gynecology: A Practical Approach*. This book is an essential resource for healthcare professionals, including obstetricians, gynecologists, and other specialists who deal with women's health.

The use of drugs in obstetrics and gynaecology is an ever-evolving field, and the correct use of drugs is crucial for successful outcomes. This book provides an in-depth discussion of the pharmacological management of various conditions that are encountered in obstetrics and gynecology. The book is structured in a way that enables healthcare professionals to quickly and easily access of the information they need to make informed decisions about the use of drugs.

The authors have provided a comprehensive review of the use of drugs in obstetrics and gynecology, including information on drug interactions, dosages, and potential side effects. The book covers a range of topics, including contraception, menstrual disorders, infertility, preterm labor, and postpartum hemorrhage. The authors have also provided practical advice on how to manage adverse drug reactions, which is essential in clinical practice.

I highly recommend this book to all healthcare professionals who deal with women's health. It is a valuable resource that will help clinicians to provide safe and effective pharmacological management for their patients.

The book is written in a clear and concise style, making it accessible to healthcare professionals at all levels of training and experience including postgraduate students and busy practitioners.

This is a well-written and comprehensive guide for the use of drugs in women's health. I commend the authors for their excellent work and am confident that this book will become a widely used reference for healthcare professionals in this field.

JB Sharma

MD FRCOG (London) MFFP FAMS PhD FICOG FIMSA

Professor, Department of Obstetrics and Gynaecology
All India Institute of Medical Sciences
Dr BC Roy Awardee, Labhsetwar Awardee
Chairperson, Urogynaecology FOGSI Society (2020-22)

Co-ordinator Delhi PG Forum
Ansari Nagar, New Delhi
jbsharma2000@gmail.com

Foreword

The practice of obstetrics and gynecology requires a deep understanding of the unique physiological and anatomical features of the female reproductive system. The use of drugs in this field is equally complex and requires a thorough understanding of the potential risks and benefits associated with different medications. This book, *Drugs in Obstetrics and Gynecology: A Practical Approach* provides a comprehensive and practical guide to the safe and effective use of drugs in the management of conditions specific to women's health.

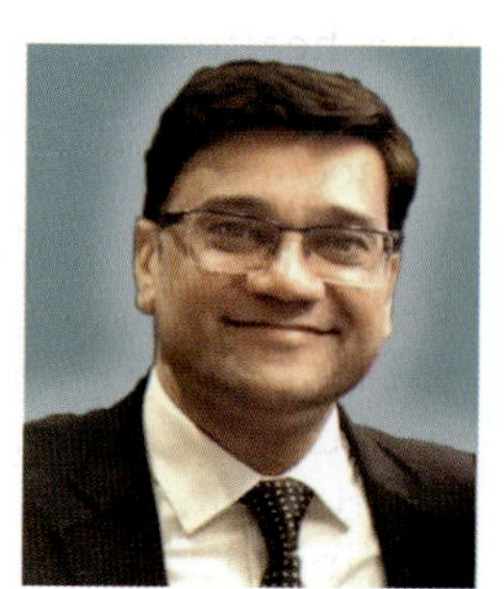

Prashant Gupta
Principal and Dean
SN Medical College, Agra

Foreword

As a healthcare professional, it is crucial to have a comprehensive understanding of drugs and their implications in obstetrics and gynaecology. The field of obstetrics and gynaecology is constantly evolving, and staying up-to-date with the latest drug therapies and their practical applications is essential.

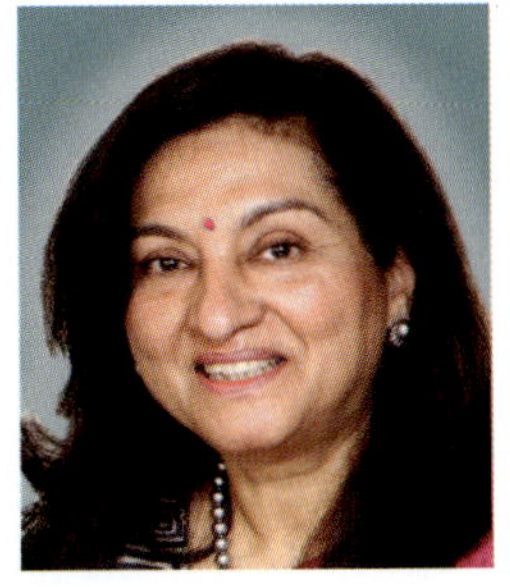

This book, *Drugs in Obstetrics and Gynaecology: A Practical Approach,* provides a thorough examination of the drugs commonly used in obstetrics and gynaecology, and how they can be effectively employed in clinical practice. The authors have put together a concise yet comprehensive guide to equip healthcare providers with the knowledge and skills necessary to provide safe and effective care to their patients.

The book is written in a clear and concise manner, and is organized to provide readers with a thorough understanding of each drug category. Each chapter includes an overview of the drug, its mechanism of action, indications, contraindications, and potential side effects. In addition, practical guidance on dosing, administration, and monitoring is provided, making this book an invaluable resource for healthcare professionals in their daily practice.

The book is an essential resource for undergraduates, postgraduate students, any healthcare provider, midwifery, homeopathic and Ayurvedic students looking to expand their knowledge and stay up-to-date with the latest drug therapies and practical applications in obstetrics and gynaecology. Dr Ruchika Garg has a teaching experience of 18 years as a undergraduate and Postgraduate teacher. She is a popular teacher, researcher and surgeon par excellence. She has provided exhaustive literature in this book. It will be useful to solve MCQs too.

I highly recommend this book to any healthcare provider looking to improve the understanding and skills in the field of obstetrics and gynaecology.

Jaideep Malhotra
Consultant Rainbow IVF, Agra
Ex-President FOGSI
Ex-President ASPIRE 2014–2016

Preface

Having the passion for reading can be the biggest sign of a successful clinician. The book *"Drugs in Obstetrics and Gynaecology: A Practical approach"* is an exclusive book, unique of its kind, as it covers practical aspects of prescribing various drugs used and approach to management of obstetric and gynaecological cases. As postgraduate students and busy consultants often do not remember pharmacokinetics, common and important side effects and contraindications of various commonly used drugs and may land up in trouble due to missed diagnosis.

This book has emphasized on this often forgotten and important points. It covers the latest evidence-based guidelines to help clinicians keep themselves abreast with the latest advances in obstetrics and gynaecology. The book will help the readers take rational decisions for managing different conditions in obstetrics and gynaecology. The addition of various trials is an icing on the cake. The book has two parts, one covering drugs in obstetrics including tocolytics, $MgSO_4$ drugs for induction of labour, ectopic pregnancy, etc. The second part covers gynaecological disorders like premenstrual syndrome, thin endometrium, drugs in PCOS, ovulation induction, contraception, contraceptive vaginal rings, etc. The book will be helpful to postgraduate students, busy practitioners as a guide in OPD for tackling tricy situations and the latest drugs available.

We thank our contributors who are all doyens in the subject. They have penned down their vast experiences in this book.

Without the love and support of our family members: Husband Dr Prabhat Agrawal, kids Pratham, Palakshi, parents Dr Anuradha and Dr JK Garg, this hurculine task would not have seen the light of day. We express our gratitude to the learned faculty of the department of Obstetrics and Gynaecology SNMC, Agra, with Prof Richa Singh, Prof Nidhi Gupta, Prof Shikha Singh, for their support and cooperation.

We are indebted to Dr Abhijit Thakur, Arya and Anushka for letting us do the task from stealing their time. We thank CBS Publishers & Distributors Pvt. Ltd. for their support and cooperation throughout the publication of this book.

Happy Reading!

Ruchika Garg
Priya Vora Thakur

Contents

PART I OBSTETRICS

PART II GYNECOLOGY

Anticoagulants in Pregnancy and Postpartum

• Mansi Medhekar • Anahita Chauhan

Introduction

Anticoagulants use in modern obstetrics and gynecology is not very uncommon. In this chapter, we will discuss the various anticoagulants and their use in pre-conceptional period, pregnancy and puerperium.

As a treating clinician, it is very important that we should know the four basic concepts—which is the right anticoagulant, what is the right timing and dose, how to prevent the potential teratogenic effect of the drug and the fine-tuning during labour and delivery to prevent antepartum hemorrhage/postpartum hemotrrhage (APH/PPH) and its complications. Use of anticoagulants in pregnancy requires an expert balancing act, as both the mother and the baby should be protected.

The common indications of anticoagulant use in pregnancy are:

1. Antiphospholipid syndrome (APS)
2. To prevent deep venous thrombosis (DVT)
3. To prevent venous thromboembolism (VTE)
4. Treatment of DVT and VTE
5. Prosthetic heart valve
6. Inherited thrombophilia
7. Atrial fibrillation.

CHOICE OF ANTICOAGULANT

- Low molecular weight heparin (LMWH) and unfractionated heparin (UFH) are the preferred anticoagulants in pregnancy as they do not cross the placenta.[1] Both these molecules are equally effective and extensively studied. LMWH is commonly recommended as it is easy to administer, do not require routine monitoring and the incidence developing heparin-induced thrombocytopenia (HIT) is also less.[2] The advantage of UFH is however its cost and that its effects can be rapidly reversed. Moreover, in patients with renal dysfunction, UFH is advised as it is excreted by both kidney and liver against LMWH which is primarily excreted by kidney.
- We will discuss more about these two drugs further in the chapter.
- Warfarin crosses the placenta leading to fetal embryopathy if given in first trimester and intracranial hemorrhage (ICH) later in pregnancy. Women receiving warfarin should be converted to LMWH/UFH prior to conceiving.
- Synthetic anticoagulants which act as indirect inhibitor of factor Xa like fonda-parinux,[4] heparinoids like danaparoid and synthetic thrombin inhibitors like

argatroban are less studied in pregnancy and their effects on fetus are not known.[3–5] This limits their use in pregnancy but can be used rarely as alternative drug in women where LMWH and UFH are not tolerated.

- Direct anticoagulants such as rivaroxaban, dabigatran, edoxaban, and apixaban are not used in pregnancy as fetal safety is not yet proven.

This leaves us with two most common drugs—LMWH and UFH with occasional exceptional use of warfarin.

LOW MOLECULAR WEIGHT HEPARIN (LMWH)

Initiation of treatment: Can be started soon as patient conceive. However, the initiation depends on the indication and risk factors. **Table 1.3** explains the details on initiation of treatment. When started in first trimester it is advisable to confirm the pregnancy via urine pregnancy test or serum β-hCG. There is no role of starting LMWH prior to conception. In women, who are already on chronic coagulation a change from oral anticoagulants to LMWH is advisable.

Administration: Subcutaneous injection is usually very well-tolerated. Local ice application prior to injection may reduce bruising, however this is not necessary.

Baseline laboratory testing: The incidence of heparin-induced thrombocytopenia (HIT) is very less during pregnancy. However, it is prudent to do a baseline CBC followed by a CBC test after 4 weeks of commencing treatment with LMWH. If no decline in platelet count there is no need for further monitoring. Monitoring of Xa levels is not indicated.[6] If monitoring needs to be done, peak anti-factor Xa activity levels should be measured 4 to 6 hours after the last dose. The dosage should be titrated to maintain a target peak anti-factor Xa activity of approximately 0.6–1.2 units/ml.[7] There is not much data supporting the need for laboratory monitoring of therapeutic dose of LMWH.

Pharmacology: LMWH is metabolised in liver and excretion happens via kidney. Individuals with chronic renal disease may have higher plasma levels and therefore need monitoring with subsequent use of lower dosage. Peak drug levels are reached 3–5 hours after subcutaneous and 2 hours after intravenous administration. Half-life varies from 5 to 7 hours. It is only after 2–3 days of treatment that drug levels reach on steady state.

The preferred interval between prophylactic dose of LMWH and any form of regional anaesthesia is 12 hours.[8]

Advantages

- Monitoring not required
- Incidence of HIT is lower
- Dose to response relationship is predictable.

Limitation

- Dose may have to be reduced in patients with renal impairment.
- Antidote not available
- Rapid reversal not possible in case of early delivery or APH.

Dosing

Dosing of LMWH **(Table 1.1)** depends on mainly two factors:
1. Risk of thromboembolism
2. Anticoagulation desired.

Contraindications

- Patients who have active bleeding or are at high risk of having bleeding (APH, PPH)
- Patients with known bleeding disorders (hemophilia)
- Patient with past history of LMWH-induced HIT or skin allergy
- Thrombocytopenia (platelet $<75 \times 10^9$/L)
- Severe liver and renal disorders
- Uncontrolled hypertension (blood pressure >200 mmHg systolic or >120 mmHg diastolic).

UNFRACTIONATED HEPARIN (UFH)

Initiation of treatment: As soon as intrauterine pregnancy confirmed. Details of the initiation of treatment are mentioned in **Table 1.2.**

Table 1.1: LMWH dosing

Prophylactic dosing Minimal dose required to prevent thromboembolism without risk of bleeding	40 mg, enoxaparin, subcutaneous, OD 5000 units dalteparin, subcutaneous, OD
Intermediate dosing	40 mg enoxaparin, subcutaneous, OD, to be increased as pregnancy progresses up to 1 mg/kg, OD*
This refers to the need of increase in dose with increasing weight in pregnancy, and certain special situations (Table 1.3)	5000 units dalteparin, subcutaneous, OD, to be increased as pregnancy progresses up to 100 units/kg, OD*
Therapeutic dosing To be used in women with high risk of thromboembolism or to treat VTE	1 mg/kg enoxaparin, subcutaneous, BD 100 units/kg dalteparin, subcutaneous, BD

*There is no evidence to suggest that the dosage may be altered as per the weight of pregnant women. However, few studies have reported risk of VTE when pregnant women were given low prophylactic doses. LMWH: Low molecular weight heparin; VTE: Venous thromboembolism

Table 1.2: UF dosing

Prophylactic	5000 units, subcutaneous, BD
Intermediate	1st trimester: 5000 to 7500 units, subcutaneous, BD 2nd trimester: 7500 to 10,000 units, subcutaneous, BD 3rd trimester: 10,000 units, subcutaneous, BD
Therapeutic	Can be given as a continuous IV infusion or subcutaneous, BD. Should be titrated to maintain the aPTT in the therapeutic range.

Administration: Subcutaneous injection. UFH can also be given intravenous, especially during labour and delivery or situations where strict monitoring and rapid anticoagulation are desired.

Baseline laboratory testing: Baseline CBC may be suggested as mentioned above. Baseline prothrombin time (PT) and aPTT to rule out underlying coagulopathies. Monitoring of prophylactic dose of UFH is not recommended. When given in therapeutic dose aPTT to be monitored 6 hours after injection and dose adjusted to maintain aPTT at 1.5–2.5 times the baseline aPTT of the patient. Daily aPTT is recommended till the desired effect achieved and then to be repeated every 1 to 2 weeks.

Pharmacology: UFH is metabolized mainly in the liver and the reticuloendothelial system, and it is excreted in the urine. Elimination is not dependent on kidney function, however in individuals with high-dose requirement, dose may need adjustment. Action of UFH when given intravenous is instantaneous, peak action happens 2–4 hours after subcutaneous administration. Half-life of the UFH is 45 minutes to 1 hour.

The advisable interval between prophylactic dose of UFH and any form of regional anaesthesia is 4 hours.[8]

Advantages
- Rapid onset, so can be used when immediate anticoagulation needed.
- Shorter half-life. This is especially important in obstetrics to prevent APH.
- Ability to monitor with aPTT, a test which is easily available.
- Action can be reversed as antidote present in the form of protamine sulphate.

Table 1.3: Obstetric thromboprophylaxis risk assessment and management[15]

Risk	Antenatal risk factors	Postnatal risk factors
High risk • Antenatal prophylaxis with LMWH • Minimum 6 weeks postpartum LMWH	Any previous history of VTE	• Previous history of VTE • Women who are on LMWH antenatally and with high-risk thrombophilia
Intermediate risk • Consider antenatal prophylaxis with LMWH • At least 10 days postnatal LMWH	• Pregnant women who need hospital admission • Previous VTE after a major surgery • High-risk thrombophilia • Medical diseases, e.g. heart failure, IBD, active SLE, sickle cell disease, nephrotic syndrome, type-1 diabetes with nephropathy • Any surgical procedure during pregnancy • OHSS (first trimester only)	• Caesarean section • BMI ≥40 kg/m² • Readmission or prolonged admission (≥3 days) required in postpartum period • Any surgical procedure in the puerperium except postpartum perineal repair • Medical diseases, e.g. heart failure, IBD, active SLE, sickle cell disease, nephrotic syndrome, type-I diabetes with nephropathy
Low risk *Initiation of treatment antenatally:* • Four or more risk factors—prophylaxis from first trimester • Three or more risk factors—prophylaxis to be started from 28 weeks • Fewer than three risk factors • Early mobilization • Avoid dehydration • No anticoagulation *Initiation of treatment postnatally:* • Two or more risk factors—anticoagulation same as in intermediate risk • Less than two risk factors—early mobilization • Avoid dehydration • No anticoagulation	• Age >35 • Parity ≥3 • Obesity (BMI >30 kg/m²) • Pre-eclampsia • Multiple pregnancy • IVF pregnancy • Smoker • Gross varicose veins • Family history of VTE in first-degree relative • Low-risk thrombophilia *Transient risk:* • Dehydration/hyperemesis • Infection • Long-distance travel	• Age >35 years • Parity ≥3 • Smoker • Obesity (BMI ≥30 kg/m²) • Elective caesarean section • Current pre-eclampsia • Multiple pregnancy • Preterm delivery • Stillbirth in this pregnancy • Mid-cavity rotational or operative delivery • Prolonged labour (>24 hours) • PPH with >1 litre or blood transfusion • Family history of VTE • Low-risk thrombophilia • Gross varicose veins • Current systemic infection • Long-distance travel

SLE: Systemic lupus erythematosus; IBD: Inflammatory bowel disease; OHSS: Ovarian hyperstimulation syndrome; IVF/ART: *In vitro* fertilization/assisted reproductive techniques

Limitations

- Shorter half-life may be an advantage as well as limitation. More dosages may be needed
- Dose to response is unpredictable
- Long-term use is associated with HIT, skin reactions and osteoporosis.

***Dosing:* Table 1.2**

Contraindications: Same as mentioned with LMWH.

WARFARIN

It is best to convert women on warfarin to UFH/LMWH, preconceptionally. Warfarin use in pregnancy is best avoided, in view of its teratogenicity, exception being women with high risk of thrombosis like presence of mechanical heart valve. In such situations, the benefits and risks of continuing warfarin are weighed in each trimester, and conversion to alternative agent is done towards the end of third trimester to avoid bleeding complications.

For preterm labour in an women taking warfarin, it is important to remember risk to the fetus in view of the anticoagulation. Cardiologist, neurologist and obstetrician should be involved in the decision-making. Caesarean delivery should be considered to prevent risk of fetal intracranial hemorrhage. Antidotes of warfarin are vitamin K and fresh frozen plasma (FFP), to be given to the neonate post-delivery, as per the situation.

Warfarin can be restarted postpartum once the risk of haemorrhage is reduced, approximately 5–7 days after delivery. Warfarin is generally safe in breastfeeding.

Warfarin Teratogenicity

The teratogenic effect of warfarin is dose-dependent. Doses <5 mg/day are associated with high-safety margins. Overall incidence of warfarin embryopathy/fetal warfarin syndrome/Di Sala syndrome is estimated to be <10%. The common developmental abnormalities affect bones and cartilage, characterized by short limbs and digits (brachydactyly), nasal hypoplasia, skeletal abnormalities and stippled epiphyses. The risk is maximum when fetus is exposed to warfarin in the first trimester between 6th and 12th week of gestation.[14] There are a few reports of central nervous system abnormalities (ventriculomegaly, microcephaly, microphthalmia, intellectual disability, hypotonia, etc.) associated with warfarin use at any stage during pregnancy. Besides the risk of neonatal cerebral haemorrhage remains due to the anticoagulation effect.

COMPLICATIONS OF ANTICOAGULANTS

Bleeding

Spotting or minor bleeding which stops spontaneously does not warranty the stoppage of anticoagulants. In women with subchorionic hematoma (SCH) but with no active bleeding, anticoagulants continuation will depend on benefit versus risks.

Women with active bleeding or imminent bleeding, *e.g.* vaginal/caesarean delivery, placenta previa, placental abruption or expanding SCH, protamine sulphate can be used to reverse the effect of UFH. It may not be an effective antidote when LMWH is used, nevertheless its administration does reduce bleeding by neutralising the high molecular weight fractions of heparin.[9]

Administration of protamine sulphate
- Slow IV infusion started at 5 mg/min
- Total dose should not exceed 50 mg which has to be given over 10 min.

UFH	• Dose 1 mg protamine sulphate/100 units heparin • It may be difficult to estimate amount of heparin in plasma at that given moment • Single dose 25–50 mg as described above and aPTT monitored
LMWH	• LMWH administered within 8 hours: 1 mg protamine/1 mg of enoxaparin. • LMWH administered >8 hours ago: 0.5 mg protamine/1 mg of enoxaparin.

Potential adverse effects of protamine sulphate include hypotension and anaphylactoid-like reactions.[10]

Heparin-induced Thrombocytopenia

The incidence of heparin-induced thrombocytopenia (HIT) is up to 5% in patients who are on UF or LMWH. It is a life-threatening complication, that occurs, regardless of the dose, schedule, or route of administration. It is more common with UFH compared to LMWH. HIT during pregnancy is extremely rare.[11]

A small decrease in platelet count in pregnancy is not an indication to investigate the HIT. On the other hand, if there is a significant fall, it is prudent to investigate other causes of thrombocytopenia in pregnancy before coming to the diagnosis of HIT. If the situation of HIT arises in pregnancy, a multidisciplinary management in tertiary care centre is warranted. Anticoagulation agents such as warfarin or synthetic anticoagulants (danaparoid, argatroban or fondaparinux) may be used to achieve desired results. The 2012 American College of Chest Physicians (ACCP) guidelines recommend danaparoid as an alternative drug for pregnant patients with HIT. The choice of non-heparin anticoagulant depends on urgency, cost, availability, hepatic and renal function and the potential need of reversal.

Local Allergic Reaction and Skin Necrosis

Allergic reactions are more common with UFH compared to LMWH. Local allergic skin reaction at the site of subcutaneous injections may manifest as itching and rash 2 weeks after starting the dose. Delayed reactions are rare. Risk factors include obesity and prolong use. The treatment is to shift to another heparin product.

Hyperkalemia

It is a rare but not unknown complication with use of heparins. As such does not need any treatment. However, in patients who have chronic renal disease it could be more serious.

Osteoporosis

Long-term use of UF (>6 months) is associated with irreversible risk of bone demineralization. Osteoporosis risk with LMWH is rare. In situations, where there is need to take heparin over prolong period, supplementation with calcium, vitamin D_3 and regular weight-bearing exercise is encouraged.

LABOUR AND DELIVERY

- Women with low risk of peripartum bleeding and preterm labour: LMWH till 38–39 weeks of gestation or until 24 hours prior to anticipated lower segment cesarian section (LSCS/induction or normal delivery.[12]
- Women at high risk of preterm labour or antepartum hemorrhage (APH): Shift from LMWH to UFH at 35–36 weeks of gestation or earlier. This minimises the risk that labour or delivery will happen within 24 hours of LMWH. Beside protamine sulphate is a better antidote for UFH as against LMWH.

If spontaneous labour starts when women are still taking UFH/LMWH, anticoagulation should immediately stop. The risk of bleeding when women undergo normal delivery within 24 hours of LMWH dose is very rare. Caesarean delivery may have increased incidence of blood loss and wound hematomas. It is important to electively plan the delivery of women who are at increased risk of thrombosis such as with mechanical heart valve and who are on warfarin. Multidisciplinary team of cardiologist, intensivist, anaesthesiologist and obstetrician should be available at the time of delivery and management should be individualised. Vaginal delivery is preferred. LSCS is indicated for obstetric reasons only.

NEURAXIAL ANAESTHESIA

Neuraxial anesthesia techniques (spinal, epidural, etc.) are contraindicated if a patient is anticoagulated due to the risk of spinal or epidural hematoma.

The duration for which anticoagulation has to stop prior to neuraxial anaesthesia is as follows:

- Prophylactic dose LMWH—after at least 12 hours since the last dose.
- Intermediate and therapeutic dose LMWH—after at least 24 hours since the last dose.

- Prophylactic and therapeutic dose of UFH—once the aPTT has normalized following discontinuation. In patients on therapeutic doses of unfractionated heparin, the aPTT is usually normal 6 hours after stopping intravenous administration but can take 24 hours to normalize after stopping subcutaneous administration.

It is possible that in the future, thrombo-elastography (TEG) may be used to determine when neuraxial anaesthesia can be initiated following discontinuation of LMW heparin, but more data are needed before this approach can be used.[13]

Routine use of protamine sulphate is not indicated unless there is excessive or unexpected bleeding due to the anticoagulant drug.

SPECIAL SITUATIONS

If an elective procedure such as cervical os tightening or any other minor surgical procedure needs to be done when patient is on anticoagulants, heparin discontinuation is enough to prevent bleeding complications. Stopping UFH 4–6 hours prior and LMWH 24 hours prior to procedure is enough. If the procedure needs to be done urgently, monitoring of aPTT or anti-factor Xa activity level can be monitored to confirm the resolution of the effect UFH or LMWH.

POSTPARTUM AND BREASTFEEDING

With the exception of patients who are receiving anticoagulation for recurrent pregnancy loss, all women on anticoagulants during pregnancy should be restarted on the treatment post delivery.

- *Therapeutic dosing:* For acute VTE within 3 months of active treatment or women with high risk of thromboembolism, the recommended drug is UFH/LMWH in therapeutic dose to be started immediately postpartum. Alternatively overlap of UFH/LMWH with warfarin for 5 days or till the desired anticoagulation is achieved,

followed by continuation of only warfarin. UFH or LMWH can be started after 4–6 hours of vaginal delivery or 6–12 hours after caesarean delivery. The decision of when to start depends on the clinical scenario, risk of VTE and the clinician judgement.

- *Prophylactic dose:* In women who were taking prophylactic dose during antenatal period or in women who were not on anticoagulants before but need anticoagulation postpartum, the urgency of starting anticoagulation is less. UFH/ LMWH can be started 6–12 hours and 12–24 hours post-vaginal delivery and caesarean delivery, respectively.

Duration of anticoagulation depends upon the indication of why the anticoagulant was started at the first place and the risk of VTE in future. When given for obstetric indication, the anticoagulants can stop 6 weeks postpartum. As a general rule, women who were on anticoagulants prior to pregnancy will have to continue the same for a prolong period in consultation with the hematologist, refer to **Table 1.3**.

As per the 2018 American Society of Hematologist Guidelines, in addition to UFH and LMWH, warfarin or vitamin K antagonist, danaparoid and fondaparinux are also safe in breastfeeding.

References

1. Cosmi B, Hirsh J. Low molecular weight heparins. Curr Opin Cardiol 1994; 9:612.

2. Litin SC, Gastineau DA. Current concepts in anticoagulant therapy. Mayo Clin Proc 1995; 70:266.

3. Lindhoff-Last E, Kreutzenbeck HJ, Magnani HN. Treatment of 51 pregnancies with danaparoid because of heparin intolerance. Thromb Haemost 2005; 93:63.

4. Elsaigh E, Thachil J, Nash MJ, et al. The use of fondaparinux in pregnancy. Br J Haematol 2015; 168:762.

5. Tanimura K, Ebina Y, Sonoyama A, et al. Argatroban therapy for heparin-induced thrombocytopenia during pregnancy in a

woman with hereditary antithrombin deficiency. J Obstet Gynaecol Res 2012; 38:749.

6. Bates SM, Rajasekhar A, Middeldorp S, et al. American Society of Hematology 2018 guidelines for management of venous thromboembolism: venous thromboembolism in the context of pregnancy. Blood Adv 2018; 2:3317

7. American College of Obstetricians and Gynecologists' Committee on Practice Bulletins—Obstetrics. ACOG Practice Bulletin No. 196: Thromboembolism in Pregnancy. Obstet Gynecol 2018; 132:e1.

8. Harrop-Griffiths W, Cook T, Gill H, Hill D, Ingram M, Makris M, et al. Association of Anaesthetists of Great Britain & Ireland; Obstetric Anaesthetists' Association; Regional Anaesthesia UK. Regional anaesthesia and patients with abnormalities of coagulation. Anaesthesia 2013;68:966–72.

9. Lu C, Crowther MA, Mithoowani S. Management of intentional overdose of low-molecular-weight heparin. CMAJ 2022; 194:E122.

10. Harenberg J, Gnasso A, de Vries JX, et al. Inhibition of low molecular weight heparin by protamine chloride *in vivo*. Thromb Res 1985; 38:11.

11. Greinacher A. Clinical practice. Heparin-induced thrombocytopenia. N Engl J Med 2015; 373:252.

12. American College of Obstetricians and Gynecologists' Committee on Practice Bulletins—Obstetrics. ACOG Practice Bulletin No. 196: Thromboembolism in Pregnancy. Obstet Gynecol 2018; 132:e1.

13. Griffiths S, Woo C, Mansoubi V, et al. Thromboelastography (TEG®) demonstrates that tinzaparin 4500 international units has no detectable anticoagulant activity after caesarean section. Int J Obstet Anesth 2017; 29:50.

14. Cotrufo M, De Feo M, De Santo LS, et al. Risk of warfarin during pregnancy with mechanical valve prostheses. Obstet Gynecol 2002; 99:35.

15. RCOG Green-top Guideline No. 37a

Antiepileptic Drugs in Pregnancy

• Mukta Agarwal • Indira Prasad

Introduction

Epilepsy is the most frequent major neurological disorder encountered during pregnancy with a prevalence of 0.5–1%. The risk of death is increased ten-fold in pregnant women with epilepsy compared to those without the condition.

CLASSIFICATION OF EPILEPSY

Based on clinical type of seizure and specific electroencephlogram (EEG) features, epilepsy is broadly divided into:

- *Primary generalised epilepsy* (including tonic-clonic, absence and myoclonic seizures)
- *Partial (focal) seizures* with or without loss of consciousness or secondary generalization (complex partial seizures).

Generalised seizures are seen in 85% of all seizure cases and involve both brain hemispheres spontaneously. These are preceded by an aura before an abrupt loss of consciousness and are often related with a strong hereditary component. These are broadly of two types:

1. *Grand mal seizures:* These present with loss of consciousness, tonic contraction of the muscles, rigid posturing and clonic contraction of all extremities. These may complicate into status epilepticus.

2. *Petit mal seizures:* These are also called absence seizures and involve a brief loss of consciousness without disturbance in muscle activity followed by immediate recovery of consciousness and orientation. These are generally of short duration, have a rapid recovery and are precipitated by hyperventilation. Absence seizures are associated with 3 Hz spike and wave discharge on EEG.

Partial seizures are seen in 15% of all seizure cases. These are usually secondary to trauma, abscess, tumor, or perinatal factors.

1. *Simple motor seizures:* These can affect sensory function or produce autonomic dysfunction or psychological changes. In these, consciousness is usually not lost and recovery is rapid.

2. *Complex partial seizures:* These are also called temporal lobe or psychomotor seizures and involve clouding of consciousness. These are often associated with aura, a duration of 1 minute or more and confusion after the event.

Conditions that Mimic Seizure Disorders

1. *Pseudoseizures:* These are also called non-epileptic attack disorders or dissociative seizures. These are usually distinguished from true epilepsy by the following features:

- Prolonged/repeated seizures without cyanosis
- Resistance to passive opening
- Down-going plantar reflexes
- Persistence of a positive conjunctival reflex.

2. *Syncope:* Some cases may be associated with jerking movements that may be mistaken for seizure. Such cases include:
- Syncope associated with cardiac arrhythmias/aortic stenosis.
- Vasovagal syncope.

PATHOGENESIS

Most cases are idiopathic with family history of epilepsy seen in 30% cases and are referred to as primary epilepsy. Secondary epilepsy is seen in patients who may have certain underlying pathologies as enumerated in **Box 2.1**.

CONCERNS DURING PREGNANCY

Major concerns with epilepsy in pregnancy are increased seizure frequency and risks of fetal malformation due to antiepileptic drugs (AEDs) and pathophysiology of the same is described as follows:

a. *Increased seizure frequency* during pregnancy has been related to sub-therapeutic anticonvulsant levels and lower seizures threshold causes for increased seuzure rates in pregnancy are given in **Box 2.2**.

b. *Increased risks for fetal malformation:* Untreated epilepsy is not associated with increased malformations but the fetus of an epileptic mother who takes anticonvulsant medications has an indisputably increased risk of congenital malformation, pregnancy losses, growth restriction, impaired postnatal development, behavioral problems and fetal anticonvulsant syndrome. The risk of recurrence of major congenital malformations was increased to 16.8% in women with epilepsy with a previous child with a major congenital malformation. There was no significant association between epilepsy type and tonic-clonic seizures in the first trimester and major malformations. Teratogenic effects of antiepileptic drugs are summarized in **Table 2.1**. Following mechanisms have been described with respect to teratogenicity:

a. Some anticonvulsant medication forms intermediate oxide metabolites that are known to be embryotoxic. These free active

---

Box 2.1: Causes of secondary epilepsy

- Previous surgery done in cerebral hemisphere
- Intracranial mass lesions (cavernomas, meningiomas, arteriovenous malformations)
- Antiphospholipid syndrome
- Eclampsia
- Thrombotic thrombocytopenic purpura (TTP)
- Posterior reversible leucoencephalopathy
- Stroke
- Subarachnoid haemorrhage
- Drug and alcohol withdrawal
- Hypoglycemia (diabetes, hypoadrenalism, hypopituitarism, liver failure)
- Hypocalcemia (magnesium sulphate therapy, hypoparathyroidism)
- Infections (tuberculoma, toxoplasmosis)
- Post-dural puncture (though rare, seen typically 4–7 days after dural puncture)
- Gestational epilepsy (seizures that are confined to pregnancy)

Box 2.2: Possible causes for increased seizure rates in pregnancy

- Increased nausea and vomiting
- Decreased gastrointestinal motilily
- Use of antacids that diminish drug absorption
- Pregnancy hypervolemia offset by protein binding
- Induction of hepatic, plasma, and placental enzymes that increase drug metabolism
- Increased glomerular filtration
- Discontinue medication
- Pregnancy-related sleep deprivation
- Hyperventilation and pain during labor

Table 2.1: Teratogenic effects of common anticonvulsant medications

Drug	Abnormalities described	Affected	Pregnancy drug category
Valproate	Neural tube defects, skeletal abnormalities, developmental delay	1–2% with monotherapy 9–12% with polytherapy	D
Phenytoin	Fetal hydantoin syndrome, craniofacial defects, fingernail hypoplasia, growth deficiency, cardiac defects	5–11%	D
Carbamazepine	Fetal hydantoin syndrome, spina bifida	1–2%	D
Phenobarbital	Clefts, cardiac anomalies, urinary tract malformations	10–20%	D
Lamotrigine	Inhibits dihydrofolate reductase, lowers fetal folate levels. Registry data suggest increased risk for clefts	4-Fold with monotherapy	C
Topiramate	Registry data suggest increased risk for clefts	2%	C
Levetiracetam	Theoretical-skeletal abnormalities and impaired growth in animals at doses similar to or greater than human therapeutic doses	Too few cases reported to assess risk	C

oxide radicals bind to proteins and nucleic acids and interfere with DNA and RNA synthesis. Critical amounts of free radicals may increase the risk of perinatal death, cause intrauterine growth retardation, and malformations.

b. Another mechanism that has been implicated in AED-induced folate deficiency. Up to 90% reduction of serum folate levels have been described.

c. Genetic predisposition that causes decreased epoxide hydrolase activity has also been illiustrated as a third mechanism.

PHARMACOKINETICS OF ANTIEPILEPTIC DRUGS DURING PREGNANCY

Carbamazepine: It is relatively slowly absorbed as 70–80% remains bound to albumin. Main route of its elimination is hepatic metabolism. The drug levels and bioavailability tend to be lower in pregnancy. Carbamazepine-10,11-epoxide increases during pregnancy due to impaired conversion of carbamazepine and due to increased carbamazepine metabolism.

Phenytoin: It is highly bound to protein, about 90–93% is protein bound. Main route of its elimination is hepatic metabolism. Process of its 8-hydoxylation is substantially increased during increased clearance rate and during pregnancy resulting in its decreased serum concentration. The fall in total serum phenytoin concentration results in lack of seizure control.

Phenobarbital: It causes sedation and impaired cognitive function. It has high oral bioavailability, *i.e.* 90%. Fifty percent are protein-bound. It induces hepatic microsomal oxidative enzymes. Its main route of elimination is hepatic metabolism and it has long elimination half-life.

Valproic acid: It is rapidly absorbed and is highly bound to plasma albumin (88–92%). Its pharmacokinetics is limited by large fluctuations in concentration and wide therapeutic index. It shows concentration-dependent protein binding and its dose needs adjustments during pregnancy.

Newer Antiepileptic Drugs

Topiramate, felbamate, oxcarbazepine, gabapentin, vigabatrin, lamotrigine are newer antiepileptic drugs and are much safer for pregnancy as they have no antifolate

Table 2.2: Common side effects of antiepileptic drugs

Drug	Maternal effects	Fetal effects
Phenytoin	Nystagmus, ataxia , hirsutism, gingival hyperplasia, megaloblastic anaemia	Possible teratogenesis Possible carcinogenesis Coagulopathy, hypocalcemia
Carbamazepine	Drowsiness, leucopenia, ataxia, hepato-toxicity, thrombocytopenia	Possible craniofacial and neural tube defects
Valproate	Ataxia, drowsiness, alopecia, hepatotoxicity, thrombocytopenia	Neural tube defects and craniofacial and skeletal defects
Lamotrigine	Rashes, headache, ataxia, diplopia, blurred vison, dizziness	Possible increase in oral clefts

effects, no arene oxide metabolites and no effects on the cytochrome P-450 enzyme system **(Table 2.2)**. These are eliminated from the body through renal clearance and so are free from first pass metabolism.

MANAGEMENT OF EPILEPSY IN PREGNANCY

Major goals of management are:
1. Seizure prevention
2. Treatment for nausea and vomiting
3. Prevention of seizure provoking stimuli
4. To ensure medication compliance
5. Anticonvulsants should be maintained at the lowest dosage associated with seizure control

Components of Management

Pre-conceptional Counseling

Adverse outcome of an epileptic woman's pregnancy depends on AED-induced teratogenicity, patient's genetic disposition, severity of patient's convulsive disorder and potential risk of increased seizure activity during pregnancy. Pre-conceptional counseling and treatment should begin at least 3 months before conception to allow review of AED medications and advise any changes to minimize the risk of neural tube defects and other malformations like institution of folic acid therapy, decreasing the dose of sodium valproate or substitution with an alternative AED details of which are illustrated in **Box 2.3**. All these should ideally

Box 2.3: Preconceptional counselling of women with epilepsy

- Supplementation of folic acid at 5 mg/day from at least 3 months before conception until the end of first trimester and may be continued throughout pregnancy as there is a small risk of folate deficiency anaemia.
- Women must be encouraged to maintain good nutrition, get enough sleep and to stop smoking and alcohol if relevant.
- They must also undergo genetic counseling.
- Counseling about concerns of epilepsy during pregnancy with regards to increased risks of seizure frequency and teratogenic effects of AEDs to the fetal CNS system.
- To ensure that the women do not avoid taking their medications and that they are on safer AEDs.
- Review of AED medication should be done and if there are any issues with fertility, association between valproate, weight gain and polycystic ovarian syndrome must be remembered.
- Women who have been seizure free for >2 years may wish to discontinue AEDs at least preconception and for the first trimester. This should be an informed decision after counseling by a neurologist.
- It is usually not appropriate for women with juvenile myoclonic epilepsy to discontinue AEDs.

be made pre-conception since the neural tube closes at gestational day 26.

The risk of recurrent seizures is about 25% by 1 year after drug withdrawal (80% of which occur within 4 months after tapering of the dose begins). The risk of recurrence is about 40% by 2 years after drug withdrawal. Recurrence risk increases to over 50% in women with a known structural lesion, an abnormal EEG, wherein onset of seizures is in adolescence and in those with a history of frequent seizures requiring more than one AED. Factors associated with a low risk of recurrence are normal EEG, onset in childhood and seizures controlled on monotherapy. The current recommendation is to stop driving from the commencement of period of drug withdrawal and for a period of 6 months after cessation of treatment even if there is no recurrence of seizures.

Antenatal Care

AED related: If epilepsy is well-controlled with carbamazepine, lamotrigine or levatiracetam, there is no need to change the AED in pregnancy. Women must be counselled not to stop AEDs prior to conception and to restart the AED if it has been discontinued as they may stop their AEDs on their own due to fears about teratogenesis. If the woman is seen after the first trimester she may be reassured that the risk of congenital abnormalities has passed.

After careful counseling, women receiving valproate may wish to be weaned off or changed under close supervision to a different AED. If this is not deemed appropriate, dose must be reduced to 600 mg per day or less to avoid risk of congenital abnormalities even at later gestation. If continued, valproate during pregnancy, therapy should be changed to a three or four times daily regimen or a modified release preparation to lower peak concentrations and reduce risk of neural tube defects. The altered pharmacokinetics in pregnancy mean that for most drugs the concentration of free drug falls because of increased plasma volume and enhanced renal and hepatic drug clearance. There is therefore a need in many patients to increase the dosage of AED during pregnancy. A baseline drug level is useful to establish compliance and inform future changes in drug dosages.

In women with regular seizures, it is a common need to increase the dose of carbamazepine, levetiracetam and especially lamotrigine may need to be increased 2–3-fold starting early in pregnancy and frequently above accepted maximum nonpregnant doses.

If a woman is seizure-free on an AED other than lamotrigine, there is no need to measure drug levels serially or adjust the dose unless she has seizure. In women who have regular seizures and who are dependent on critical drug levels, it is worth monitoring drug levels since they are likely to fall. Dose increases of AED should be guided by serum concentrations of the free drug and seizure frequency and severity. There is no consensus as to the frequency that drug levels should be drawn during pregnancy. However, a reasonable approach could be to draw AED levels monthly and then modify this schedule appropriately based on seizure frequency.

In general, it is preferable to be guided by the patient and her seizure or aura frequency and severity rather than by drug levels.

General measures: Women should be advised to bathe in shallow water or take a shower and family must be advised on how to place a woman in the recovery position to prevent aspiration in the event of a tonic-clonic seizure event.

All women receiving AEDs should be advised folic acid 5 mg daily for 12 weeks prior to conception and to be continued throughout pregnancy as there is a small risk of folate deficiency anaemia.

Prenatal screening for congenital abnormalities with nuchal translucency scanning and detailed ultrasound to rule out congenital anomalies must be offered. Scanning should also include cardiology assessment.

An increased dose of corticosteroids to induce fetal lung maturation is not recommended if steroids are required to compensate for increased metabolism in women receiving hepatic enzyme inducing drugs like carbamazepine, phenytoin, phenobarbitone.

There is insufficient evidence to support the use of oral vitamin K in the mothers to prevent postpartum hemorrhage.

Serial growth scans need to be advised to detect small for gestational age babies and there is no role for routine antepartum fetal surveillance with cardiotocography in women on AEDs.

Pregnancy in women with epilepsy may often get complicated with pre-eclampsia, postpartum hemorrhage, postpartum depression, increased cesarean section rate, nonproteinuric hypertension increased incidence of labor induction and development of seizure disorder in children.

Intrapartum Management

About 1–2% of women with epilepsy will have a seizure during labor and same proportion will have one in the first 24 hours postpartum. The risk of seizures increases around the time of delivery. Women with major convulsive seizures should deliver in hospital.

Women should continue their regular AEDs in labor. If cannot be tolerated orally in labor, parenteral alternatives should be administered.

Early epidural analgesia should be considered to limit the risk of precipitating a seizure due to pain and anxiety. Other methods of pain relief may be transcutaneous electrical nerve stimulation (TENS) and Entonox (nitrous oxide and oxygen). Pethidine should be avoided and diamorphine may be used instead.

If seizures that are not rapidly self-limiting occur in labor, oxygen and intravenous (IV) lorazepam (4 mg over 2 minutes) or diazepam (10–20 mg rectal gel) or 10–20 mg, IV, at 2 mg/ min) should be given.

Most women with epilepsy have normal vaginal deliveries and cesarean section is only required if there are recurrent generalized seizures in late pregnancy.

Seizures in labor should be terminated as soon as possible to avoid maternal and fetal hypoxia and fetal acidosis. Benzodiazepines are the drugs of choice. Continuous fetal monitoring is recommended in women at high risk of a seizure in labor and following an intrapartum seizure.

Postnatal Management

Neonates born to women taking hepatic enzyme inducing AEDs should be offered 1 mg intramuscular vitamin K to prevent hemorrhagic disease of the newborn risk of which is increased due to degradation of vitamin K by enzyme inducing AEDs such as carbamazepine, phenytoin, phenobarbital, primidone. Breastfeeding should be encouraged in all women with epilepsy. Mothers on AEDs should be informed that the risk of adverse cognitive outcomes is not increased in children exposed to AEDs through breast milk.

Most AEDs are secreted into breast milk, but for most drugs the dose received by the baby is only a fraction (3–5%) of the therapeutic level for neonates, and in any case is less that received *in utero*. However, lamotrigine and phenobarbitone cross in significant amounts (30–50%) to breastmilk.

Withdrawal symptoms may be experienced by babies whose mothers received phenobarbitone in pregnancy and although this is rare with the newer AEDs, it provides a logical reason to encourage breastfeeding in all mothers with epilepsy.

Due to slow elimination, phenobarbitone, primidone and lamotrigine can get accumulated in a breastfed baby. Lamotrigine is metabolized mainly glucuronidation and the capacity to glucuronidate is not fully developed in newborn. Lamotrigine should not be initiated in breastfeeding mothers.

If the mother's dose of AED was increased during pregnancy, the dose may be gradually decreased again over a few weeks in the puerperium. Blood levels of phenytoin and lamotrigine increase rapidly following delivery but carbamazepine and valproate takes longer to return to pre-conception levels. Therefore, if doses of lamotrigine has been increased in pregnancy, they should be rapidly decreased postpartum.

The mother should be encouraged to feed before taking her AED. This would avoid peak serum and therefore breast milk levels.

The mother should be advised of strategies to minimize the risk to her and her baby should she have a major convulsive seizure. This includes changing nappies with the baby on the floor and bathing the baby in very shallow water or with supervision.

Women on antiepileptic drugs should be screened for depressive disorder in the puerperium. They must be informed about the symptoms and provided with contact details for any assistance.

Management of Newly Diagnosed Epilepsy in Pregnancy

The annual incidence of new cases of epilepsy in women of childbearing age is 20–30 per 100,000.

It is important to exclude all the secondary causes of seizures. It is not obligatory to treat one isolated primary seizure. If treatment is required, lamotrigine or carbamazepine is appropriate for partial seizures and levetiracetam for primary generalized epilepsy as it is desirable to avoid valproate.

Contraception

Women taking hepatic enzyme inducing drugs (phenytoin, primidone, carbamazepine, phenobarbitone) require higher doses of estrogen to achieve adequate contraception details of which are summarized in **Table 2.3**. Valproate, clonazepam, vigabatrin, levatiracetam, gabapentin and tiagabine do not induce hepatic enzymes and all methods of contraception are suitable. Estrogen can induce the metabolism of lamotrigine so lowering drug levels and combined oral contraceptives (COCs) are not appropriate as may precipitate seizures. The risks of contraceptive failure and the short and long-term adverse effects of each contraceptive method should be carefully explained to the woman. Effective contraception is extremely

Table 2.3: Contraceptive advise for women on antiepileptic drugs (AED)

Contraceptive method	Effectiveness in women with epilepsy
Combined oral contraceptive pills (COCPs)	Efficacy lowered due to enzyme inducing AED COCPs with 50 µg ethinyl estradiol or 2 COCPs containing 30 µg may be advised
Progesterone-only pills (POPs)	Efficacy lowered due to enzyme inducing AED 2 POPs may be advised
Emergency pills with levonorgestrel and ulipristal acetate	Efficacy lowered due to enzyme inducing AED Double dose to be advised
Contraceptive implants	Efficacy lowered due to enzyme inducing AED and an alternative method of contraception may be appropriate
Contraceptive rings	Efficacy lowered due to enzyme inducing AED and an alternative method of contraception may be appropriate
Contraceptive patches	Efficacy lowered due to enzyme inducing AED and an alternative method of contraception may be appropriate
Medroxyprogesterone injection (depo-provera)	Is effective and larger doses are not needed since elimination is dependent on hepatic first-pass rather than enzyme activity
Intrauterine system (Mirena)	Is not affected by AEDs as the progesterone is released locally and may be advised

important with regard to stabilization of epilepsy and planning of pregnancy to optimize outcomes.

SUMMARY

- Optimizing epilepsy treatment prior to conception, choosing the most effective AED to control seizures, using monotherapy and lowest effective dose if possible, and supplementing with folate are the key elements in the management.
- Valproate has been associated with impaired neurodevelopment, reduced IQ, increased risk of autistic spectrum disorder and ADHD in the children. Hence, guidelines suggest to avoid valproate when possible.
- Screening for congenital abnormalities should be offered.
- In most women, the frequency of seizures is not altered by pregnancy provided there is adherence with AED regimens.
- Patient must be informed of the relative risks and guided appropriately in her therapy. Delineation of these risks should be placed in the context that most children born to women with epilepsy (WWE) are normal.
- Breastfeeding should be encouraged.
- Hepatic enzyme inducing AEDs reduce the efficacy of most hormonal methods of contraception, especially COCs.

Suggested Reading

1. Davanzo R Dal Bo S, Bua J, Copertino M, Zanelli E, Matarazzo L. Antiepileptic drugs and breastfeeding. Ital J Paediatr 2013:39–50.
2. Edey S, Moran N, Nashef L. SUDEP and epilepsy-related mortality in pregnancy. Epilepsy 2014;55:e72–4.
3. Faculty of Sexual and Reproductive Healthcare. Faculty of Sexual and Reproductive Healthcare Clinical Guidance: Combined Hormonal Contraception (London): FSRH; 2011 (updated 2012).
4. National Institute for Health and Care Excellence. The epilepsies: the diagnosis and management of the epilepsies in adults and children in primary and secondary care. NICE clinical guideline 13. (Manchester). NICE 2012.
5. Penell PB. Antiepileptic drug pharmacokinetics during pregnancy and lactation. Neurology 2003; 61 Suppl 2:S35–42.
6. RCOG. Green Top Guideline no 68. Epilepsy in pregnancy. https://www.rcog.org.uk/globalassets/documents/guidelines/green-top-guidelines/gtg68_epilepsy.pdf. (2016)
7. Teratogenicity of Newer Antiepileptic Drugs—Australian Experience Lancet Neurol 2012; 11:803–11.
8. Tomson T, Battino D, Bonizzoni E, Craig J, Lindhout D, Sabers A, Perucca E, Vajda F. EURAP Study Group. Dose dependent risk of malformations with antiepileptic drugs: An analysis of data from the EURAP epilepsy and pregnancy registry. Lancet Neurol, 2011;10: 609–617.

Hypertensive Disorders of Pregnancy

• Reena Bansiwal

Introduction

Hypertensive disorders in pregnancy still remain a global problem. It complicates 5–10% of all pregnancies and poses a threat on both mother and fetus. Hypertensive disorders in pregnancy (HDP) were classified by the American College of Obstetrician and Gynecology (ACOG) in 2013 into four categories: Gestational hypertension, pre-eclampsia/eclampsia, chronic hypertension, and chronic hypertension complicated with pre-eclampsia/eclampsia.[1] The International Society of Hypertension in 2020, also accepted the ACOG 2013 classification of HDP but haemolytic anaemia, elevated liver enzymes and low platelet count syndrome (HELLP syndrome) were classified as a separate category.[2] This condition requires close monitoring, optimal management and timely intervention to improve maternal and fetal outcome and thereby decreasing their morbidity and mortality. The ultimate goal of this HDP classification is to prevent and treat seizures and hypertension which are the major cause of maternal and fetal adverse outcomes. Hence, this chapter mainly emphasizes on the treatment of hypertension and seizures.

Antihypertensives in Pregnancy

Severe hypertension can cause congestive heart failure, myocardial ischaemia, renal injury or failure, ischaemic or haemorrhagic stroke and liver injury. So, there lies the importance of timely intervention. Antihypertensives should be started in acute-onset, severe hypertension (blood pressure ≥160/110 mm Hg, confirmed on repeat BP monitoring at 15 minutes or more.[3] Antihypertensives should be administered within 30–60 minutes of its onset to prevent adverse outcome. Most common drugs used for hypertensive crisis are intravenous hydralazine or labetalol and oral nifedipine. A recent Cochrane review involving 3,573 women found no significant differences regarding either efficacy or safety between hydralazine and labetalol or between hydralazine and calcium channel blockers (Table 3.1).[4] Oral labetalol and calcium channel blockers are often used in expectant management for treatment of hypertension (systolic blood pressure of ≥160 mm Hg or diastolic blood pressure of ≥105 mm Hg or both).[5]

The antihypertensives used in pregnancy are classified under sympathomimetics, adrenergic receptor blocking agents, vasodilators and calcium channel blockers.[3,6]

SYMPATHOMIMETICS

Alpha methyl dopa: It is a centrally-acting antihypertensive.

Table 3.1: Antihypertensive drugs in hypertensive crisis

Drug	Dose	Onset of action
Labetalol	10–20 mg, IV, then 20–80 mg every 10–30 minutes to a maximum cumulative dosage of 300 mg; or constant infusion 1–2 mg/min, IV	1–2 minutes
Hydralazine	5 mg IV or IM, then 5–10 mg, IV, every 20–40 minutes to a maximum cumulative dosage of 20 mg; or constant infusion of 0.5–10 mg/hr	10–20 minutes
Nifedipine	10–20 mg, orally, repeat in 20 minutes if needed; then 10–20 mg every 2–6 hours; maximum daily dose is 180 mg	5–10 minutes

Mechanism of Action

It is an α_2-agonist acts centrally. It decreases efferent sympathetic activity and also reduces the total peripheral resistance with lesser effect on heart rate and cardiac output.

Pharmacokinetics

Per oral administration: Only one-third drug is absorbed.

Metabolism: In liver

Excretion: Kidney

Its action starts in 3–6 hours and total duration of action is 12–24 hours.

Dose: Orally 500 mg–2 g daily in divided doses. Maximum 3 g/day.

Tablet: 250 mg, 500 mg

IV infusion: 250–1000 mg infusion over 30–60 minutes q6–8hrs PRN; not to exceed 4 g/day
Injectable solution: 50 mg/ml.

Adverse Effects

Maternal

Common: Sedation, lethargy, reduced mental capacity, dryness of mouth, nasal stuffiness, headache, and retention of fluid.

Rare: Postural hypotension, positive Coombs' test in one-sixth of women, haemolytic anaemia, fever, flu-like symptoms, thrombocytopenia and lupus syndrome.

Fetal: Intestinal ileus.

Contraindication: Hepatic disorders, psychiatric patient, congestive heart failure and postpartum (risk of postpartum depression).

Interaction: Caution with tricyclic antidepressants as it may block its active transport to adrenergic neurons making the drug ineffective.

Note: Methyl dopa was the drug of choice for hypertension in pregnancy as it is safe and effective for both mother and fetus but since 2015, it is not available in the market due to non-production from the manufacturer.

ADRENERGIC RECEPTOR BLOCKING AGENTS

Labetalol: Drug of choice for hypertension in pregnancy. It equalizes to methyl dopa both in efficacy and safety.

Mechanism of Action

It is both α- and β-adrenergic receptor blocker. It blocks β receptors 3–5 times more than α-receptors. Orally, it blocks in the ratio 3:1. Decrease in blood pressure is due to α_1- and β_1-receptors blockade and also due to β_2 agonism causing vasodilation. At high dose it also reduces the cardiac output and total peripheral resistance. There is little effect on heart rate which can be same, decrease or increase. It has no effect on plasma lipid levels.

Pharmacokinetics

On oral administration the bioavailability is around 30% due to significant first pass metabolism. Route of elimination is mainly through liver.

Half-life: 4–6 hours

Dose: Orally starting 100 mg, bid to maximum 2400 mg/day.

Hypertensive Crisis

Injectable route: Its effect on beta receptor is more in comparison to α-receptors and blocks in the ratio of 6.9:1.

Dose: 10–20 mg, IV, then 20–80 mg every 10–30 minutes to a maximum cumulative dosage of 300 mg; or constant infusion 1–2 mg/min, IV.

Onset of action: 1–2 minutes.

Adverse effects: Tremors, headache, tingling sensation of scalp, asthma, congestive cardiac failure, bronchospasm, elevation of blood urea nitrogen, creatinine and liver enzymes, pruritis and rarely ventricular arrhythmia.

Contraindications and caution: Hepatic disorders, asthma, pre-existing myocardial disease, congestive heart failure, heart block, bradycardia, depression and glaucoma.

VASODILATORS

a. Hydralazine

Mechanism of Action

It was introduced in 1950. It directly acts on arteriolar dilation with little effect on venous capacitance vessels. It reduces total peripheral resistance and causes greater decrease in diastolic than systolic blood pressure. This elicits a reflex mechanism causing tachycardia, increase in cardiac output and renin release leading to increase sodium and water retention. Thus, a state of hyperdynamic circulation is produced which may precipitate angina. However, the renal flow is not compromised in spite of decrease in BP.

Pharmacokinetics

Orally, well-absorbed but subject to first pass metabolism in liver through acetylation. It gets completely metabolized in liver and plasma. Excreted through urine.

Half-life: 1–2 hours but the hypotensive effect lasts for 12 hours, probably due to its persistence in vessel wall.

Tablet: 10 mg, 25 mg

Injectable solution: 20 mg/ml

Dose: Hydralazine is used during pregnancy in hypertensive crisis only, in injectable form due to its hypotensive property.

Dose (hypertensive crisis): 5 mg IV or IM, then 5–10 mg, IV, every 20–40 minutes to a maximum cumulative dosage of 20 mg; or constant infusion of 0.5–10 mg/hr.

Onset of action: 5–10 minutes.

Adverse Effects

Facial flushing, conjunctival injection, throbbing headache, dizziness palpitation, nasal stuffiness, fluid retention, edema, CHF, gastrointestinal symptoms. Angina and MI can be precipitated in patients with coronary artery disease. Paraesthesia, muscle cramps and rarely peripheral neuritis. Rarely lupus erythematosus and rheumatoid arthritis symptoms may occur with prolonged use of high dose 100 mg/day. This usually occur in slow acetylators.

b. Nitroglycerine

It is a nitrate vasodilator and should be used as last resort in hypertensive crisis only in pregnancy for short time. It is also the drug of choice in pulmonary edema.

Mechanism of Action

It relaxes mainly the venous but arterial smooth muscle is also relaxed to some extent. It reduces both cardiac preload and afterload as well as coronary artery spasm. It decreases systemic vascular resistance as well as systolic and diastolic blood pressure.

Pharmacokinetics

Half-life

- 3 min in intravenous route
- 6 min in sublingual route

Metabolism

It is a protein bound drug and metabolizes in liver. Nitroglycerin is metabolized to nitrite, 1,2-glyceryl dinitrate, and 1,3 glyceryl dinitrate in mitochondria with the help of enzyme aldehyde dehydrogenase. These metabolites 1,2- and 1,3-dinitroglycerols are less potent in strength than nitroglycerin, but they have longer half-lives, which explain prolonged effects of nitrates. They ultimately metabolized to mononitrates that are not active and to glycerol and carbon dioxide at last.

Dose: IV infusion 5 µg/min to be increased at every 3–5 min up to 100 µg/min.

Interactions

Caution while taking acetaminophen (paracetamol) with nitroglycerin as the risk or severity of methemoglobinemia can be increased. Acetylsalicylic acid (asprin) increases the concentration of nitrogycerin if taken together and potentiate the effects.

Food interactions: Avoid alcohol.

Adverse Effects

Hypotension, dizziness, flushing, irritability, nervousness and paraesthesia. Contra-indicated in hypertensive encephalopathy as it increases blood flow and intracranial pressure.

c. Sodium Nitroprusside

It is used as the last resort in hypertensive crisis for a short time in pregnancy due to its toxic effects on fetus. It is fast-acting and consistent vasodilator.

Mechanism of Action

Nitric oxide (NO) is generated at endothelial cell level as RBCs split it, which causes smooth muscle relaxation. This occurs both enzymatically and non-enzymatically. It relaxes both resistance and capacitance vessels, thereby reducing total peripheral resistance as well as resistance. Though, it reduces the myocardial work but ischaemia may be accentuated due to coronary steal. It causes mild tachycardia in supine position. Plasma renin is also increased.

Pharmacokinetics

Onset of action within seconds but the effect lasts only for 2–5 min, so it needs to be given as infusion. It is metabolized to cyanmethaemoglobin and cyanide ions after reacting with haemoglobin. One molecule of sodium nitroprusside is metabolized by combination with haemoglobin to produce one molecule of cyanmethaemoglobin and four CN^- ions, thiosulfate reacts with cyanide to produce thiocyanate, which is eliminated in the urine.

Dose: 50 mg is added to 500 ml of NS/glucose solution and given as IV infusion @0.25–8 µg/kg/min, titrated according to response.

Caution: The infusion bottle needs to be covered with black paper as it decomposes at alkaline pH and exposure to light.

Adverse effects

Maternal: Nausea, vomiting, severe hypotension and palpitations.

Fetal toxicity due to metabolites—cyanide and thiocyanate.

Interactions: Its hypotensive effect is accentuated with simultaneous use of other antihypertensives including ganglionic blocking agents, negative inotropic agents, and inhaled anaesthetics.

CALCIUM CHANNEL BLOCKER

Nifedipine: It belongs to subgroup dihydropyridines and a direct arteriolar dilator.

Mechanism of Action

Direct arteriolar vasodilatation is by inhibition of slow inward calcium channels in vascular smooth muscle. They decrease peripheral resistance without compromising cardiac output. There is no fluid retention.

Pharmacokinetics

Oral bioavailability: About 56–77%.

Metabolized: Liver

Excreted: Through urine liver

Onset of action: 5–10 min, with duration of action 6–8 hours.

Half-life: 2 hours.

Dose

Expectant management: 5–10 mg TDS, maximum 180 mg/day.

Hypertensive crisis: 10–20 mg orally, repeat in 20 minutes if needed; then 10–20 mg every 2–6 hours; maximum daily dose is 180 mg.

Adverse Effects

Flushing, hypotension, headache, tachycardia and inhibition of labour.

Interactions

Synergistic effect with magnesium sulphate, so should be avoided. Strong CYP3A inducers therefore, caution while using rifampin, rifabutin, phenobarbital, phenytoin, carbamazepine along with it as it reduces its bioavailability and efficacy.

ANTICONVULSANT

Magnesium Sulphate (MgSO$_4$)

It is the drug of choice for eclampsia and for prophylaxis in severe pre-eclampsia.

Mechanism of Action

It acts as a membrane stabilizer and neuro-protector. It decreases the acetylcholine release from the nerve endings and reduces the motor end-plate sensitivity to acetylcholine. It also blocks the calcium channels. It induces vasodilatation and increases cerebral, uterine and renal blood flow. It decreases intracranial edema. It is safe for the fetus within therapeutic level. It has no antihypertensive property.

Pharmacokinetics

Absorption: Intravenously administered magnesium is immediately absorbed.

Distribution: Approximately 1–2% of total body magnesium is located in the extracellular fluid space. Magnesium is 30% bound to albumin.

Half-life: 5.2 hours.

Metabolism: Magnesium is not metabolized.

Excretion: Solely by the kidney at a rate proportional to the serum concentration and glomerular filtration, therefore caution with renal impairment, can leads to toxicity.

Dose

- 2 ml 50% = 1 g vial
- 10 ml 50% = 5 g vial

Regimes

Pritchard

Loading dose intramuscular, 4 g (20% solution), IV, over 3–5 minute followed by 10 g (50%), deep IM, 5 g in each buttock (**Note:** 8 ml of 50% magnesium sulphate solution + 12 ml sterile water makes 4 g, 20% solution; the medication can be mixed with 1 ml of xylocaine 2% solution to reduce the pain at the intramuscular administration).

Maintenance dose = 5 g (50%), IM, 4 hourly in alternate buttock

Repeated dose of MgSO$_4$ given only when:

1. The knee jerks are present
2. Urine output exceeds 30 ml/hr
3. Respiration rate is >12/minute

Zuspan/Sibai = Intravenous 4–6 g, IV, slow, over 15–20 minutes, 1–2 g/hr, IV infusion.

The therapeutic level of serum magnesium is 4–7 mEq/L. Serum magnesium levels may be monitored in selected cases (renal insufficiency, absent deep tendon reflexes). To control fits, optimum serum magnesium level is 4.8–8.4 mg/dl (4–7 mEq/L) to be maintained.

Magnesium toxicity and serum Mg level is seen when it exceeds the therapeutic levels **(Table 3.2)**.

Table 3.2: MgSO$_4$ serum concentration and their toxicity

Effect	mEq/L	mg/dl	mmol/L
Therapeutic range	4–7	5–9	2–3.5
Loss of patellar reflexes	>7	>9	>3.5
Respiratory paralysis	>10	>12	>5
Cardiac arrest data	>25	>30	>12.5

Data from Duley L magnesium sulphate regimens for women with eclampsia: messages from the Collaborative Eclampsia Trial. Br J Obstet Gynaecol 1996;103:103–5 and Lu JF, Nightingale CH. Magnesium sulfate in eclampsia and pre-eclampsia: pharmacokinetic principles. Clin Pharmacokinet 2000;38:305–14.

Magnesium sulfate is continued for 24 hours after the last seizure or delivery whichever is later. For recurrence of fits, further 2 g, IV bolus, is given over 5 minutes in the above regimens. If the patient seizes, despite magnesium therapy, midazolam 1–2 mg, IV, is given (and may be repeated in 5–10 minutes time). In case of MgSO$_4$ toxicity, emergency correction with calcium gluconate 10% solution, 10 ml, IV, over 3 minutes, along with furosemide intravenously to accelerate the rate of urinary excretion should be done.

Other regimens used before were: (1) Lytic cocktail (Menon, 1961) using chlorpromazine, promethazine and pethidine, (2) diazepam (lean) and (3) phenytoin.

Magnesium sulphate has many advantages over other regimes as follows:

i. It controls fits effectively without any depression effect to the mother or the infant.

ii. It reduced risk of recurrent convulsions (9%).

iii. It significantly reduced maternal death rate (3%).

iv. It reduced perinatal mortality rate.

Adverse Effects

It is relatively safe for mother and fetus, if used in therapeutic range. Calcium gluconate is used as antidote in case of toxicity. It is contraindicated in myasthenia gravis. Caution in renal disease as it is excreted from kidneys.

Interaction

Nifedipine to be avoided as it synergizes its action. It has serious drug interaction with doxycycline, minocycline and tetracyclines. Caution, if patient is in pulmonary edema as it can cause further respiratory depression. IV labetalol is to be avoided along with MgSO$_4$ in pulmonary edema as it may aggravates the condition. Timely management of hypertension, seizure prophylaxis and management and timely delivery can reduce maternal and fetal morbidity and mortality significantly.

References

1. Hypertension in pregnancy. Report of the American College of Obstetricians and Gynecologists' Task Force on Hypertension in pregnancy. Obstet Gynecol. 2013;122(5):1122–31.
2. Unger T, Borghi C, Charchar F, Khan N, Poulter N, Prabhakaran D, et al. 2020 International Society of Hypertension Global Hypertension Practice Guidelines. Hypertension (Dallas, Tex: 1979). 2020;75(6):1334–57.
3. ACOG Practice Bulletin Gestational Hypertension and Pre-eclampsia. VOL 133, NO 1, JANUARY 2019.
4. Duley L, Meher S, Jones L. Drugs for treatment of very high blood pressure during pregnancy. Cochrane Database of Systematic Reviews 2013, Issue 7. Art. No.: CD001449. (Systematic Review and Meta-analysis.
5. Report of the National High Blood Pressure Education Program Working Group on High Blood Pressure in Pregnancy. Am J Obstet Gynecol. 2000; 183: S1–S22.
6. Essentials of medical pharmacology. Eighth edition. Daryaganj, New Delhi. Jaypee Brothers Medical Publishers (P) Ltd. 2019. 41. Antihypertensive drugs; 604-621.

Viral Infections and Antivirals in Pregnancy

• Kiran Guleria • Priyanka Mathe • Niharika Sethi

Introduction

Viruses are obligate intracellular parasites which comprise of mainly two components: Nucleic acid and a protein coat. This nucleic acid can be either single or double stranded, DNA or RNA enclosed in a protein coat called capsid. Few viruses also possess a lipid envelope (derived from infected host cells) outside this protein coat which contains antigenic glycoproteins (virus proteins).

DNA viruses include herpesvirus (chickenpox, shingles, oral and genital herpes), hepadnavirus (hepatitis B), adenovirus (conjunctivitis, sore throat) and poxvirus (smallpox). These DNA viruses use host cell polymerase for transcription of viral DNA into mRNA which takes place in host nucleus followed by translation into viral specific proteins. On the other hand, RNA viruses use enzymes present in their virion for translation which takes place in host cell cytoplasm.

CLASSIFICATION OF ANTIVIRALS (Flowchart 4.1)

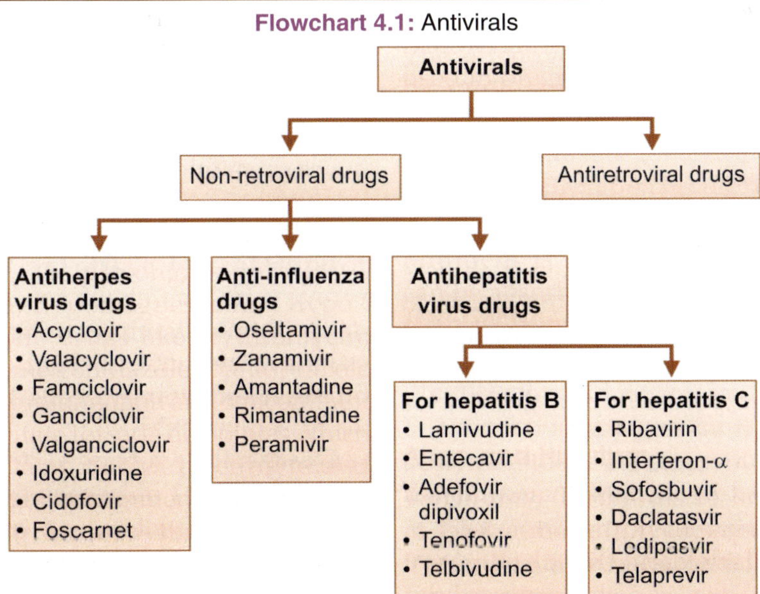

Flowchart 4.1: Antivirals

Exception being influenza virus in which transcription takes place in host cell nucleus. Various RNA viruses include; rubella virus (German measles), coronaviruses (common cold, SARS), flaviviruses (yellow fever, hepatitis C, Zika virus), orthomyxoviruses (influenza), picornaviruses (poliomyelitis, meningitis, colds, hepatitis A), rhabdoviruses (rabies), paramyxoviruses (measles, mumps).

There are two main challenges with antiviral drugs, first being that viruses use host cell nutrition as well as their enzymes for replication. Second, during symptomatic period the viral load is already at its peak thus, to control the infection antivirals should be commenced during the incubation period itself.

ANTIHERPES DRUGS

Herpes virus are of two types; herpes simplex virus-1 (HSV-1) and herpes simplex virus-2 (HSV-2). HSV-1 causes herpes labialis, gingivostomatitis, and keratoconjunctivitis while HSV-2 causes genital infection which less frequently involves skin and hands. The incidence of new HSV-1 or HSV-2 infection during pregnancy is approximately 2%. Anti-herpes drugs are effective against HSV-1, HSV-2, Varicella-Zoster virus (VZV), Epstein-Barr virus (EBV), and Cytomegalovirus (CMV).

Acyclovir

FDA: Category B

Mechanism of Action

It is a deoxyguanosine analogue which uses virus specific enzyme thymidine kinase to convert into its active metabolites: Acyclovir monophosphate and acyclovir triphosphate which then incorporate in viral DNA thus inhibiting DNA polymerase irreversibly preventing DNA synthesis. Acyclovir does not affect the host cells. It is highly active against HSV-1 infection followed by HSV-2, VZV and EBV. It is not effective against CMV infection.

Pharmacokinetics

Oral bioavailability is only 20% and very little is bound to plasma protein. It is widely distributed in plasma of which nearly 50% is found in CSF. Plasma $t_{1/2}$ is 2–3 hours. Drug is excreted in urine via glomerular filtration and tubular secretion. Renal dose modification is required in case of renal compromise. There is no need to modify drug dose in pregnancy and is generally well-tolerated.[1]

Side Effects

Renal dysfunctions: Acute kidney injury (>10%), obstructive nephropathy, renal tubular necrosis and interstitial nephritis. Risk of renal injury increases with IV route of administration, especially in third trimester,[2] however it is reversible after dose reduction or cessation. Risk factors for renal impairment include—higher dose, IV route administration, pre-existing renal disease, diabetes, hypertension and concurrent use of nephrotoxic drugs. Neuropsychiatric symptoms like confusion, agitation, motor disturbances, impaired consciousness can be dose related. Thrombotic microangiopathies like thrombotic thrombocytopenic purpura (TTP) and hemolytic-uremic syndrome (HUS) have also been reported. Nausea, vomiting, headache, injection site phlebitis, deranged bilirubin and transaminase levels can also be found. Although acyclovir is secreted in breastmilk, it is considered safe in breastfeeding.

Uses

1. Genital herpes: During first trimester primary HSV infection is associated with microphephaly, chorioretinitis and skin lesions. Maternal treatment decreases both duration and severity of disease and thereby decreased viral shedding.

Dosage: Recommended dose of acyclovir in management of herpes in pregnancy is shown in **Table 4.1**.[3]

2. Varicella (chickenpox): Uncomplicated varicella infection should be treated with oral

Table 4.1: Dose recommendation of acyclovir

Indication	Acyclovir
Primary infection	400 mg, oral, TDS, for 7–10 days*
Symptomatic recurrent infection	400 mg, oral, TDS, for 5 days or 800 mg, oral, BD, for 5 days
Daily suppression	400 mg, oral, TDS, from 36 weeks until delivery
Severe or disseminated disease	5–10 mg/kg, IV, q8h, for 2–7 days, then oral therapy for primary infection to complete 10 days

*Treatment may be further continued if no response till 10 days of therapy. BD: Twice daily, TDS: Thrice daily, IV: Intravenous, q8h: every 8 hours

acyclovir 800 mg, five times a day for 7 days. It is recommended to start this therapy within 24 hours of onset of symptoms. Complicated varicella infection (varicella pneumonia) have a high mortality rate of nearly 35–40%.[4] Thus, intravenous acyclovir 10 mg/kg every eight hours is preferred.

3. Mucocutaneous herpes simplex: It is caused by HSV-1 infection and is localised to lips and mouth. Topical acyclovir application is useful. In spreading lesions, 10 days oral acyclovir therapy is recommended.

4. Herpes simplex encephalites: It is caused by HSV-1 infection and early treatment is recommended to avoid neurological complications. Drug of choice remains injection of acyclovir, 10 to 20 mg/kg every 8 hourly for 10 days or more.

Drug interaction: Tenofovir, foscarnet may increase serum concentration of acyclovir/ valacyclovir and vice versa. Hence, these drugs should be used with caution if used in combination and need close monitoring.

Valacyclovir:

FDA: Category B

Valacyclovir is the valyl ester form (prodrug) of the acyclovir which is active against HSV-1,2, VZV and CMV. It undergoes first pass metabolism in hepatic and/or intestinal cells by enzyme esterase and is converted into acyclovir. Oral bioavailability is higher than acyclovir (55–70%), so daily dose needed is less and hence patient compliance may be more compared with acyclovir. However, valacyclovir is generally more expensive than acyclovir. It is the drug of choice for herpes zoster infection. It is excreted in urine and have a $t_{1/2}$ of around 3 hours. The recommended dose of valacyclovir in management of herpes in pregnancy is shown in **Table 4.2**.[5]

Table 4.2: Dose recommendation of valacyclovir

Indication	Valacyclovir
Primary infection	1 g, oral, BD, for 7–10 days
Symptomatic recurrent infection	500 mg, oral, BD, for 3 days or 1 g, oral, daily, for 5 days
Daily suppression	500 mg, oral, BD, from 36 weeks until delivery

Ganciclovir and Valganciclovir

FDA: Category C

Due to their potential fetotoxic effects primary indication of these drugs remain maternal or fetal life-threatening CMV infection. Ganciclovir is indicated as intraocular plus intravenous injections in cases of severe CMV retinitis where vision loss is suspected. The main side effects are leukopenia, renal toxicity, and bone marrow suppression.[6]

ANTI-INFLUENZA DRUGS

Oseltamivir

FDA: Category C

This is a broad-spectrum anti-influenza drug active against influenza A, influenza B, H1N1 (swine flu), H5N1 (bird flu) and others. Pregnant women with either suspected or confirmed influenza infection should receive antiviral medication without any delay. CDC also recommends post-exposure chemoprophylaxis in those who are postpartum unto 2 weeks.[7]

Mechanism of Action

It is a viral neuraminidase enzyme inhibitor which prevents the virion release from the host cells .

Pharmacokinetics

It is metabolized in liver and intestine into its active metabolite oseltamivir carboxylate. Oral bioavailability of this drug is high (80%). It is excreted primarily through kidneys and thus dose modifications are required with renal impairment. $t_{1/2}$ of oseltamivir is 6–10 hours.

Side Effects

Nausea, gastric irritation (should be taken with food), headache, insomnia, rarely neuropsychiatric effects (delirium, hallucinations, confused state) and severe skin reactions (including toxic epidermal necrolysis and Stevens-Johnson syndrome).

Uses

It is effective for both prophylaxis and treatment of influenza A, B, swine flu and bird flu as it decreases duration and severity of these infections. It should be started as soon as possible after illness, preferably within 48 hours of onset of symptoms without waiting for laboratory confirmation of diagnosis.

Dosing

75 mg BD for 5 days. May be continued longer in case of severely ill patients. Higher dose of 150 mg BD can also be opted in severely ill cases.

Zanamivir

It is also a neuraminidase inhibitor with a very low oral bioavailability. This is used as inhalational powder. It is excreted by kidneys. $t_{1/2}$ is 2–5 hours. Given in dose of 10 mg as two 5 mg inhalations BD for 5 days which can be further extended in severe illness. It is relatively contraindicated in bronchial asthma and chronic obstructive pulmonary diseases as it can precipitate bronchospasm in these conditions. Also, to be avoided in those with milk protein allergy. Headache, nausea and dizziness are the other side effects. Not recommended for use in nebulisers or mechanical ventilators.

Amantadine and Rimantadine

FDA: Category C

It is effective against influenza A only. It interacts with transmembrane M2 protein of virus cells and inhibits virus assembly as well as release of viral nucleic acid into the host cells. Amantadine is well-absorbed orally with $t_{1/2}$ life of nearly 16 hours. It can be used in treatment of influenza A but not as a first line of treatment as its teratogenic effects are not yet established and thus it is better to avoid these drugs in first trimester.[8] It is contraindicated in patients with untreated angle closure glaucoma and should be used with caution in patients with history of epilepsy.

ANTIHEPATITIS DRUGS

These drugs mainly constitute antihepatitis B and antihepatitis C drugs. Hepatitis B virus is a partially double-stranded DNA virus which has some unusual features similar to retrovirus and incorporates itself into host cells thus leading to persistent lifelong infection **(Table 4.3)**. While, hepatitis C is a single-stranded RNA virus which does not incorporate into host cell and thus does not cause incurable infection but can lead to chronic hepatitis. It is recommended in case of hepatitis C positive pregnant females that the treatment should be deferred till delivery as perinatal mode of transmission is not very efficient and antiretrovirals (peginterferon and ribavirin) are teratogenic. New direct-acting anti-retroviral (sofosbuvir) is a potential hope due to the safety but is still not recommended.[9] Also, preconception

Table 4.3: Drugs for viral hepatitis

	Adefovir dipivoxil	*Tenofovir disoproxil fumarate*
Mechanism of action	Phosphorylated into its diphosphate form and inhibits viral DNA polymerase leading to termination of DNA chain formation	Nucleoside diester analog of adenosine monophosphate with 2 oral formulations available as tenofovir disoproxil fumarate (TDF) and tenofovir alafenamide (TAF)
Pharmacokinetics	Metabolised by esterase in intestine and liver and excreted by kidneys. Oral bioavailability is nearly 60%. Plasma $t_{1/2}$ is 7 hours, the intracellular $t_{1/2}$ of its diphosphate metabolite is up to 18 hours	
Uses	HBV-induced hepatitis, chronic hepatitis, lamivudine-resistant cases and patients with concurrent HIV infection	Chronic HBV hepatitis and HIV treatment and is efficacious regardless of HBeAg status, coexisting cirrhosis or concomitant use of any other nucleotide.
Side effects	Headache, weakness, abdominal pain and flu-like syndrome. At higher doses, nephrotoxicity may occur. Lactic acidosis may occur in patients on anti-retroviral therapy	Renal tubular dysfunction, fatty liver, lactic acidosis and decreased bone mineral density; consider ALT levels monitoring; less with tenofovir alafenamide
Dosing	10 mg per day	TDF 300 mg daily while TAF is more potent form and is given in dose of 25 mg daily

counselling is essential in females with hepatitis C to delay the conception for 6 months after discontinuing drugs.

ANTIRETROVIRAL DRUGS

These drugs include various categories which are active against human immunodeficiency virus (HIV), an RNA retrovirus. Normally, RNA is transcribed into a DNA. HIV causes reverse transcription of its RNA into proDNA which gets incorporated into host DNA leading to Acquired Immuno-Deficiency Syndrome (AIDS). The main target cells are the CD4+ helper T-lymphocyte and later macrophages **(Flowchart 4.2)**. The main aim of ART therapy in pregnancy is to decrease the risk of perinatal transmission, morbidity, and mortality even in females with high CD4 counts. While selecting antiretroviral drugs during pregnancy one should keep in mind drug safety, efficacy, resistance profile, dose modification due to pharmacodynamic changes of pregnancy and interaction with other drugs. Various combination therapies are available, most popular is 3-drug therapy [usually a combination of 2 nucleoside reverse transcriptase inhibitor (NRTIs) and a protease/integrase inhibitor] **(Table 4.4)**. antiretroviral therapy (ART) must be given lifelong and may have to be changed from time to time, if the virus develops resistance. The therapy response is monitored through CD4 cell counts and HIV-RNA levels in the body **(Tables 4.5 and 4.6)**. According to BHIVA pregnancy registry, fetal safety of various antiretroviral drugs can be classified as follows:

- No increased risk: Zidovudine, lamivudine, nevirapine, ritonavir, atazanavir
- Slight increased risk: Darunavir, efavirenz, raltegravir
- Insufficient data: Dolutegravir
- Women who become pregnant on dolutegravir should be counselled about slight increased risk of neural tube defects and advised to start preconception folic acid 5 mg OD immediately, switchover to another drug is generally not needed.[10]

WHO recommendations for ART therapy.[11]

Table 4.4: Preferred and alternative first-line ART regimens

Population	Preferred first-line regimen	Alternative first-line regimen
Adults and adolescents	TDF + 3TC (or FTC) + DTG	TDF + 3TC + EFV 400 mg

Remdesivir

FDA: Not approved

Mechanism of Action

It is a nucleotide reverse transcriptase inhibitor and is effective against majority of single stranded RNA virus like severe-acute-respiratory-syndrome related coronavirus-2 (SARS-CoV2), middle-east respiratory syndrome related coronavirus (MERS-CoV), respiratory syncytial virus and ebola virus. After entering the host cells, it inhibits RNA-dependent RNA polymerase (RdRp) thus reducing SARS-CoV, MERS-CoV and delta coronavirus replication. It has also found to reduce the severity of disease, time of recovery and the amount of lung damage.

Pharmacokinetics

After IV administration, bioavailability of remdesivir is 100%. It is metabolised by enzyme hydrolases into its intermediate metabolites GS-441524 and GS-704277. The elimination $t_{1/2}$ is nearly 1 hour while the peak plasma concentrations of these metabolites are reached after 1–3 hours of the infusion. Remdesivir is nearly 88–93.6% protein bound with a difference in plasma and cellular distribution of its metabolites. GS-441524 has mainly cellular distribution while GS-704277 is plasma distributed. Remdesivir is predominantly metabolised by liver enzymes carboxyesterase-1 (80%), cathepsin A (10%) and CYP3A (10%). The major route of elimination of remdesivir

Table 4.5: Preferred and alternative second-line ART regimens

Population	Failing first-line regimen	Preferred second-line regimen	Alternative second-line regimens
Adults and adolescents	TDF + 3TC (or FTC) + DTG	AZT + 3TC + ATV/r (or LPV/r)	AZT + 3TC + DRV/r
	TDF + 3TC (or FTC) + EFV (or NVP)	AZT + 3TC + DTG	AZT + 3TC + ATV/r (or LPV/r or DRV/r)
	AZT + 3TC + EFV (or NVP)	TDFb + 3TC (or FTC) + DTG	TDFb + 3TC (or FTC) + ATV/r (or LPV/r or DRV/r)

3TC: Lamivudine; ABC: Abacavir; AZT: Zidovudine; DTG: Dolutegravir; EFV: Efavirenz; FTC: Emtricitabine; LPV/r: Lopinavir/ritonavir; NVP: Nevirapine; PI/r: Protease inhibitor boosted with ritonavir; RAL: Raltegravir; TAF: Tenofovir alafenamide; TDF: Tenofovir disoproxil fumarate

Flowchart 4.2: Antiretroviral drugs

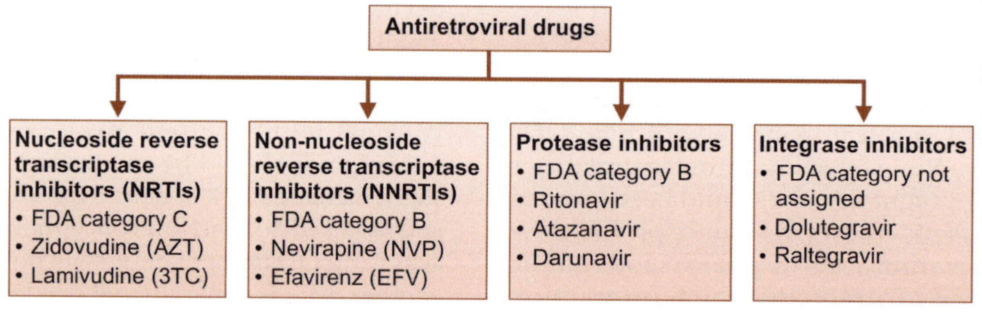

Table 4.6: Antiretroviral drugs

	Zidovudine (AZT)	Lamivudine (3TC)	Nevirapine (NVP) and Efavirenz (EFV)	Ritonavir	Dolutegravir and raltegravir
Mechanism of action	AZT is a thymidine analogue, undergoes phosphorylation in the host cell to form zidovudine triphosphate which inhibits reverse transcriptase enzyme, thus inhibiting formation of proviral DNA and ultimately chain elongation. However, it does not affect proviral DNA which has been already incorporated in host DNA.	3TC inhibits both nucleoside reverse transcriptase and HBV DNA polymerase. It gets incorporated in host DNA and thus halt the viral chain formation.	It inhibits reverse transcriptase without intracellular phosphorylation. Effective only against HIV-1. There is a high tendency of resistance if used alone.	It acts at late step of viral replication where it binds to protease molecules and inhibits the cleavage function leading to formation of immature virions which are non-infective. They act both on new and old infected cells thus are highly effective in preventing further infection.	Integrase enzyme helps to nick the host chromosomal DNA and incorporate proviral DNA, this step is inhibited by integrase inhibitors, active against both HIV-1 and HIV-2 infection.
Pharmaco-kinetics	Bioavailability of nearly 65%. It is metabolised by hepatic glucuronidation with $t_{1/2}$ of 1 hour and excreted in urine. It is 30% plasma protein bound, crosses placenta and secreted in milk.	Bioavailability is high with $t_{1/2}$ of 6–8 hours and intracellular $t_{1/2}$ of nearly 12 hours. It is excreted in urine.	$t_{1/2}$ of nearly 30 hours. The bioavailability of EFV is nearly 50% with $t_{1/2}$ of 48 hours.	$t_{1/2}$ of 2–8 hours, metabolised by CYP3A4 and can also induce their own metabolism, highly protein bound.	Generally, well-tolerated.
Uses	Used in ART therapy in combination with other drugs and in post-exposure prophylaxis of HIV and to reduce mother to child transmission.	First line of management in ART therapies and in chronic HBV hepatitis	WHO recommended EFV as alternative first line regimen in HIV pregnant females treated in limited resource settings has now been replaced by dolutegravir.[12]	Ritonavir-boosted atazanavir combination is recommended by WHO and is safe in all trimesters although the dose should be titrated in later two trimesters. Generally, added in those failing initial therapy, mostly used as boosting agents	Dolutegravir: It is now recommended by WHO as first-line regimen in pregnant and reproductive age as it is found to be more effective and rapid in suppressing viral load as compared to previously used efavirenz.[11] More effective in decreasing viral transmission risk as well.

Contd...

Table 4.6: Antiretroviral drugs (*Contd..*)

	Zidovudine (AZT)	Lamivudine (3TC)	Nevirapine (NVP) and efavirenz (EFV)	Ritonavir	Dolutegravir and raltegravir
Side effects	Anaemia, neutropenia, nausea, anorexia, headache, myalgia; less frequent side effects are myopathy, lactic acidosis, peripheral neuropathy	Nausea, anorexia, fatigue, rashes, abdominal pain, pancreatitis, neuropathy.	Nausea, headache, hyperlipidemia, increased transaminases, hepatic dysfunction. Hypersensitivity reaction (severe skin rash) and liver toxicity is a concern with NVP, more common in women who have higher CD4 cell count (greater than 250 cells/mm^3)	Insulin resistance, hyperglycemia, diabetes, hyperlipidemia, lipodystrophy, hepatotoxicity	Nonspecific with myopathy being the most common.
Dosing	Oral formulation, 300 mg, two times a day, IV, 10 mg per mL in 20 mL vial solution for infusion.	ART therapy—oral tablets, 300 mg, OD or 150 mg, BD	NVP used in dose of 200 mg once a day and then titrated to 200 mg twice daily after 2 weeks due to auto-reduction	Administered in dose of 300 mg atazanavir plus 100 mg ritonavir once daily which can be escalated to 400 mg atazanavir plus 100 mg ritonavir in females already receiving ART.[13]	Dolutegravir—dose of 50 mg, orally per day, increased to twice daily in those with suspected resistance. Reltegravir—dose of 400 mg, orally, twice daily
Interactions	ketoconazole, fluconazole, paracetamol and stavudine decreases AZT metabolism thus enhances drug toxicity.		Both drugs are enzyme inducers and increase their own metabolism. Rifampicin induces NVP metabolism but not that of EFV thus in patients with concomitant HIV and TB infection, EFV is preferred with rifampicin.	Drug combination avoided with proton pump inhibitors. Also, avoided with methergin/ergot alkaloids due to exaggerated vasoconstrictive response	Dolutegravir dose adjustment is required if co-administered with rifampicin/carbamazepine where the dose is 50 mg twice daily. Both these drugs should be avoided with iron and calcium containing formulas; thus a gap of 2–6 hours should be ensured.[14]

is nonrenal while that of the metabolite GS-441524 is via glomerular filtration and active tubular secretion with only minimal faecal excretion.[15]

Side Effects

Hypersensitivity reactions, nausea, rash, increased transaminases, increase in prothrombin time, although renal effects of the drug have not been studied yet, thus to be used with caution in renal impairment. There is insufficient data to conclude the feto-maternal side effects in humans, although animal studies have shown no adverse effects on embryo–foetal development. Also, animal studies have detected remdesivir metabolites in nursing pups mostly due to milk excretion.

Uses

It is used in treatment of Covid-19 infection in hospitalized females if benefit outweighs the risk as there are not sufficient clinical trials to support the use. The National Institutes of Health (NIH) covid-19 Treatment Guidelines Panel and Society of Maternal Fetal Medicine both recommend remdesivir for treatment of Covid-19 pregnant females with decreased oxygen saturation (SpO_2 <94%) or increased oxygen requirement.[16,17] RCOG, however, recommends clinician determined use in pregnant females only if benefits outweigh risks due to uncertain fetal safety profile data.[18]

Dosage

The drug comes in a single dose vial of 100 mg/20 ml (5 mg/ml) IV preparation to be given slow intravenous infusion over 30–120 minutes. 200 mg, IV, on day 1, followed by 100 mg IV(OD), for 5 days or till hospitalization whichever is earlier although may be given up to 10 days [in patients on invasive mechanical ventilation and/or extra-corporeal membrane oxygenation (ECMO)] depending upon severity of disease and clinical improvement.[19]

Caution

Pharmacokinetics of remdesivir is not studied in renal impairment and thus should only be commenced in patients with eGFR ≥30 ml/min. This is due to the fact that the excipient betadex sulfobutyl ether sodium present in the formulation is excreted renally thus gets accumulated in kidney leading to renal toxicity. Also, it is mandatory to keep a check on liver transaminases levels as AST/ALT levels ≥10 times, the lab value is an indicator to discontinue the treatment.[20]

Drug Interaction

Due to antagonism effect, remdesivir should not be used with chloroquine or hydroxychloroquine, CYP3A4 inducers can reduce the effect of this drug.

Bariticinib

FDA: Category not assigned in pregnancy.

It is reversible and selective Janus kinase-1 and -2 inhibitor (JAK inhibitor). It has immonumodulator, anti-inflammatory, antineoplastic along with some antiviral property and interferes with entry of virus in host cells. It binds to JAK receptors and decreases the level of cytokines and inflammatory response. It can be used in pregnancy with SARS-CoV2 infection but should be considered on case-to-case basis after assessing maternal and fetal risks. It is used as a combination drug with remdesivir in hospitalized patients who have rising oxygen demand despite steroid therapy. There is sparse data on tetratogenicity of this drug. Although emergency use authorization (EUA) has been issued for baricitinib and remdesivir combination. It is used in doses of 4 mg oral tablets once daily for 14 days.[21] It is contraindicated in renal insufficiency patients with glomerular filtration rate (eGFR) <15 ml/min per 1.73 m². The side effects include nausea, hepatoxicity, neutropenia, muscle ache, more prone to herpes infection.

SUMMARY WITH KEY POINTS

The common infections in pregnancy which need antiviral drug treatment include herpes, hepatitis, influenza, HIV and now SARS-CoV-2 infection. These drugs reduce the adverse effect of virus on mother and fetus and decrease perinatal transmission. These drugs are most effective when started in incubation period when the viral load is the least and this is the biggest challenge in treatment. None of the drugs is completely safe in pregnancy and most are category-C. Hence, both mother and fetus should be closely monitored throughout the duration of treatment. The newer repurposed drugs should be used with caution only for life-saving indications.

References

1. Royal College of Obstetricians and Gynaecologists. Management of Genital Herpes in Pregnancy, October-2014. https://www.rcog.org.uk/globalassets/documents/guidelines/management-genital-herpes.pdf (Accessed on May 23, 2016).

2. Boujenah J, Cohen E, Carbillon L. Intravenous acyclovir-induced nephrotoxicity. Is pregnancy a risk factor? J Gynecol Obstet Hum Reprod. 2020 Oct;49(8):101783. doi: 10.1016/j.jogoh.2020.101783. Epub 2020 Apr 28. PMID: 32360486.

3. Management of Genital Herpes in Pregnancy: ACOG Practice Bulletin, Number 220. Obstet Gynecol. 2020 May;135(5): e193–e202.

4. Reiff-Eldridge R, Heffner CR, Ephross SA, Tennis PS, White AD, Andrews EB. Monitoring pregnancy outcomes after prenatal drug exposure through prospective pregnancy registries: a pharmaceutical company commitment. Am J Obstet Gynecol. 2000 Jan;182(1 Pt 1):159–63. doi: 10.1016/s0002-9378(00)70506-0. PMID: 10649172.

5. Antiviral drugs for varicella-zoster virus and herpes simplex virus infections. Med Lett Drugs Ther. 2018; 60:153–7.

6. Seidel V, Feiterna-Sperling C, Siedentopf JP, et al. Intrauterine therapy of cytomegalovirus infection with valganciclovir: review of the literature. Med Microbiol Immunol 2017; 206:347.

7. Centers for Disease Control and Prevention. Influenza antiviral medications: summary for clinicians. Atlanta (GA): CDC; 2018. Available at: https://www.cdc.gov/flu/pdf/professionals/antivirals/antiviral-summary-clinician.pdf. Retrieved June 12, 2018.

8. Greer LG, Sheffield JS, Rogers VL, Roberts SW, McIntire DD & Wendel GD Jr. Maternal and neonatal outcomes after antepartum treatment of influenza with antiviral medications. Obstet. Gynecol, 2010;115:711–716.

9. Society for Maternal-Fetal Medicine (SMFM). Electronic address: pubs@smfm.org, Hughes BL, Page CM, Kuller JA. Hepatitis C in pregnancy: screening, treatment, and management. Am J Obstet Gynecol. 2017 Nov;217(5): B2–B12.

10. British HIV. Association guidelines for the management of HIV in pregnancy and postpartum 2018. HIV Med. 2019 doi: 10.1111/hiv.12720

11. World Health Organization. Update of recommendations on first- and second-line antiretroviral regimens. https://apps.who.int/iris/bitstream/handle/10665/325892/WHO-CDS-HIV-19.15-eng.pdf?ua=1 (Accessed on March 19, 2021).

12. Kintu K, Malaba TR, Nakibuka J, et al. Dolutegravir versus efavirenz in women starting HIV therapy in late pregnancy (DolPHIN-2): an open-label, randomised controlled trial. Lancet HIV 2020; 7: e332.

13. Eley T, Bertz R, Hardy H, Burger D. Atazanavir pharmacokinetics, efficacy and safety in pregnancy: a systematic review. Antivir Ther. 2013; 18:361.

14. Blonk MI, Colbers AP, Hidalgo-Tenorio C, et al. Raltegravir in HIV-1-Infected Pregnant Women: Pharmacokinetics, Safety, and Efficacy. Clin Infect Dis 2015; 61:809.

15. Veklury (remdesivir): US prescribing information. https://www.accessdata.fda.gov/drugsatfda_docs/label/2020/214787Orig1s000lbl.pdf. Accessed 7 Dec 2020.

16. COVID-19 Treatment Guidelines Panel. Remdesivir. National Institutes of Health 2020. Nov 3, 2020. Accessed Dec 19, 2020; Available from: https://www.covid19treatmentguidelines.nih.gov/antiviral-therapy/remdesivir/

17. SMFM Society for Maternal-Fetal Medicine, Halscott T, Vaught J. Management considerations for pregnant patients with COVID-19. 2020. Available at: https://s3.amazonaws.

com/cdn.smfm.org/media/2336/SMFM_ COVID_Management_of_COVID_pos_preg_ patients_4-30-20_final.pdf. Retrieved May 18, 2020.

18. RCOG Royal College of Obstetricians & Gynaecologists. Coronavirus (COVID-19) infection in pregnancy - Version 9 [4 June 2020] London, UK. RCOG 2020. https://www.rcog. org.uk/coronavirus-pregnancy

19. Bhimraj A, Morgan RL, Shumaker AH, et al. Infectious Diseases Society of America (IDSA) guidelines on the treatment and management of patients with COVID-19. https://www. idsociety.org/practice-guideline/covid-19-guideline-treatment-and-management/. Updated April 14, 2021. Accessed April 22, 2021.

20. WHO Solidarity Trial Consortium, Pan H, Peto R, et al. Repurposed antiviral drugs for COVID-19—interim WHO Solidarity Trial results. N Engl J Med. 2020. Available at: https:// www.ncbi.nlm.nih.gov/pubmed/33264556.

21. Fact sheet for healthcare providers: Emergency use authorization (EUA) of baricitinib. https:// www.fda.gov/media/143823/download (Accessed on November 20, 2020)

Drugs in Recurrent Pregnancy Loss: Aspirin and Low Molecular Weight Heparin

• Ganpat Sawant • Madhuri Mehendale

Introduction

When women have two or more consecutive pregnancy losses, it is labelled recurrent pregnancy loss or RPL. Approximately, 0.8–1.4% women have RPL. Fifty percent of women with RPL is unexplained. Multitude of treatments have been made available to patients with unexplained RPL, such as preimplantation genetic diagnosis, lifestyle changes and human menopausal gonadotropin. Recently, Brenner, et al. and Dolitizky, et al. showed anticoagulants and thromoboprophylaxis could be the possible preventive therapy for RPL.[1,2] 50% cases have no specific cause, the anticoagulants and thromoboprophylaxis therapy has been recommended for this group of patients.[3]

ASPIRIN

Aspirin (acetylsalicylic acid) belongs to nonsteroidal anti-inflammatory drug (NSAID) group. Mechanism of action is mainly by inhibition of two cyclo-oxygenase isoenzymes (COX-1 and COX-2), which are necessary for prostaglandin biosynthesis. The COX-1 isoform exists in the vascular endothelium. It regulates the synthesis of prostacyclin and thromboxane-A2 prostaglandins. It has opposing effects on vascular homeostasis and function of platelet. Prostacyclin is a potent vasodilator and inhibitor of platelet aggregation. Thromboxane-A2 (TXA2) is a potent vasoconstrictor and promotes platelet aggregation. The COX-2 isoform can be induced. It is produced entirely post-exposure to cytokines or other inflammatory mediators. The effect of aspirin on COX-dependent prostaglandin synthesis is dependent on its dose. Lower dosages (60–150 mg/day) aspirin irreversibly acetylates COX-1. This decreases platelet synthesis of TXA2. It does not affect vascular wall production of prostacyclin . At higher doses, aspirin inhibits both COX-1 and COX-2. Thus, effectively blocking all prostaglandin production.

RISKS OF ASPIRIN USE IN PREGNANCY

Maternal Risks

Most of systematic reviews of randomized controlled trials (RCTs) have concluded that there was no increase in hemorrhagic complications during pregnancy with the low-dose aspirin.[4–6]

Fetal Risks

- Using low-dose aspirin for prevention of pre-eclampsia showed no increase in risk of congenital anomalies, as seen in various systematic reviews of trials.
- There is concern about possible association between aspirin use during pregnancy and gastroschisis.[7–9]

- Low-dose aspirin (60–150 mg) in the third trimester has not shown any association with ductal closure.[10,11]
- Recent most Cochrane meta-analysis did not find an increased risk of neonatal intracranial hemorrhage [10 trials (26, 184 infants)]. Neither did it show any other neonatal hemorrhagic complications [eight trials (27,032 infants)] associated with maternal intake of low-dose aspirin during the last trimester.[4]

Contraindications to Aspirin Use during Pregnancy

1. History of aspirin allergy (*e.g.* urticaria) or hypersensitivity to other salicylates.
2. Patients with known hypersensitivity to NSAIDs.
3. Patients with nasal polyps, asthma may result in life-threatening broncho-constriction and hence should be avoided.
4. Relative contraindications to include a history of gastrointestinal bleeding, active peptic ulcer disease, other sources of gastrointestinal or genitourinary bleeding, and severe hepatic dysfunction. Reye syndrome has been reported rarely (<1%) in children <18 years who are given aspirin while recovering from viral illnesses, particularly influenza and chickenpox.

Aspirin in Early Pregnancy Loss

- The risk of early pregnancy loss in women with antiphospholipid syndrome has shown decline with usage of combination of low-dose aspirin and unfractionated or low molecular weight heparin.
- Low-dose aspirin has not been effective in preventing unexplained early pregnancy loss in women not suffering from anti-phospholipid syndrome.
- The use of low-dose aspirin prophylaxis is not recommended for the prevention of early pregnancy loss.

LOW MOLECULAR WEIGHT HEPARIN

Low molecular weight heparin (LMWH) has been studied enough for its use during pregnancy. The biology and the pharmacology is well-studied and well-understood. It can be summated in three main mechanisms of action: Anticoagulant, anti-inflammatory, and immunomodulant. The clinical significance of these drugs during pregnancy is mainly because of its action on the placenta. Owing to the presence of specific molecular and cellular targets of these, particularly at the trophoblast-endometrial interface. It is well-documented for the prevention and treatment of thromboembolism. LMWH have been immensely investigated for the improved chances of embryo implantation and for the prevention of placenta-related complications such as pre-eclampsia, fetal growth restriction, and intrauterine fetal death.

Are LMWHs safe for women with RPL? Evaluating the possible adverse events is important. Various studies have been done and most of them reported that thromboprophylaxis during pregnancy was safe for both the fetus and patients. Moreover, Bazzan, et al. found that the LMWHs could not pass through the blood–placental barrier, thus the safety of using it for pregnant patients.[12] However, it has been noticed that there is increase in skin reactions at the injection site after the LMWH.

LMWHs have shown greater benefit for women with either congenital or acquired thrombophilias in terms of live births, miscarriage rates and late obstetrical complication rates.

Conclusions

In accordance to current evidences and results, it shows that the LMWH therapy may increase the live births and decrease the miscarriage rates in patients with RPL compared with control groups. Also, most of the recent RCTs have proven the safety and efficacies of the LMWH treatment in patients with unexplained RPL. Owing to the small sample sizes of currently available publications and the limitations in this study, further more high-quality studies which have larger sample size and are multicentric are needed.

COMBINATION OF ASPIRIN AND HEPARIN

Recurrent pregnancy loss (RPL) is the most commonest presentation and worry of anti-phospholipid syndrome (APS). Activated CD4+ T cells are involved in its pathogenesis. Treatment with low-molecular weight heparin (LMWH) and aspirin combination improves pregnancy outcome, however, its mechanism of action is still to be well-understood. On evaluating the effect of this therapy on Th1/Th2 cells showed that serum cytokine levels, T cell phenotypes, and transcription factors' gene expression levels representing Th1 responses were higher, whereas those representing Th2 responses were lower in patients with APS-RPL at the time of early pregnancy. This Th1-bias was reversed in patients who had live birth after receiving the combination therapy at the time of delivery. Patients with miscarriages continued to exhibit Th1-bias. In conclusion, these data support a role of Th1-bias in the pathogenesis of APS-RPL and suggest restoring T-cell phenotype as a new immunomodulatory mechanism of LMWH/aspirin combination.

References

1. H. Qublan, Z. Amarin, M. Dabbas, A.E. Farraj, Z. Beni-Merei, H. Al-Akash, et al.Low-molecular-weight heparin in the treatment of recurrent IVF-ET failure and thrombophilia: a prospective randomized placebo-controlled trial [J] Hum Fertil (Camb), 2008;11(4):246–253[24].

2. B Brenner, R Hoffman, H Carp, M Dulitsky, J Younis, Investigators L-EEfficacy and safety of two doses of enoxaparin in women with thrombophilia and recurrent pregnancy loss: the LIVE-ENOX study [J] J Thromb Haemostasis, 2005;3(2):227–229[25].

3. M Dolitzky, A Inbal, Y Segal, A. Weiss B. Brenner, H. Carp A randomized study of thrombo-prophylaxis in women with unexplained consecutive recurrent miscarriages [J] Fertil Steril, 2006;86(2):362–366.

4. Duley L, Henderson-Smart DJ, Meher S, King JF. Antiplatelet agents for preventing pre-eclampsia and its complications. Cochrane Database of Systematic Reviews 2007, Issue 2. Art. No.: CD004659.

5. Askie LM, Duley L, Henderson-Smart DJ, Stewart LA. Antiplatelet agents for prevention of pre-eclampsia: a meta-analysis of individual patient data. PARIS Collaborative Group. Lancet 2007;369:1791–8.

6. Henderson JT, Whitlock EP, O'Connor E, Senger CA, Thompson JH, Rowland MG. Low-dose aspirin for prevention of morbidity and mortality from preeclampsia: a systematic evidence review for the U.S. Preventive Services Task Force. Ann Intern Med 2014;160:695–703.

7. Kozer E, Nikfar S, Costei A, Boskovic R, Nulman I, Koren G. Aspirin consumption during the first trimester of pregnancy and congenital anomalies: a meta-analysis. Am J Obstet Gynecol 2002;187:1623–30.

8. Sibai BM, Mirro R, Chesney CM, Leffler C. Low-dose aspirin in pregnancy. Obstet Gynecol 1989; 74:551–7.

9. Wyatt-Ashmead J. Antenatal closure of the ductus arteriosus and hydrops fetalis. Pediatr Dev Pathol 2011;14:469–74.

10. Bujold E, Roberge S, Lacasse Y, Bureau M, Audibert F, Marcoux S, et al. Prevention of preeclampsia and intrauterine growth restriction with aspirin started in early pregnancy: a meta-analysis. Obstet Gynecol 2010;116:402–14.

11. Roberge S, Bujold E, Nicolaides KH. Aspirin for the prevention of preterm and term preeclampsia: systematic review and metaanalysis. Am J Obstet Gynecol 2017;218:287–93.e1.

12. M. Bazzan, V. Donvito Low-molecular-weight heparin during pregnancy [J] Thromb Res, 2001; 101 (1):V175–V186.

Atosiban

• Priyanka H Vora • Kairavi H Gokani • Kedar N Ganla

Introduction

Atosiban was developed in Sweden and foremost described in the literature in 1985. It has now been licensed for use as evidenced by Royal College of Obstetricians and Gynecologists (RCOG), Cochrane and randomized controlled trials (RCTs). Its systemic name is 1-(3-mercaptopropionic acid-2-(o-ethyl-D-ornithine)-4-L-threonine-8-L-ornithine-oxytocin.

Molecular formula	$CH_{43}H_{67}N_{11}O_{12}S_2$
Molecular weight	994.2 g/mol

Pharmacokinetics

Atosiban is a synthetic peptide with a structure similar to oxytocin except in positions 1, 2, 4, 8 **(Figs 6.1 and 6.2)**.

It is a nona-peptide, desamino-oxytocin analogue (1-[3-Mpa, 2-D-Tyr (Et), 4-Thr, Orn]-oxytocin), and a competitive mixed vasopressin V1a/oxytocin receptor antagonist (VOTra).

Two metabolites of atosiban have been identified:

- M1 (main metabolite) (des-(Orn , Gly-NH2)-[Mpa , D-Tyr(Et) , Thr]-oxytocin) and
- M3 in the plasma and urine of women.

The ratios of the main metabolite M1 to atosiban concentrations in plasma were 1.4 and 2.8 at the second hour and at the end of the infusion respectively. It is indeterminate whether M1 accumulates in tissues. Atosiban

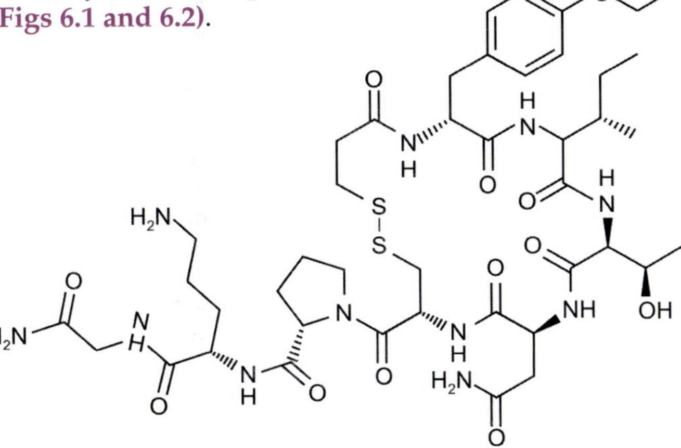

Fig. 6.1: Molecule of atosiban acetate

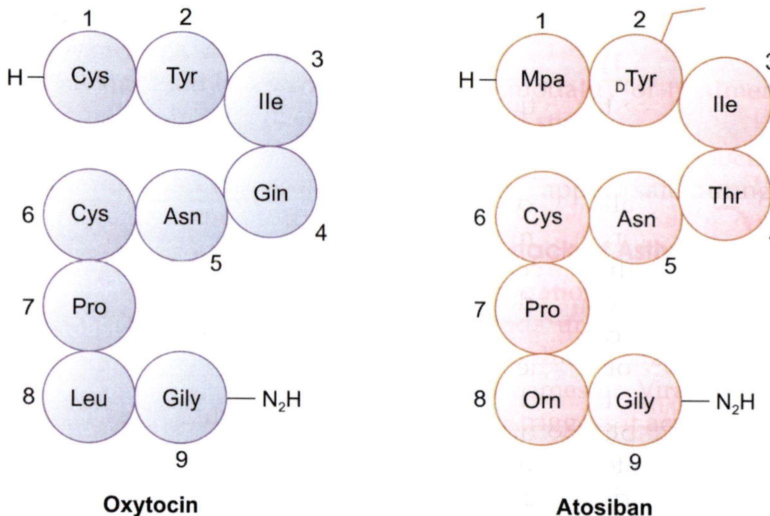

Fig. 6.2: Peptide structures of oxytocin and atosiban

has been found in small quantities in urine, its urinary concentration is about 50 times lower than that of M1. M1 is approximately 10 times less potent than atosiban in inhibiting contractions *in vitro* and is excreted in breast milk.

In pregnant women plasma protein binding of atosiban is 46 to 48%. It is undetermined whether the free fraction in the maternal and fetal compartments differs substantially. Atosiban does not seperate into red blood cells. Peak plasma concentrations are achieved within 2–8 minutes after intravenous administration. Once the infusion is stopped, plasma concentrations decline rapidly with an initially half-life of 0.21+/–0.01 hours and terminal half-life of 1.7+/–0.3 hours, respectively.[1]

COMPOSITION

One vial of solution for injection contains 0.9 ml solution, equivalent to 6.75 mg atosiban.

Colourless glass vials, clear borosilicated (type I) sealed with grey siliconized bromo-butyl rubber stopper, type I, and flip-off cap of polypropylene and aluminium.

It is stored between 2–8°C. Shelf life of atosiban is 4 years. It has a protective covering in order to shield it from light. Once, the vial is opened, it has to be used immediately. The solution once diluted should be used within 24 hours after preparation for intravenous administration.

It is available as the brand name Tractocile (Ferring)/Tosiban (Zuventus).

INDICATIONS OF ATOSIBAN

1. The main indication of use is in uterine contractions when
   - They are regular lasting for at least 30 seconds with cervical dilatation of 1–3 cm in multiparous women or 0–3 cm in nulliparous women with 50% effacement.
   - Between 24–33 weeks of pregnancy.
   - A normal foetal heart rate
2. It is the safest drug of choice in spontaneous pre-term labor, multiple pregnancies, anemia and expanded blood volume.
3. It is also used in recurrent implantation failures, uterine fibroids and patients of endometriosis.
4. It also increases the implantation and pregnancy rates in patients post-embryo transfer.
5. In the non-pregnant uterus, in patients with dysmenorrhea.

MECHANISM OF ACTION
(Fig. 6.3 and Flowchart 6.1)

a. Atosiban is an effective tocolytic as it is uterospecific.

b. It blocks the increase in intracellular calcium and does not allow oxytocin to activate the V1a receptor. As a result, the stored calcium from the sarcoplasmic reticulum of myometrial cells is decreased leading to less influx of calcium from the extracellular space through the voltage gated channels.[2] This, thus, decreases the frequency and amplitude of uterine contractions leading to uterine quiescence.

c. It inhibits the endometrial production of prostaglandin $F_{2\alpha}$, which improves the endometrial perfusion thereby increasing the live birth rate.[3]

d. It relaxes the uterine arteries through improved perfusion of the endometrium and muscular wall of the uterus.

e. It decreases the intensified uterine contractions, endomyometrial ischemia and pain, caused by glandular endometrial cells in a non-pregnant uterus.

f. It causes less thrombocyte aggregation.[4]

How should atosiban be used?

A. In Pre-term Labour

Step	Dose	Infusion rate	Regimen
1	0.9 ml (6.75 mg)	Not applicable	Intravenous bolus injection– over 1 min
2	7.5 ml in 100 ml normal saline (54 mg)	24 ml/hour (300 µg/min)	Intravenous loading infusion– over 3 hours
3	7.5 ml in 500 ml Ringer Lactate (up to 270 mg)	8 ml/hour (100 µg/min)	Subsequent intravenous infusion––up to 45 hours

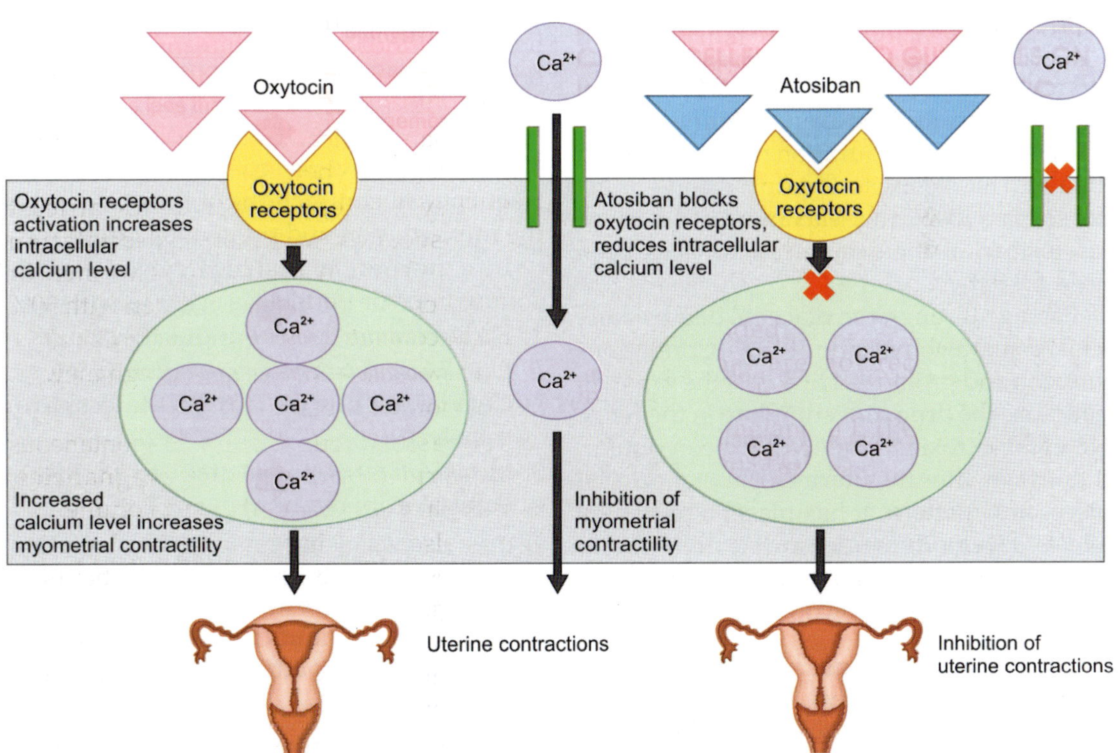

Fig. 6.3: Mechanism of action

Flowchart 6.1: Mechanism of action

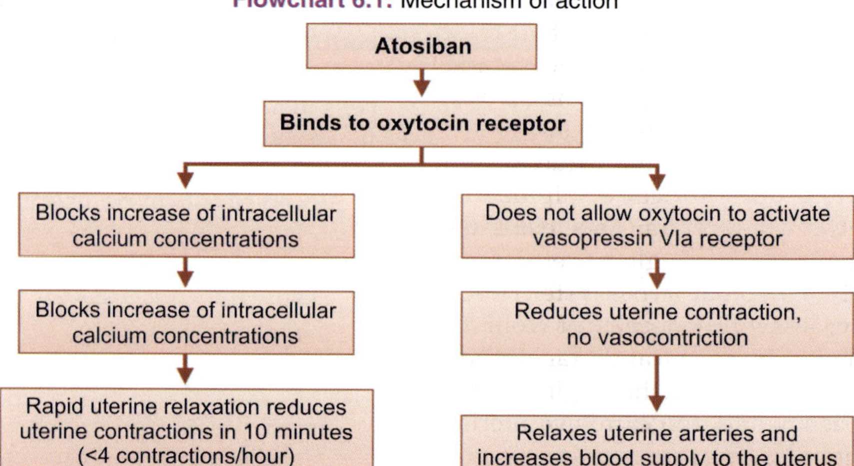

Within 10 minutes of administration of atosiban, the number of contractions are lessened to <4 in 24 hours. Between 24 and 27 weeks of gestation, there is limited clinical research in multiple pregnancy patients, because of a limited patient population.

The effectiveness of atosiban is gestation dependent since more receptors are available with increasing gestation. There is a decline in almost 75% of the uterine contractions in the first three hours post-drug administration. The total treatment duration must not exceed 2 days. The complete therapy dosage must not surpass 330.75 mg. Maximum of 4 reusage of atosiban in the same gestation has been used till date.[5]

Passage through the placenta of atosiban–fetal versus maternal ratio of 0.124. Continuous infusion and prolonged hours of the same do not cause the drug to accumulate in the fetus. No embryo toxic influence has been noted.[3] It does not alter the uterine or foetal arterial blood flow pattern. It has placebo level side effects. Haemodynamic cardiac activities in fetuses remains unaffected.

Rationale of Tocolysis[6]

- There is a time frame savior for cortico-steroid administration.
- Buys time for patient shift with fetus in utero to a tertiary care center where neonatal intensive care unit (NICU) facilities are available. Permits further growth and maturation of the fetus.
- Number of days gained *in utero* increases.
- Reduces the NICU stay of the neonate.
- Cuts cost/burden of the couple
- Reduces the risk of perinatal morbidity and mortality.
- Best maternal and fetal safety profile.

B. In Embryo Transfer (ET)

There is an inverse co-relation between frequency of contractions of the uterus with the implantation and pregnancy rates.[3]

In a normal menstrual cycle, uterine contractions or peristalsis occur as follows:[7]

1. *Early follicular phase:* Fundus to cervix
2. *Late follicular and peri-ovulatory phase:* Cervix to fundus (to facilitate sperm transfer)
3. *Luteal phase:* Quiescence (to facilitate embryo implantation)

Hyperperistalsis: More than 2 waves per minute.

Dysperistalsis: Contractions arising from the middle portion and advancing to both fundal and cervical region.

Excessive uterine contractions: More than 5 contractions per minute.

Two main causes of embryo transfer (ET) failure have been noted—one is failure of embryo-endometrial dialogue and second is wave of myometrial contractions causing the embryo to expel out of the uterine cavity.[8] Factors influencing uterine contractions in ET patients include cervical manipulation, rigid catheters, difficult transfers, excessive catheter tip movement, high concentrations of estradiol in fresh embryo transfer cycles. Studies have shown that <50% of embryos transferred remain *in utero* after transfer and about 15% are found in the vagina.[4] This could probably be due to excessive uterine contractions.

Step	Dose	Infusion rate	Regimen
1	0.9 ml (6.75 mg)	Not applicable	Intravenous bolus injection, 30 min. prior to ET
2	18 mg	2.4 ml/ hour	Intravenous infusion continued after the loading dose
3	12 mg (up to 37.5 mg)	0.8 ml/ hour	Intravenous infusion continued for 2 hours post-ET

Et: Embryo transfer

Side Effects

Very common	Common	Infrequent	Rare
Nausea	Hyper-tension	Pruritis	Uterine atony (post-partum)
	Headache	Rash	Uterine hemorrhage (postpartum)
	Dizziness	Insomnia	
	Tachycardia	Pyrexia	
	Vomiting		
	Hot flush		
	Hypotension		
	Reaction at the injection site		

The cardiovascular side-effects are less than ten times.

Contraindication

- Pregnant women <24 weeks or >33 weeks of gestation
- Premature membrane rupture >30 weeks of gestation
- *Fetal heart rate:* Irregularity or abnormality
- Eclampsia
- Pre-eclampsia
- Intra-uterine fetal death
- Suspected chorioamnionitis
- Placenta previa and abruptio placenta
- Hypersensitivity to atosiban

Precautions

- Renal or hepatic impairment patients.
- Pregnant woman <18 years of age.
- Multiple pregnancy or a 24 and 27 weeks gestation pregnancy.

Drug Interactions

Atosiban has no role in drug-to-drug interactions mediated by CYP450.

No interactions have been found between atosiban and betamethasone or labetalol which are of clinical relevance.

Pharmacovigilance

Till date no safety issues have been reported on routine monitoring of drug safety.[9]

REVIEW OF LITERATURE

A. Strong Evidence in Spontaneous Preterm Labour

- >350 research articles, earliest 1985 compared to nifedipine (poor quality evidence) and β-agonist (isoxsuprine, ritodrine, terbutaline, fenoterol)[10]
- From its clinical introduction in open-label pilot studies through Phase II, Phase III, world-wide comparative studies and Phase IV studies a robust evidence base for atosiban has been established.[10]

- Open label comparative study concluded that atosiban reduces uterine electrical activity in women with preterm labor. Atosiban showed 79% success with regards to its effectiveness as a tocolytic agent among 208 patients after 48 hours of treatment.[11]
- Cochrane meta-analysis concluded that oxytocin antagonists appear to be effective and safe for tocolysis in preterm labor.[12]
- RCOG recommended that if tocolytics are to be used atosiban or nifedipine are preferable. Atosiban is licensed and nifedipine is not. β2-agonists should not be used.
- According to a meta-analysis of 9 randomized studies infants born after tocolysis with atosiban revealed no ill-effects on their psychosocial and motor development up to the age of 2 years.[13]

B. Evidence in Embryo Transfer and Recurrent Implantation Failures

- A randomized controlled trial showed that atosiban increases the implantation rate and pregnancy rate after *in vitro* fertilization (IVF)—embryo transfer.[14]
- A randomized placebo-controlled multi-center trial evaluated effects of the selective oxytocin antagonist and the mixed oxytocin/vasopressin V1a antagonist, atosiban and placebo on luteal phase uterine contractions after controlled ovarian stimulation and luteal phase support with progesterone in 125 oocyte donors suggested that atosiban and barusiban reduced uterine contractility in luteal phase.[15]
- In recurrent implantation failure, when atosiban was used in 71 women, the frequency of uterine contractions reduced, thus improving the implantation rate per cycle to 13.9% and clinical pregnancy rate per cycle to 43.7%.[16]
- Comparison between effect of atosiban and piroxicam in 60 patients before embryo-transfer showed higher pregnancy, implantation and live birth rates in atosiban group than piroxicam group.[17]

CONCLUSIONS

- Atosiban is recommended as a first line new advent agent in spontaneous preterm labor management.
- Atosiban acts only on myometrium/myoepithelial tissues.
- Most of the tocolytics are not uterospecific and have multiorgan side-effects.
- The aim for tocolysis in cases of preterm delivery is to curb the contractions of the uterus and delay preterm labor to allow *in utero* transfer to an appropriate level facility with NICU facilities and to allow for administration of corticosteroids to induce lung maturation. In addition, this allows to delay in delivery and permit *in utero* growth, maturation of fetus and to reduce perinatal mortality and morbidity of the fetus.
- In patients with threatened preterm birth, repeated usage of atosiban in the same gestation stops labour. This is useful in twin pregnancy, however there must not be any fetal compromise or underlying maternal infection.
- Atosiban does not have side effects even when reused multiple times in the same pregnancy.
- Since its mechanism of action is relaxation of the uterus, postpartum blood loss as a potential side effect must be kept in mind, however no such case has been reported in literature till date.[18]
- In certain cases of embryo transfer, an excessive peristaltic activity may be the cause of recurrent implantation failure. Atosiban may help reduce the implantation rates in these subset of patients.

References

1. Gail M Fullerton, Mairead Black, Ashalatha Shetty and Sohinee Bhattacharya. Atosiban in the management of preterm labour. Clinical Medicine insights: Women's health 2011;4:9–16.
2. Katie M Groom Philip. R.Bennet. Tocolysis for treatment of preterm labour-a clinical based review. Review The Obstetrician and Gynaecologist 2004; 6:1.

3. Ozlem Moralogul, Esra Tongu, Turgut Var, Tugba Zeyrek, Sertac Batioglu et al. Treatment with oxytocin antagonist before embryo transfer may increase implantation rates after IVF. J of Reproductive Healthcare 2010;04:009.

4. Decleer et al. Osmanagoaglu. Role of oxytocin antagonist is repeated implantation failure FVV in OBGYN. 2012;4(4):227–229.

5. Dr. Priyanka Vora, Dr. Kedar Ganla. Multiple re-treatments with Atosiban, an oxytocin receptor antagonist helps to delay preterm labor successfully. Acta Scientific Women's health. MAY 2021:2582–3205(3):5.

6. Romero R, et al. An oxytocin receptor antagonist (atosiban) in the treatment of preterm labor: a randomized, double-blind, placebo-controlled trial with tocolytic rescue. American journal of obstetrics and gynecology 182.5(2000):1173–83.

7. Ernest Hung Yu Ng, Raymond Hang Wun Li, Leining Chen, A randomized double blind comparison of Atosiban in patients undergoing IVF treatment. J of Human Reprod 2014. 29(12):2687–2694.

8. SA Hebisha, Hisham MA del. Impact of the oxytocin receptor antagonist atosiban administered shortly before embryo transfer on pregnancy rates after ICSI, Clinical Exp. Obstet. Gynecol 2018. 0390–6663:V(4).

9. Ronald F Lamont EXPERT REVIEW OBSTET. GYNECOL. 2008;3(2):163–174.

10. Lyndrup J, Lamont RF. The choice of tocolytic for the treatment of preterm labor: a critical evaluation of nifedipine versus atosiban. Expert opinion investigation drugs. 2007 Jun;6(6):843–53.

11. Hadar E. BJOJ An journal of obstetrics and Gynecology 2013 June 2015. 9378(13):00542–5.

12. Coomarasamy A.Med Sci Monit. 2002 November; 8(11):RA268–73.

13. The world wide Atosiban versus beta-agonists study group. BJOG.2001 Feb ;108(2):133–42.

14. Moraloglu O. Moralglu O.Reprod Biomed Online. 2010 Sep;21(3):338–43.

15. C Blockeel, R Pierson Effects of barusiban and atosiban on frequency of uterine contractions in luteal phase after stimulation; Human Reprod 2009 ESHRE Amsterdam.

16. Vuong Thi Ngoc lan, Vu Nhat Khang Reproductive Biomedicine online Sept 2012;25 (3), 254–260.

17. Kadhim BH, Salman MO. Comparison between the effect of Atosiban and piroxicam administration before embryo transfer on in vitro fertilization outcome: Pharmacology online; 2021;1:511–516.

18. Husslein P, et al. Clinical Practice evaluation of atosiban in preterm labour management in six European countries. BJOG; an international journal of obstetrics and gynaecology 2006; 113(3): 105–10.

Augmentation of Labour

• Nishita Shah • Sarita Bhalerao

Introduction and Definition

Augmentation of labour is indicated when spontaneous contractions are not adequate this for the labour to progress, if not corrected can lead to prolonged labour and increase the rate of caesarean section, as well as increase the risk of adverse maternal and fetal outcomes.

In this chapter, we will discuss the various methods for labour augmentation along with their benefits and side effects. Labour augmentation can be done by various methods ranging from artificial rupture of membranes to the use of uterotonic drugs-like oxytocin.

The aim of augmentation of labour is to help the contractions increase in intensity (if <25 mm Hg) or frequency (if <3 contractions in 10 minutes) or duration or both.

WHO has given some Guiding Principles, which overall highlights the precautions to be taken while augmenting labour, including the patients wish, risks *vs* benefits, indications and contra-indications, monitoring, previous scars, malpresentations and the set-up.[1]

In a nulliparous woman, the diagnosis of a prolonged second stage should be considered when the second stage exceeds 3 hours, if regional anesthesia has been administered or 2 hours, if no regional anesthesia is used. In multiparous women, the diagnosis can be made when the second stage exceeds 2 hours with regional anesthesia or 1 hour without.[12]

Indications: The type of arrest in labour, whether it is primary or secondary, can determine to some extent the success of labour augmentation.

Primary arrest is when progression in the early part of active labour (between 3–7 cm dilatation) is <1 cm/h in multiparas and 0.5 cm/h in nulliparas. Most common causes for this are poor uterine activity, malposition or malrotation or deflexed head. Augmentation works well for most of these patients for labour to progress.

Secondary arrest is in the later half of cervical dilatation; between 7–10 cm. In these patients there is a higher risk of instrumental delivery, most common reason being a mechanical problem-like malposition, malrotation or deflexed head. Yet 60% of nulliparas and 70% of multiparas respond to oxytocin augmentation due to adequate uterine contractions.[2]

METHODS OF AUGMENTATION

Amniotomy[3] (Table 7.1)

- Is defined as artificially rupturing of the membranes
- Benefits—it increases the uterine contractions and helps in early meconium detection

Table 7.1: Effects of amniotomy

Study	Number	Effects of amniotomy					
		Mean dilatation at amniotomy	*Mean shortening of labor*	*Need for oxytocin*	*Cesarean delivery rate*	*Abnormal tracing*	*Neonatal effects*
Fraser (1993)	925	<5 cm	125 min	None	None[a]	None	None
Garite (1993)	459	5.5 cm	81 min	Decreased	None	Increased[b]	None
UK amniotomy group (1994)	1463	5.1 cm	60 min	None	None	NA	None

[a]No effect on overall rate; cesarean delivery for fetal distress significantly increased
[b]Increased mild and moderate umbilical cord compression patterns
NA = Not assessed

- Recommended prior to commencing oxytocin augmentation
- The procedure hastens the labour and can also reduce the oxytocin usage.[12,13]

Drugs (Table 7.2)

1. Oxytocin

Introduction

- Nonapeptide CNS neuropeptide which is made in the paraventricular nuclei of hypothalamus and stored there. It is released from posterior pituitary gland.
- Oxytocin is a recombinant hormone, which needs to be maintained in cold chain.
- It helps in labour augmentation by increasing the intensity of uterine contractions.
- It was discovered in 1906 by Sir Henry Dale, who also gave it the name Oxytocin- from Greek words (swi birth).

Pharmacodynamics

- Stimulates labour and delivery as well as lactation
- Physiological influences on metabolic and cardiovascular functions.

Indications

1. Antepartum for induction of labour. Medical indications for induction of labor include Rh isoimmunisation, maternal diabetes, pre-eclampsia, PROM
2. Intrapartum, it is used for labour augmentation. It is also used in cases of incomplete or inevitable abortion.
3. Postpartum usage is to control postpartum hemorrhage.

Contraindications

- Allergy to the drug
- Malpositions or malpresentations or cephalopelvic disproportion

Table 7.2: Methods of use drug regimen for augmentation of labour

Regimen	Starting dose (mU/min)	Incremental increase (mU/min)	Interval (min)
Low-dose	0.5–1.5	1	15–40
	2	4, 8, 12, 16, 20, 25, 30	15
High-dose	4	4	15
	4.5	4.5	15–30
	6	6[a]	20–40[b]

[a]With uterine tachysystole and after oxytocin infusion is discontinued, it is restarted at the previous dose and increased at 3 mU/min incremental doses.
[b]Uterine tachysystole is more common with shorter intervals.
Data from Merril, 1999; Satin, 1992, 1994; Xenakis, 1995

- Fetal distress in early labour
- Hypertonic uterus
- Contraindications to vaginal birth-cord presentation, cord prolapse, complete placenta previa and vasa previa

Administration[3]

Methods of use

The bed-side method is to dilute 5 IU in 500 ml of Ringer lactate or 0.9% sodium chloride (10 milliunits per ml), and start the drip at 2–8 drops/minute which is 1–4 milliunits/minute; to be titrated over 20–30 mins as per uterine contractions and fetal heart rate monitoring, by 1–2 milliunits/min, till uterine contractions increase in intensity and duration and labour progress.

Always rule out all the contraindications and the patients' general health is of utmost priority.

Monitoring is the most crucial part of labour augmentation, as high doses can lead to complications like fetal distress, precipitate labour, uterine rupture or perineal tears; and hence to use it in a set-up where adequate facilities are available.

Mechanism of action (Flowchart 7.1)

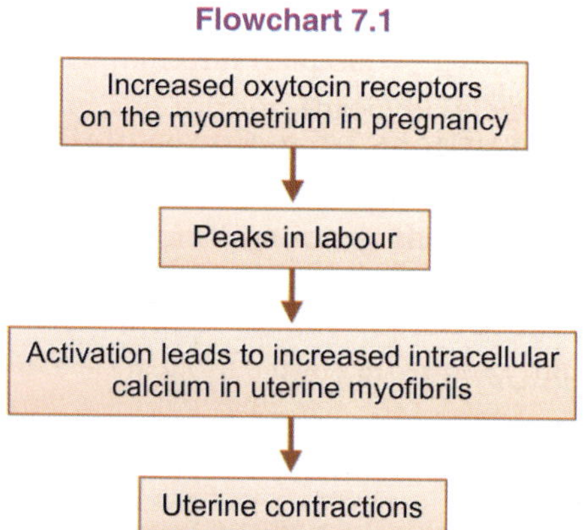

Flowchart 7.1

Oxytocin is regulated by positive feedback mechanism continuing until parturition: Fetal head engagement and cervical dilatation signals the release of oxytocin from the posterior pituitary of the mother—stimulates uterine contractions—increasing amounts of oxytocin released—positive feedback loop continues.

Absorption: It is fully bioavailable.

After parenteral administration, it takes approximately 40 minutes for oxytocin to reach steady-state concentrations in the plasma.

Metabolism and route of elimination: By the enzyme oxytocinase (major source being placenta); while small percentage is excreted in the urine unchanged.

Half-life: From 1–6 minutes in the plasma; decreased in late pregnancy and during lactation.

Toxicity: High doses can lead to uterine spasms, hypertonicity, or rupture.

It can also cause myocardial ischemia, tachycardia, and arrhythmias in high doses.

Being an antidiuretic; water intoxication at larger doses of 40–50 milliunits/minute, can result in maternal convulsions, coma, and even death.

Adverse reactions can range from nausea and vomiting to severe drug reactions due to allergies. Fetal cardiac arrhythmia and premature ventricular contractions have also been noted; permanent fetal CNS damage and death are some of the serious adverse reactions. Others include neonatal retinal hemorrhage, low Apgar score at 5 minutes and neonatal jaundice.

2. Valethamate

Valethamate is an anticholinergic medication used to symptomatically manage conditions involving smooth muscle spasms. It works by blocking the effect of acetylcholine, thereby relaxing the smooth muscles of cervix and intestine.

Mechanism of action: It works by its effect on cervical ripening and dilatation, and hence augmenting the progress of labour.

Side effects: Some patients complain of dry mouth and flushed face.

In a few, feto-maternal tachycardia has been noted.[4–8]

3. Drotaverine

It is used to decrease the smooth muscle spams, hence relieves the gastrointestinal and genitourinary spasmodic pain. It is structurally related to papaverine.

Pharmacodynamics: Drotaverine is a spasmolytic agent decreasing the visceral spasms and thus helping in cervical dilation

Mechanism of action: Increased levels of cyclic adenosine monophosphate (cAMP) leads to smooth muscle relaxation. Phosphodiesterase-4 (PDE_4) is an enzyme responsible for the degradation of cAMP.

Drotaverine selectively inhibits PDE_4, which causes levels of cAMP to increase; thus leading to smooth muscle relaxation.

Metabolism and route of elimination: Liver and biliary excretion contributes maximum elimination with excretion in feces, and lesser in urine.

Half-life: By oral or intravenous administration of 80 mg dose, the mean half-life was about 9.11 or 9.33 hours ± 1.29 or 1.02 hours.

Drotaverine has been seen to accelerate labor more rapidly with lesser side effects as compared to valethamate bromide.[9]

4. Meperidine (Pethidine)

Being an opioid agonist, it helps in labour and postoperative analgesia, especially for moderate to severe pain. It has sedative properties.

Pharmacodynamics: Chemically this synthetic opiate agonist is similar to local anesthetics.

Mechanism of action: Opiate receptors are coupled with G-protein receptors and function as both positive and negative regulators of synaptic transmission via G-proteins that activate effector proteins. Binding of the opiate stimulates the exchange of guanosine triphosphate (GTP) for guanosine diphosphate (GDP) on the G-protein complex. As the effector system is adenylate cyclase and cAMP located at the inner surface of the plasma membrane, opioids decrease intracellular cAMP by inhibiting adenylate cyclase. Subsequently, the release of nociceptive neurotransmitters such as substance P, GABA, dopamine, acetylcholine and noradrenaline, is inhibited. Opioids also inhibit the release of vasopressin, somatostatin, insulin and gluca-gon. Opioids close N-type voltage-operated calcium channels (OP2-receptor agonist) and open calcium-dependent inwardly rectifying potassium channels (OP3 and OP1 receptor agonist). This results in hyperpolarization and reduced neuronal excitability.

Absorption: Meperidine has better effect with parenteral administration as compared oral, due to extensive first-pass metabolism.

Route of elimination: It is excreted in the urine.

Half-life: Initial distribution 2–11 minutes in healthy individuals; is prolonged to 7–11 hours in patients with hepatic impairement.

Administering antispasmodics during labour could lead to faster dilatation of the cervix thus decreasing the incidence of prolonged labour.

5. Camylofin (Anafortan)

It helps in faster cervical dilatation, reducing the first stage of labour; thus helps in labour augmentation. It does not seem to have any effect during second and third stages of labour.[10,11]

The side effects of antispasmodics like tachycardia are lesser with camylofin.

6. Misoprostol

Misoprostol is a prostaglandin E_1 analogue.

Mode of administration: It can be used by any mode like oral, vaginal, sublingual or rectal.

Misoprostol has its action by stimulating uterine contractions.

There have been numerous studies on misoprostol use for labour induction and augmentation, trying different dosages and frequencies of dose titration. It has been especially studied in low resource settings, where the facilities for electronic oxytocin infusion are not available, as it prevents the risk of hyperstimulation with uncontrolled oxytocin usage.

It has a safer side effect profile and has been found to be an effective drug for labour augmentation. Sublingual misoprostol has been used in some studies.[14,15]

KEY POINTS

1. WHO recommendations are quite compre-hensive to guide about the precautions to be taken during augmentation of labour.
2. Active phase partograph should be charted in every labour to monitor progress.
3. There are various methods of augmentation of labour, which should be individualized as per the patients' health, fetal monitoring, the set-up where the labour is monitored with keeping a detailed contraindication list.
4. Labour outcomes improve when monitored correctly and augmented under supervision.
5. Correct and adequate labour augmentation helps reduce the risk of prolonged labour and caesarean sections.

References

1. World Health Organization, 2014.
2. Pinas-Carrillo A, Chandraharan E, Glob. libr. women's med., ISSN: 1756-2228; DOI 10.3843/GLOWM.413013.
   The Continuous Textbook of Women's Medicine Series – Obstetrics Module; Volume 11 LA-BOR AND DELIVERY.
3. Williams Obstetrics, 24th Edition.
4. Valethamate bromide: Conflicting evidence and continuing use; Thirunavukkarasu Arun Babu, Vijayan Sharmila.
5. Madhu C, Mahavarkar S, Bhave S. A randomised controlled study comparing Drotaverine hy-drochloride and Valethamate bromide in the augmentation of labour. Arch Gynecol Obstet 2010;282:11–5.
6. Sharma JB, Pundir P, Kumar A, Murthy NS. Drotaverine hydrochloride vs. valethamate bro-mide in acceleration of labor. Int J Gynaecol Obstet 2001;74:255–60.
7. Batukan AC, Özgün MT, Türkyılmaz C, Dolanbay M, Müderris II. The effect of valethamate bromide in acceleration of labor: A double-blind, placebo-controlled trial. J Turkish German Gy-necol Assoc 2006;7:202–5.
8. Ajmera SK, Shah PK, Shinde GA. Comparative Study of Drotaverine v/s Valethamate in Cer-vical Phase of Labour. Bombay hospital journal. Available from: http://www.bhj.org/journal/2006_4802_april/html/org_res_305-309. html [last cited on 2010 Sep 7].
9. A randomised controlled study comparing Drotaverine hydrochloride and Valethamate bro-mide in the augmentation of labour; Chendrimada Madhu 1, Suvarna Mahavarkar, Sudhir Bhave; Randomized Controlled Trial Arch Gynecol Obstet 2010 Jul.
10. J Clin Diagn Res. 2013 Sep; 7(9):1897–1899. Published online 2013 Jul 22.
11. Effectiveness and Safety of Camylofin in Augmentation of Labor: A Systematic Review and Meta-Analysis; J Obstet Gynaecol India 2020 Dec.
12. ACOG practice bulletin clinical management guidelines for obstetrician–gynecologists number 49, DECEMBER 2003.
13. Garite TJ, Porto M, Carlson NJ, Rumney PJ, Reimbold PA. The influence of elective amniotomy on fetal heart rate patterns and the course of labor in term patients: a randomized study. Am J Obstet Gynecol 1993;168: 1827–31; discussion 1831–2. (Level I).
14. Cochrane Database Syst Rev 2013 Sep 23; Titrated oral misoprostol for augmenting labour to improve maternal and neonatal outcomes Joshua P Vogel, Helen M West, Therese Dowswell.
15. Sublingual Misoprostol for labour augmentation Aruna Verma, Abhilasha Gupta, Monika Kashyap; International Journal of Reproduction, Contraception, Obstetrics and Gynecology Verma A, et al. Int J Reprod Contracept Obstet Gynecol. 2019 Apr.

Common Problems in Pregnancy

• Shilpa Agrawal   • Purnima Satoskar

Drugs should be prescribed with caution in pregnancy as maternal drug intake can reach the fetus and may affect the fetus causing malformations and side effects.

CLASSIFICATION BY FOOD AND DRUG ADMINISTRATION

In 1979, a system was developed by Food and Drug Administration (FDA) that determines the teratogenicity of drugs by considering the quality of data from human and animal studies.[1] FDA classifies various drugs used in pregnancy into five categories—categories A, B, C, D and X. Category A is considered the safest category and category X is absolutely contraindicated in pregnancy. This provides therapeutic guidance for the clinician.[1,2]

A: No risk demonstrated by controlled studies in pregnant women in all three trimesters.

B: 1) No fetal risk demonstrated by animal reproduction studies but there are no controlled studies in pregnant women.

Or

(2) Adverse effects in animal studies which were not proven in controlled studies in pregnant women across trimesters.

C: 1) Adverse effects seen in animal studies and there are no controlled studies in pregnant women.   Or

(2) No studies in animals and pregnant women to be prescribed only if benefit outweighs risk.

D: Positive evidence of risk of fetal adverse effects in human pregnancy. However, may need to be prescribed in life-threatening situations or for serious illness where a safer alternative is unavailable.

X: Clearly teratogenic in animal and human studies or with experience after use in humans. Contraindicated in pregnancy.

The fetal effect of any drug depends on the gestational age, dose of the drug and drug levels achieved in maternal blood. There is limited information on the drug effects during the period of fertilization and implantation. It is recommended that women who are planning pregnancy should avoid unnecessary medications during preconception period, mainly 3 to 6 months preconception.

In early period of pregnancy up to 2 weeks after fertilization (blastogenesis), the effect is all or none. It can either be very severe to kill the embryo or not affect the pregnancy at all. The embryonic period, 3rd to 8th week of gestation (organogenesis) is the most vulnerable. It can cause a miscarriage, a birth defect, or a permanent but subtle damage which can be seen later in the life. From 9th week onwards, the embryo is referred to as a fetus. Drug effect can cause disturbances in the maturation and growth and usually not associated with major malformations.

PHARMACOKINETIC CHANGES IN PREGNANCY

1. During pregnancy, there is a 30% expansion in plasma volume and a proportionate increase in cardiac output and glomerular filtration rate. This may reduce the circulating levels of certain drugs to subtherapeutic range.
2. An increase in body fat increases the volume of distribution of fat-soluble drugs.
3. Plasma albumin concentration decreases in pregnancy due to hemodilution. Consequently, the unbound fraction of drugs which are highly protein bound increases.
4. Gastric emptying time is increased (progesterone effect), especially in late pregnancy, thereby onset of action is delayed.
5. Concurrent use of common medications like antacids, vitamins and iron can alter the effect by binding and making the drug inactive.

SAFE MEDICATION DURING PREGNANCY

Taking medicines for minor ailments without advice can be harmful. However, in patients with chronic ailments, *e.g.* epilepsy, or acute problems, *e.g.* high fever, the risk of not taking a medication be more serious than the potential risk associated with taking it. A physician's advice regarding safety of any drug should ideally be sought preconception, including herbal and topical preparations. Most pregnant women use over the counter medications.[3]

The woman should be counselled as follows:

1. Minimum effective dose
2. Minimum duration
3. Not to try new medications in pregnancy
4. Not to stop medications on their own
5. Avoid medications in first trimester as far as possible
6. Avoid self-medication, including herbal preparations

Safety and effectiveness of natural remedies and alternative therapies have not been studied in pregnancy and lactation and hence their safety is not known and should be advised with caution.

Antihistamines

Histamine is released from mast cells in inflammatory processes and type I hypersensitivity allergic reactions. Antihistamines antagonize their actions.

Antihistamines are categorized as 'classic' or first-generation antihistamines and 'newer' or second-generation antihistamines. This classification is based on the presence of side effects on the central nervous system (CNS) at standard dose levels.

The duration of action in second-generation antihistamines tends to be longer (>24 hours) and they can be administered once a day. First-generation antihistamines must be administered 2–3 times a day. Most antihistaminics belong to either category B or category C of US FDA classification.[4]

Precautions
- Administer topically if possible
- Assess if systemic use is required despite the risk
- Preferably use category B agents (chlorpheniramine, diphenhydramine, cetirizine, levocetirizine, and loratadine)
- Avoid using them in first trimester.

They are generally used for allergic rhinitis or nausea.

First generation antihistaminics are safe, *e.g.* diphenhydramine, brompheniramine, chlorpheniramine, pheniramine. No significant fetal malformation with use in first trimester has been shown.

Second generation antihistaminics, *e.g.* loratadine, cetirizine, fexofenadine, do not appear to increase overall fetal risk **(Table 8.1)**.

Table 8.1: FDA categories of various antihistaminics

First generation	Category	Second generation	Category
Diphenhydramine	B	Cetirizine	B
Brompheniramine	C	Loratadine	B
Chlorpheniramine	C	Fexofenadine	C
Pheniramine	C		

One study showed slightly higher incidence of hypospadias with loratadine use but was not found in other study. In animal studies, Fexofenadine has been associated with early pregnancy loss. Though not studied in human pregnancy, it should be avoided.

Topical antihistamines have not been studied sufficiently. One study with topical ophthalmic agent pheniramine did not show any significant malformation. No data is available for other topical antihistamines but since there is no systemic absorption possibility of fetal risk is unlikely.

Decongestants

Phenylephrine: Safety of phenylephrine is not established in pregnancy. Data showed risk of ophthalmic, ear and minor limb malformations (RR 2.7).

Pseudoephedrine: Pseudoephedrine was previously considered safe but small associations with defects, such as gastroschisis, small intestinal atresia, and hemifacial microsomia were observed in recent case-control studies.

Overall, oral decongestants should be avoided as they may increase maternal risk of stroke and myocardial infarction.

Topical decongestants: Xylometazoline and oxymetazoline are inhaled decongestants. They may be associated with some systemic absorption.

A study of 207 women of xylometazoline use in the first trimester did not show any increased incidence of birth defects.

Topical decongestants are relatively safe in pregnancy. Women should be informed about rebound effect after overuse.

Saline nasal sprays can be used safely in pregnancy.[5]

Expectorants and Antitussives

Guaifenesin: There is insufficient evidence about its safety in pregnancy. A weak association with inguinal hernia and neural tube defects was observed. It is better to avoid in pregnancy, especially in the first trimester.

Dextromethorphan: It was not found to be teratogenic in human studies. Maximum dose should not exceed 120 mg in 24 hours.

In 2000, ACOG and the American College of Allergy, Asthma, and Immunology released a position statement regarding the use of asthma and allergy medication. Recommended antihistamines were chlorpheniramine and tripelennamine (PBZ).

Cold medications can be used in pregnancy but should not be used for extended period of time and indiscriminately.

Analgesics and antipyretics: Acetaminophen, aspirin and NSAIDs like ibuprofen or naproxen are commonly used.

Acetaminophen: Animal studies revealed a premature reduction in the diameter of ductus arteriosus, but this cannot be extrapolated to humans.

Acetaminophen for fever in pregnancy actually showed reduced risk of various craniofacial and abdominal wall defects. This may be due to reduction of fever which is associated with these defects.

The National Birth Defects Prevention Study (NBDPS), which analysed data from 16,110 children in the United States with a history of exposure to acetaminophen in utero, found no increased risk of birth defects.

Salicylates: Salicylates have been associated with fetal growth restriction, increased perinatal mortality, prolonged gestation and labour, neonatal haemorrhage and possible birth defects. They should be used only under the guidance and not as an over-the-counter medicine. Low-dose aspirin was not found to be associated with miscarriage or abruption. Aspirin has been extensively studied and is used during pregnancy for many chronic medical disorders like thromboembolism, antiphospholipid syndrome. In the third trimester, aspirin use can cause fetal growth restriction, maternal and fetal haemorrhage, hence should be avoided unless prescribed by the medical professional.

Non-steroidal Anti-inflammatory Drugs (NSAIDs)[6]

Indomethacin

Use of indomethacin in pregnancy has been widely studied. Oligohydramnios, premature closure of fetal ductus arteriosus with subsequent persistent pulmonary hypertension of the newborn may occur but this is uncommon before 30 weeks. It can also cause fetal nephrotoxicity, and periventricular haemorrhage.

Ibuprofen

Small studies did not show association of ibuprofen with fetal defects **(Table 8.2)**. No overall increase in the teratogenicity was seen in a Swedish study of nonsteroidal anti-inflammatory drug (NSAID) use in early pregnancy. Naproxen was associated with orofacial clefts, and all NSAIDs were associated with structural cardiac defects.

Antidiarrheal Agents

Oral rehydration solution (ORS) and probiotics should be recommended for diarrhoea. ORS containing sodium and glucose with osmolality and concentration similar to luminal fluid are very effective. Sorbitol-containing ORS should be avoided as they aggravate diarrhoea. Patients should avoid beverages with high sugar, alcohol and caffeine.

Lactobacillus acidophilus: It is a digestive enzyme which restores normal gut flora. Lactobacillus use has so far not been associated with congenital abnormalities.

Commonly used antidiarrheal medications include:

- Kaolin and pectin preparations
- Bismuth subsalicylate
- Loperamide

Atropine/diphenoxylate: Iron deficiency anaemia can be found in people taking kaolin preparations as iron absorption is affected. Category B in all the trimesters.

Bismuth subsalicylate in pregnancy should be avoided as it falls in Category C in first and second trimesters, category D in third trimester.

There are inadequate studies for the use of loperamide, however one study had shown association between loperamide intake in first trimester and fetal cardiac malformation. Category B in all the trimesters.

Atropine was found to be teratogenic in animals, but there are inadequate human studies. Category C in all the trimesters.

Table 8.2: FDA categories of various analgesics

Medication	Drug class	FDA category
Acetaminophen	Non-narcotic analgesic/antipyretic	B, drug of choice
Aspirin	Salicylates analgesic/antipyretic	C, in the first and second trimesters D, in the third trimester
Ibuprofen	NSAID analgesic	C, in the first and second trimesters D, in the third trimester

Laxatives[7]

Initial advice for constipation includes increasing water intake to 8–10 glasses per day and dietary fibre to about 25–30 grams per day and moderate amounts of daily exercise.

Bulk fibres: Psyllium, polycarbophil, and methylcellulose are used.

Increased dietary fibre improves regularity. It may not provide immediate relief and can cause abdominal bloating and cramping.

The dose is 3 g daily up to 10–20 g daily depending on the tolerance.

Stool softeners: Docusate sodium is used frequently due to favourable safety profile. It may cause electrolyte abnormalities. It is less effective than other laxatives.

Osmotic laxatives: Polyethylene glycol (PEG), lactulose, and osmotic salts are popular.

They retain water which improves stool frequency. Not studied extensively in pregnancy but since it is minimally absorbed, unlikely to cause fetal malformations. Lactulose is considered safe but may cause nausea, abdominal cramping and flatulence. Osmotic salts are better used for short periods as they can cause sodium retention and hypermagnesemia with prolonged usage.

Stimulant laxatives: They increase colonic motor activity and are highly effective.

They may cause dehydration and electrolyte imbalance due to inadvertent diarrhoea hence not commonly prescribed in pregnancy. They have low teratogenic potential as the systemic absorption is minimal.

This class of laxatives are only recommended if there is failure of bulk fibre and osmotic laxatives.

Rectal therapy: Enemas, sodium phosphate are generally not recommended due to the risk of inducing labour.

First-line therapies include an increase in dietary fibre, following which PEG and docusate may be employed.

Mineral oil, castor oil and saline hyperosmotic agents are avoided (Table 8.3).

Antacids (Table 8.4)

Topical antacids: Topical antacids contain alginic acid, aluminium, magnesium, and calcium.

There are sporadic reports of fetal malformations with aluminium containing antacids but insufficient data regarding the same. They can rarely cause neurotoxicity. Antacids containing aluminium and calcium are safe as compared to bismuth and bicarbonate. Antacids containing bicarbonate can cause fluid overload and metabolic alkalosis.

Magnesium sulphate is a tocolytic agent, so usually calcium containing antacids are the preferred one.

Acid reflux in later pregnancy responds better to preparations with sodium alginate which forms a raft floating on stomach contents and protects lower esophagus from acid. The dose is sodium alginate oral suspension (50 mg/ml) 20 ml administered thrice a day.

Table 8.3: FDA categories of various gastrointestinal drugs

Simethicone	Antiflatulent	C
Bismuth subsalicylate	Antidiarrheal	C
Loperamide	Antidiarrheal	C
Mineral oil	Laxative	C
Polyethylene glycol	Laxative	C Drug of choice for chronic constipation
Castor oil	Laxative	X

Table 8.4: FDA categories of various antacids

Antacids	FDA category
Containing aluminium, magnesium and calcium	None
Safe to use in pregnancy	
Containing sodium bicarbonate	None
Not safe for use in pregnancy	
Mucosal protectant sucralfate	B
Histamine-2 receptor antagonist	
Ranitidine	B
Cimetidine	B
Proton pump inhibitors	
Rabeprazole	B
Pantoprazole	B
Omeprazole	C

Table 8.5: FDA categories of various antiemetics

Ginger	C
Pyridoxine	A
Doxylamine	A
Metoclopramide	Not assigned
Ondansetron	B

H2 receptor blockers: They cross the placenta so they are used as a second-line treatment, if the patient is not better with lifestyle changes and antacids.

Cimetidine and ranitidine are the most studied drugs. Animal studies did not show any adverse effect. Nizatidine is linked to adverse effects in animal studies (intrauterine death, spontaneous miscarriage, and low birth weight in rabbits). The recommendation is to avoid them in first trimester as far as possible.

Proton pump inhibitors (PPI): In spite of best efficacy, PPIs have not been extensively studied and the data available is limited. Omeprazole is associated with higher fetal loss in animal studies. It is still categorized as category C in spite of later cohort studies demonstrating the safety profile of omeprazole in periconception and pregnancy. All other PPIs are category B **(Table 8.4)**.[8]

Nausea and Vomiting[9]

Ginger: Ginger containing foods reduce nausea. It contains gingerols and shogaols. A meta-analysis of randomized controlled trials (RCTs) with over 1000 gravidas, ginger use relieved nausea but not vomiting. Use of ginger was not found to be associated with increased risk of major malformations **(Table 8.5)**.

Pyridoxine: Vitamin B_6 acts as an important coenzyme for protein, carbohydrate and lipid metabolism. Vitamin B_6 is considered as a first-line therapy. It is safe and easily available with minimum side effects. It can be taken as a single agent or along with other antiemetics. It reduces nausea but is not effective for vomiting. The mechanism of action is not known. There is limited data on fetal safety at high doses but it is reassuring. An observational study of 96 gravidas in the first trimester administered a dose of >50 mg/day, found no increase in major fetal malformations as compared to controls.[10]

10 to 25 mg, orally, 6–8 hourly up to a maximum of 100 mg/day is advised.

Doxylamine: Doxylamine is an antihistamine which blocks H1 receptors. Direct action is by inhibiting the H1 receptors and indirect action is by reducing the stimulation of vomiting centre. It is usually given in combination with pyridoxine.

A formulation containing doxylamine 10 mg and pyridoxine 10 mg is recommended in an initial dose of two extended-release tablets at night which can take care of morning nausea and vomiting. If needed, a tablet in the morning and afternoon can be added. Side effects include giddiness, dryness of mouth, headache, sleepiness and hypersensitivity. If a woman is on central nervous system depressants like other antihistamines, opiates or sedatives, this drug is not recommended. Caution is advocated in women who have—(1) asthma,

(2) narrow-angle glaucoma, (3) peptic ulcer, (4) pyloroduodenal obstruction, or (5) bladder-neck obstruction.

Metoclopramide: One of the most commonly prescribed medicines for nausea and vomiting of pregnancy. It increases lower oesophageal sphincter tone, hastens gastric emptying and reduces nausea and vomiting by blocking dopamine in the brain. Dose is 5 to 10 mg orally, intravenous or intramuscular, thrice a day, 6–8 hourly. It is safe in pregnancy.

Adverse effects are extrapyramidal symptoms. Usage for >12 weeks may cause tardive dyskinesia, especially in older women and at higher doses.

Phenothiazines (*e.g.* prochlorperazine) are effective in reducing hyperemesis at a dose of 5 mg three times a day but may cause drowsiness. They are safe in pregnancy though unpleasant side effects such as oculogyric crises and extrapyramidal syndrome may uncommonly occur.

Ondansetron: Selective 5-HT3 serotonin antagonist. Not recommended as a first-line therapy in pregnancy more so in the first trimester of pregnancy.

The dose is 4 mg orally or intravenously by slow bolus injection or intravenous infusion up to 8 hourly. The dose may be increased, if necessary, up to 8 mg/dose.[11]

If combination of above two oral medications fail to treat nausea and vomiting of pregnancy, ondansetron to be considered. Common side effects are headache, constipation, fatigue and drowsiness. There are reports of myocardial ischemia with intravenous use. It causes QTc prolongation on ECG. Hypokalaemia, hypomagnesaemia, hypo/hyperthyroidism, drugs like erythromycin, azithromycin, metronidazole, pantoprazole also cause QTc prolongation and concomitant use may precipitate torsade de pointes which is potentially fatal. Serum electrolyte and ECG monitoring is recommended in patients with risk factor for arrhythmia. Serotonin syndrome which is rare, is a life-threatening situation.

Although use of ondansetron in early pregnancy in large studies is fairly safe, there may be a small increase in risk of cleft palate and cardiac malformations especially septal defects by about 2–3 per 10,000 births.[12]

Topical Creams

Antifungals: Commonly used are imidazoles, nystatin and terbinafine.

Systemic absorption of nystatin is negligible, whereas imidazoles are absorbed to a variable extent, 1% for miconazole and 10% for clotrimazole. Terbinafine is not studied in humans. Studies of nystatin and imidazoles showed that they are safe in pregnancy. Oral terbinafine is Category B, so can be used topically in pregnancy.

Steroids: Systemic and potent dermatological steroids may have a small increased risk of cleft lip with or without cleft palate from 1.7 to 2.7 per thousand. The risk of steroid use should be balanced with their necessity in chronic medical conditions such as autoimmune diseases. They may be used in pregnancy in the lowest dose and for the shortest time possible.

Antimicrobial creams: In smaller studies topical bacitracin is not associated with fetal malformations. Topical antimicrobials can be used in pregnancy.

Topical antimicrobial, antifungal, and steroid preparations are largely safe in pregnancy.

Analgesic ointment/balms: Diclofenac ointment is contraindicated as about 6% can be absorbed systemically with fetal side effects. Counterirritant balms in small doses are safe for common aches and pains of pregnancy.

Acne and Hirsutism

Tretinoins: Tretinoins to be discontinued at least a month preconception, preferably 3 months due to variable half-life and hence wash-out period.

Finasteride and flutamide given for hair loss affect external genitalia of male fetus.

The Endocrine Society recommends against antiandrogen monotherapy unless adequate contraception is used. Oral contraceptive monotherapy is first prescribed. If no response is obtained in 6 months of contraceptive, an antiandrogen (spironolactone, finasteride, flutamide) may be added.

Pregnancy poses a challenge for both over the counter and prescribed drugs. It is difficult to conduct well-designed prospective studies in pregnant women. Initial management should be lifestyle modifications and non-pharmacologic therapy. Patient should be evaluated by the physician regarding the pharmacologic therapy. Pregnant women should not be deprived of any treatment if it is needed for the fear of fetal effects.

References

1. Labeling and prescription drug advertising; content and format for labeling for human prescription drugs. Federal Register. 1979; 44(124):37451.

2. US. Food and Drug Administration. Summary of proposed rule on pregnancy and lactation labeling. http://www.fda.gov/Drugs/ Development Approval Process/Development Resources/Labeling/ucm093310.htm. Accessed June 28, 2014.

3. Werler MM, Mitchell AA, Hernandez-Diaz S, Honein MA. Use of over-the-counter medications during pregnancy. Am J Obstet Gynecol. 2005;193 (3 pt 1):771–777.

4. Gilboa SM, Strickland MJ, Olshan AF, Werler MM, Correa A; National Birth Defects Prevention Study. Use of antihistamine medications during early pregnancy and isolated major malformations. Birth Defects Res A Clin Mol Teratol. 2009;85(2):137–150.

5. Källén BA, Olausson PO. Use of oral decongestants during pregnancy and delivery outcome. Am J Obstet Gynecol. 2006;194(2):480–485.

6. Edwards DR, Aldridge T, Baird DD, Funk MJ, Savitz DA, Hartmann KE. Periconceptional over-the-counter nonsteroidal anti-inflammatory drug exposure and risk for spontaneous abortion. Obstet Gynecol. 2012;120 (1):113–122.

7. Brigstocke S, Yu V, Nee J. Review of the safety profiles of laxatives in pregnant women J Clin Gastroenterol. 2022;56(3):197–203.

8. Gill SK, O'Brien L, Einarson TR, Koren G. The safety of proton pump inhibitors (PPIs) in pregnancy: a meta-analysis. Am J Gastroenterol. 2009;104(6):1541–1545.

9. Smith JA, Refuerzo JS, Ramin SM. Treatment of nausea and vomiting of pregnancy (hyperemesis gravidarum and morning sickness). Up-to-date 2011. Available from: www.uptodate.com (Accessed Oct, 2011).

10. Shrim A, Boskovic R, Maltepe C, et al. Pregnancy outcome following use of large doses of vitamin B6 in the first trimester. J Obstet Gynaecol 2006; 26:749.

11. Huybrechts KF, Hernandez-Diaz S, Straub L, et al. Intravenous Ondansetron in Pregnancy and Risk of Congenital Malformations. JAMA 2020; 323:372.

12. Andrade C. Major Congenital Malformation Risk After First Trimester Gestational Exposure to Oral or Intravenous Ondansetron. J Clin Psychiatry 2020;81.

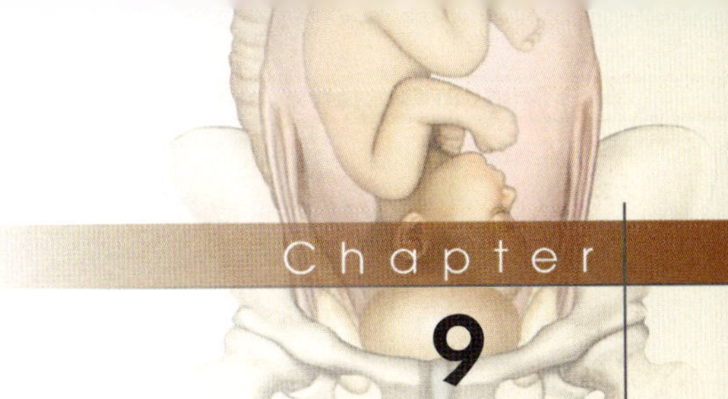

Drugs for Induction of Labour

• Moushmi Parpillewar Tadas

Introduction

Induction of labour (IOL) is one of the most common obstetric procedures done worldwide. It is widely agreed that IOL is appropriate when the outcomes for the fetus, the mother, or both are regarded to be better than with expectant management, which is waiting for the natural commencement of labour. Furthermore, IOLs should be considered when the vaginal route is regarded to be the most suited for delivery. When done correctly and for the right reasons, induction of labour is beneficial to both the woman and her fetus. Unnecessary dangers may be experienced if done inadequately or inappropriately. The objective is to facilitate natural delivery experience as much as possible. The literature on labour induction methods (*i.e.* cervical ripening and the onset of uterine contractions) analyzes the efficacy of pharmacological, mechanical, experimental, and complementary and alternative medicine methods of third trimester IOL. The pharmaceutical methods include oxytocin and prostaglandins (PGE_1: misoprostol and PGE_2: dinoprostone), which will be extensively discussed below.

Definitions

Induction: Induction is the artificial initiation of contractions in a pregnant woman for the purpose of achieving a vaginal birth within 24 to 48 hours, who is not in labour.

Augmentation: Augmentation is the enhancement of contractions in a pregnant woman who is already in labour.

Cervical ripening: Cervical ripening is the use of pharmacologic or other means to soften, efface, and/or dilate the cervix to increase the likelihood of a vaginal delivery after labour induction.

LABOUR INDUCTION METHODS

Methods for induction of labour include mechanical and pharmacologic means. Choice of this depends on the preinduction cervical score. Favourable cervix, multiparty, prior vaginal delivery, body mass index (BMI) and method used for IOL are the factors most likely to lead to success. Pre-induction cervical score is an important predictor of success, with the modified Bishop score being a widely used scoring system. **Table 9.1** shows modified Bishop's score.

Drugs for Cervical Ripening and IOL with an Unfavourable Cervix

1. Prostaglandins (PGs)

  i. E_2 (dinoprostone) is available in two forms in India for cervical ripening.

    (a) Dinoprostone gel (3 g gel/0.5 mg

Table 9.1: Bishop scoring system

Factor	0	1	2	3
Cervical dilatation (cm)	0	1–2	3–4	>4
Cervical length (cm)	≥4	3–4	3–2	<1
Consistency	Firm	Medium	Soft	
Position	Posterior	Mid	Mid	
Station in relation to ischial spine	–3 or above	–2	–1 or 0	+1 or lower

Total score: 13; Favourable score: 6–13; Unfavourable score: 1–5

dinoprostone). (b) Dinoprostone vaginal pessary (10 mg embedded in a mesh).

ii. Prostaglandin E_1 (misoprostol).

2. Low-dose Oxytocin Infusion

In this method, a low-dose oxytocin infusion is started, with an increase in dose from 1 to 4 mU/min. Because of the ease of stopping the oxytocin infusion, this method is preferred in high-risk pregnancies where foetuses are compromised.

3. Other Drugs

Mifepristone, nitric oxide donors, relaxin, hyaluronidase are presently not recommended for induction of labour in view of the availability of low quality evidence for their use.

Drug for IOL with Favourable Cervix

Oxytocin

Let us discuss these drugs in details.

PROSTAGLANDINS IN IOL

Prostaglandins, produced in the cervix, uterus and from the fetal membranes, play a critical role in cervical ripening and uterine contractility and the induction of labour.

Prostaglandins are eicosanoids, formed from the 20-carbon unsaturated fatty acid, arachidonic acid (which is widely distributed throughout the body) which is liberated from membrane phospholipids via phospholipase-A_2. In females, PGs are found in menstrual blood, endometrium, decidua and amniotic membrane.

There are five primary types of PGs: prostaglandin E_2, prostaglandin D_2, prostaglandin F_2, prostaglandin I_2, and thromboxane-A_2. PGE_2 and PGF_2 are the two main prostaglandin types involved in cervical ripening and parturition.

As they act on their local site of production, PGs are paracrine/autocrine hormones. Amnion produces PGE_2, decidua is the main source of PGF_2, and myometrium produces PGI_2. PGE_2 helps cervical ripening and PGF_2 causes myometrial contractility. PGs cause myometrial contraction irrespective of period of gestation as compared to oxytocin which acts predominantly on uterus at term or in labour.

Pharmacokinetics

Biotransformation of PGs occurs rapidly in most tissues, fastest in the lungs. Most PGs have plasma half-life of a few seconds to a few minutes. First there is a specific carrier mediated uptake into cells, the side chains are then oxidized and double bonds are reduced in a stepwise manner to yield inactive metabolites, which are excreted in urine.

Mechanism of Action

PGs (E_2 and F_2) found in amniotic membranes and fluid, diffuses in myometrium, acts on sarcoplasmic reticulum, and inhibits intracellular cAMP generation, increases local free calcium ions and causes uterine contractions. PGs also sensitise the myometrium to oxytocin. PGE_2 is 5 times more potent than PGF_2. PGF_2 acts predominantly on the myometrium, while PGE_2 acts mainly on the cervix. PGE_2 regulates the synthesis of hydrophilic glycosaminoglycans and increases the activity of elastin, both of which induce cervical ripening by separating and dispersing collagen bundles. The inflammatory response is modulated by PGE_2 that characterizes cervical ripening and remodelling.

Misoprostol (PGE_1), a synthetic analogue, is approved and marketed for the prevention and treatment of gastric ulcers. It has two primary effects when used in labour induction: Increase uterine contractility and to soften the cervix, primarily through its ability to degrade collagen in the connective tissue stroma of the cervix.

Therapeutic Uses

PGs are mainly used in:
1. Induction of abortion, termination of molar pregnancy
2. Augmentation and induction of labour
3. Cervical ripening prior to abortion and induction of labour
4. Management of atonic postpartum haemorrhage (PPH).
5. Medical management of ectopic pregnancy.

Misoprostol and PGE_2 analogues are mainly used for induction and augmentation of labour, which will be discussed in details.

PROSTAGLANDIN E₂

Dinoprostone (PGE_2) is available in the form of gel, vaginal pessary and 10 mg suppository. The gel and pessary are used for cervical ripening before induction of labour and suppository is indicated in pregnancy termination from 12 weeks to 20 weeks and evacuating uterus in fetal demise up to 28 weeks.

Dosage and Preparations

Dinoprostone: Dinoprostone is commonly used for cervical ripening. A 0.5 mg of dinoprostone in gel form Prepidil in United

States and Cerviprime in India is available in a 2.5 ml syringe for an intracervical application. With the woman lying in supine position, the tip of a prefilled syringe is placed intracervical, and the gel is deposited just below the internal cervical os. After application, the woman remains lying for at least 30 minutes. The application can be repeated in 6 hours if contractions are not adequate, not more than three doses in 24 hours.

The second is Propess in India and Cervidil pessary in the United States (Fig. 9.1), which contains 10 mg of dinoprostone embedded in a mesh and is placed in the posterior fornix of the vagina (Fig. 9.2). After the pessary is inserted, the withdrawal tape is cut with scissors ensuring there is sufficient tape

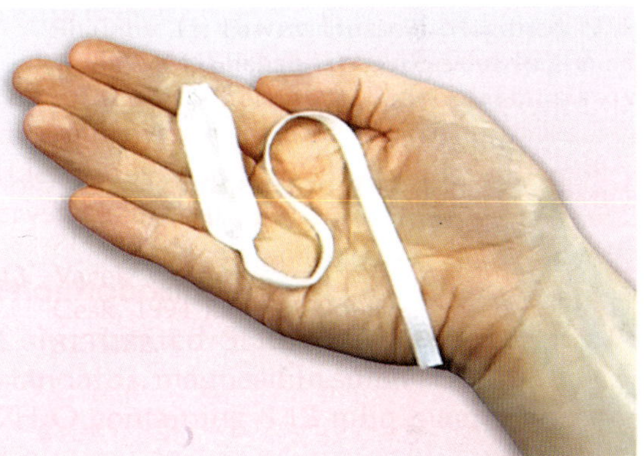

Fig. 9.1: Dinoprostone vaginal pessary

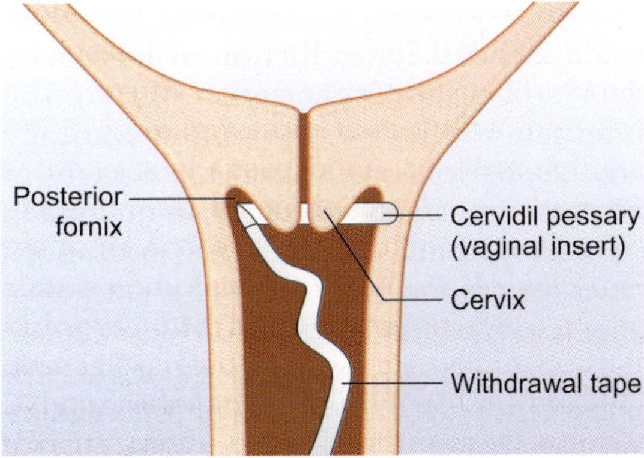

Fig. 9.2: Method of insertion of dinoprostone pessary (anterior cross-section view)

outside the vagina to allow removal. Patients should remain recumbent for 20–30 minutes to allow the pessary to hydrate and swell. It allows for controlled release of dinoprostone over 24 hours, after which it is removed. The insert provides slower release of medication 0.3 mg/hour than the gel form. Oxytocin induction that follows prostaglandin use for cervical ripening should be delayed for 6 to 12 hours following prostaglandin E_2 gel administration or for at least 30 minutes after removal of vaginal pessary. Rupture of membranes after the insertion of pessary does not necessitate removal of the pessary.

Contraindications specific to dinoprostone vaginal pessary:

1. When oxytocic drugs are being administered, pessary should not be used or left in place (the uterotonic activity of oxytocin is potentiated by dinoprostone).
2. A history of difficult or traumatic deliveries.
3. If there are more than three previous full-term deliveries.
4. If there is history of previous surgery or rupture of the cervix.
5. When there is current, or a history of pelvic inflammatory disease, unless adequate prior treatment has been instituted.

Storage

Dinoprostone pessary should be stored in a freezer (at 10° to 25°C) and gel has to be stored under 2–8°C.

Misoprostol: Oral misoprostol has been recommended for induction of labour by the World Health Organization (WHO), The International Federation of Gynaecology and Obstetrics (FIGO), and the Society of Obstetricians and Gynaecologists of Canada (SOGC). For detailed dosage and indications must refer to the FIGO chart of misoprostol only recommended regimen 2017.

Routes of Administration and Dose

Vaginal: Dose of 25 µg, every 6 hourly to a maximum of 6 doses can be given into the posterior vaginal fornix.

Oral: Dose of 50 µg every 3 hours to a maximum of 6 doses can be given or dose of 25 µg every 2 hours can be given.

Oral misoprostol when compared to vaginal misoprostol is less effective and had lower caesarean rates, without increase in fetal or maternal adverse outcomes. Other routes administration: 1. Buccal, 2. rectal, 3. sublingual

Preparations: 25 and 50 µg tablets are available for cervical ripening, induction and augmentation of labour.

Pharmacokinetics

Bioavailability: Extensively absorbed from the GIT

Metabolism: De-esterified to prostaglandin F analogues

Half-life: 20–40 minutes

Excretion: Mainly renal 80%, remainder is fecal

No specific drug interactions are observed.

PGE_1 versus PGE_2: Misoprostal when compared to dinoprostone is cheaper, cost-effective, is stable at room temperature, easily administered and less side effects. Induction to delivery interval is short. Need of oxytocin and failure of induction is less.

Risks: Meconium passage, incidence of tachysystole, rupture of uterus can occur. Misoprostol is not yet approved by the FDA for induction of labour.

Contraindications

Overall contraindications for PGs are:

1. Previous uterine scar is relatively contra-indicated
2. Established uterine activity
3. Asthma
4. Severe hepatic or renal impairment
5. Known hypersensitivity
6. Active vaginal bleeding.

Adverse Effects

1. Nausea, vomiting, uterine cramps, watery diarrhoea, flushing, shivering, fever, malaise, tachycardia, fall in BP, chest pain.
2. Tachysystole: Overall incidence of hyperstimulation is 4.8%—same as with oxytocin. In 1 to 5% of women hyperstimulation occurs following vaginal administration of prostaglandin E_2. If there is pre-existing spontaneous labour, incidence of tachysystole is more when prostaglandins are used, such use is not recommended. If tachysystole follows pessary, its removal by pulling on the tail will usually reverse this effect. Irrigation to remove the gel preparation has not been shown to be helpful. It is more with vaginal gel (5%) than intracervical (1%) and least with controlled release insert.

Preparations: As discussed above.

Drug interactions: PGs have not shown any drug interactions.

Monitoring Drug Therapy for Oxytocin

Foetal and maternal monitoring is a must as follows:

1. A non-stress test before induction of labour is recommended.
2. Intermittent foetal (foetal heart rate) and maternal monitoring must be done every hour initially.
3. In active labour continuous electronic/more frequent intermittent foetal heart rate monitoring should be done.
4. Labour progress is monitored using partogram.
5. Close watch is kept for temperature, blood pressure, pulse rate, input, output chart, foetal heart pattern, vaginal bleeding, uterine hyperstimulation, and signs of uterine rupture should looked for.

Counselling to the Patients while Prescribing the Oxytocin

Before the induction procedure is initiated, the patient and her partner should be informed. The woman should be given enough time to address her concerns and ask any questions she may have. The women and her partner should be counselled regarding:

i. Indication of drug usage
ii. Risks *vs* benefit of the drug and procedure
iii. Method of induction of labour and its advantages and disadvantages
iv. Any alternatives available
v. Method of electronic equipment for monitoring
vi. Expected duration of labour
vii. Support system available during labour
viii. Pain relief options
ix. Other options if there is failure.

When compared to placebo, both gel and pessary are successful in inducing cervical ripening, although pessary achieves ripening over a shorter period of time (11.1 h *vs* 15.2 h). Although the pessary is more expensive than gel, the time to achieve vaginal delivery is shorter, and oxytocin administration is less frequent, thus the pessary may be more cost-effective in the long run. Prostaglandin E_2 is reported to be superior to placebo in terms of boosting Bishop score, decreasing induction failures, and lowering the rate of caesarean sections. When compared to misoprostol, prostaglandin E_2 takes longer to reach active phase, has a longer induction period, and a higher risk of caesarean section.

OXYTOCIN

Oxytocin is nonapeptide hormone released from the pars nervosa of the posterior pituitary gland and secreted in the paraventricular nucleus of the hypothalamus. Most hormones produce negative feedback loops after release, whereas oxytocin is one of the few that produces positive feedback loops. This indicates that oxytocin release causes activities that trigger even greater oxytocin release. This is comparable to antidiuretic hormone (ADH) vasopressin (the second hormone stored and released by the posterior pituitary), which has a negative feedback loop following release.

Exogenous oxytocin stimulates the female reproductive system in the same way as endogenous oxytocin does. Both forms of oxytocin cause uterine contractions in the myometrium by stimulating intracellular calcium in uterine myofibrils via G-protein coupled receptors.

Pharmacokinetics

Being a peptide, it is not active orally. It is usually administered intravenous or intramuscular and rarely intranasal by spray. It gets rapidly degraded in liver and kidney; plasma half-life is 6–12 minutes. This is further shortened at term due to enzyme oxitocinase secreted by placenta.

Mechanism of Action

Exogenous oxytocin stimulates the female reproductive system in the same way as endogenous oxytocin does. Both forms of oxytocin cause uterine contractions in the myometrium by stimulating intracellular calcium in uterine myofibrils via G-protein coupled receptors. Many signals are produced by oxytocin receptor activation, which then stimulate uterine contraction by increasing intracellular calcium levels. This is what causes the contractions to become more intense and frequent, allowing a mother to deliver her baby vaginally. When the fetus' head pushes on the cervix, nerve impulses are delivered to the mothers brain, activating the posterior pituitary to secrete oxytocin.

Oxytocin has pharmacologic effects on other organs, such as the breast. It produces contractions of the myoepithelial cells in the female breasts, which drives milk from small ducts into bigger sinuses, allowing milk ejection. Positive reinforcement is also important in this milk-ejection reflex. Baby that is attempting to latch onto his mother's breast, signals oxytocin secretion into the blood in the same manner as vaginal delivery; except, instead of uterine contractions, milk is ejected from the breast. The oxytocin makes its way to the brain at the same time to increase more oxytocin secretion.

Lastly, oxytocin also has antidiuretic and vasodilator effects, increasing cerebral, coronary, and even renal blood flow.

The response of the uterus to oxytocin depends on the circulating levels of progesterone, estrogen and the gestational age. In late pregnancy, as estrogen levels rise and progesterone levels fall, the uterine response to oxytocin increases. The increase in sensitivity begins at 20 weeks, and there is a sharp rise after 30 weeks.

Therapeutic Uses

1. Oxytocin is used in the antepartum period for induction and augmentation of labour (approved by the FDA).
2. In the postpartum period, oxytocin is used for prevention and treatment of postpartum haemorrhage (approved by the FDA).

Methods of Administration and Dosage

Routes of administration:
1. Controlled intravenous method is widely used for induction of labour
2. Bolus IV or IM (usually in third stage for prevention and treatment of PPH)
3. Buccal tablets or nasal spray: limited use

Uses

Oxytocin is mainly used for induction and augmentation of labour. Principles to be followed when used for induction are:
1. Should always be started in low dose and escalated every 20–30 minutes if no response.
2. Oxytocin infusion should be charted in mU/min or drops/min with the dilution being mentioned.
3. The oxytocin infusion can be escalated until labour progress is normal or uterine activity reaches 200 to 250 Montevideo units (*i.e.* good regular uterine contractions, each lasting for 40–45 seconds duration and minimum of three contractions in 10 min).

4. It should preferably administered by infusion pump, and if it is not available, it must be manually regulated by counting of drops per minute.

Oxytocin is given as 10–20 units dissolved in 1000 ml of Ringer lactate or normal saline making it as 10–20 mU/ml and given through an infusion pump. Further increments are made according to the low dose or high-dose protocol given below **(Table 9.2)**:

Table 9.2: Protocol for oxytocin dosage in ml

Regimen	Starting dose (mU/min)	Incremental dose (mU/min)	Dosage interval (min)
Low dose	1–2	1–2 (every 30 min)	30–40
High dose	4–6	4–6 (every 15–30 min) 6, 3*, 1*	20–40

*The incremental increase can be reduced to 3 mU/min in presence of hyperstimulation and reduced to 1 mU/min with recurrent hyperstimulation.

How to prepare oxytocin infusion and calculate dose?

For fluid selection, Ringer lactate or normal saline are preferable over dextrose solution to reduce the danger of electrolyte imbalance (*e.g.* hyponatremia) and volume overload.

Each oxytocin ampoule (1 ml) contains five units. In a 10 ml syringe, 2 ml of oxytocin (two ampoules) is diluted with 8 ml of normal saline. It produces 10 mL of oxytocin-containing saline solution. This saline solution contains 1 unit of oxytocin per ml.

2 ml of this solution is added to 500 ml of Ringer lactate to make a bottle containing 2 units of oxytocin infusion. The oxytocin dose is indicated below in drops/minute and mU/minute **(Table 9.3)**.

For augmentation of labour Oxytocin can be used following cervical ripening agents, alone or in combination with amniotomy.

Monitoring during Oxytocin Infusion

1. Continuous cardiotocography is better for monitoring oxytocin infusion rate, uterine contractions, and fetal heart rate. If cardiotocography is not available, fetal monitoring should be done by intermittent auscultation every 15 minutes in the first stage and every 5 minutes in the second stage.

2. Blood pressure and pulse should be assessed hourly. Intake and output should be assessed every 4 hours.

3. Every 30 minutes and with each incremental increase in oxytocin, the frequency, strength, and duration of uterine contractions should be monitored, where gadgets are unavailable, 'finger tip' palpation for uterine tonus between contractions may be used. When using intra-uterine pressure monitoring, a peak intra-uterine pressure of 50–60 mm Hg with a resting tone of 10–15 mm Hg is ideal.

4. Cervical status should be evaluated prior to oxytocin administration and repeated after at least 4 hours of moderate contractions.

5. If the fetal heart pattern is unconvincing, a vaginal examination should be repeated

Table 9.3: Oxytocin infusion dosage in drops per min

Units of Oxytocin to be added in 500 ml of RL	Oxytocin infusion rate in drops/minute and equivalent dose in mU/minute (1 ml is equal to 16 drops)							
1 unit	8 drops	16 drops	24 drops	32 drops	40 drops	48 drops	56 drops	64 drops
	1 mU	2 mU	3 mU	4 mU	5 mU	6 mU	7 mU	8 mU
2 units	8 drops	16 drops	24 drops	32 drops	40 drops	48 drops	56 drops	64 drops
	2 mU	4 mU	6 mU	8 mU	10 mU	12 mU	14 mU	16 mU

to rule out the presence of meconium, a cord accident, abruption, uterine hyperstimulation and uterine rupture.

Contraindications

1. Contraindications to oxytocin are hypersensitivity to oxytocin or any part of its synthetic version, where vaginal delivery is itself contraindicated in conditions like active genital herpes infection, complete placenta praevia, vasa praevia, invasive cervical cancer, and presentation or prolapse of the umbilical cord.
2. Other contraindications to oxytocin are malpresentations and fetal distress when delivery is not imminent.
3. It is also contraindicated in women with contracted pelvis or when there is either hyperactive or hypertonic uterine activity.

Adverse Effects

Common side effects of oxytocin administration include the following:

1. Erythema at the site of injection, nausea, vomiting, stomach pain, and loss of appetite.
2. Tachysystole and hyperstimulation are the most common side effects of oxytocin. Tachysystole is the occurrence of >5 contractions over a period of 10 minutes. Uterine hypertonus is described as a single contraction lasting longer than 2 minutes. Uterine hyperstimulation is when either condition leads to a nonreassuring fetal heart rate pattern. It is quickly reversible by discontinuation of the oxytocin. To maximize fetal oxygenation, oxygen should be administered and the patient should be placed in the left lateral position. Injudicious use of oxytocin during labour can produce too strong uterine contractions forcing the presenting part through incompletely dilated birth canal, causing maternal and fetal soft tissue injury, rupture of uterus,

placental abruption, fetal asphyxia and death.

3. Water intoxication: This occurs due to ADH like action when large doses given along with IV fluids, especially in toxemia of pregnancy and renal insufficiency. It may be a fatal complication. It is manifested by cardiac arrhythmias, seizures, anaphylaxis, confusion, hallucinations, extreme increase in blood pressure, and blurred vision. Therefore, prolonged administration with doses higher than 40 mU of oxytocin per minute and infusion of fluids in any 10 hours should not be exceed by 1500 ml.
4. Amniotic fluid embolism is rare which may be caused by strong, tumultuous contractions. (Usually occur in 3rd stage after placenta separation and with tetanic condition of uterus).
5. *Hypotension:* Oxytocin in bolus intravenous doses causes significant hypotension. As little as 2 units given by rapid intravenous bolus can cause a 30% drop in mean arterial pressure. Oxytocin used for control or prevention of postpartum hemorrhage should be given by controlled intravenous infusion or intramuscular injection. Bolus intravenous doses should never be given.
6. *Neonatal hyperbilirubinemia:* Recent evidence suggests that infants at a higher risk of developing jaundice associated with large doses of oxytocin.
7. *Uterine atony:* In women of high parity, the use of oxytocin is thought to be associated with an increased incidence of uterine atony and postpartum hemorrhage.

Preparations

1 IU of oxytocin = 2 µg of pure hormone. Commercially available oxytocin is produced synthetically. Oxytocin, syntocinon 2 IU/2 ml and 5 IU/ml inj., pitocin 5 IU/0.5 ml inj.

Oxytocin should be stored in refrigerator at 2 to 8°C.

Drug interactions: None

Counselling to the Patients while Prescribing the Drug

Same as prostaglandins.

Pre-induction cervical softening improves the chances of a successful induction in women with an unfavourable cervix. Oxytocin is administered at least 6 to 12 hours after the last dose of dinoprostone gel, 30 minutes after the removal of the dinoprostone insert, and 4 hours after the last dose of misoprostol. In women with favourable cervix, oxytocin combined with early amniotomy is preferable to amniotomy alone.

MIFEPRISTONE

Mifepristone is a 19-norsteroid, antiprogesterone and antiglucocorticoid having affinity for progesterone receptors and blocks the action of progesterone at the cellular level.

Pharmacokinetics

Mifepristone is effective when taken orally, however its bioavailability is just 25%. It is quickly absorbed, primarily metabolized in the liver by CYP 3A4, and excreted in bile; some enterohepatic circulation occurs; half-life ranges from 20 to 36 hours. A number of key metabolites have a high affinity for progesterone receptors. It has been observed that erythromycin and ketoconazole act as CYP 3A4 inhibitors and rifampin and anticonvulsants act as inducers.

Mechanism of Action

Mifepristone blocks support of progesterone to the endometrium, unblocks PG release from it and this stimulates uterine contractions. It also sensitises myometrium to PGs.

Uses and Preparation

Mifepristone is mainly used in induction of abortion but due to its action it is being used for induction of labour and cervical ripening. Mifepristone is recommended only after intrauterine fetal death. Tablet of 200 mg is used for this purpose. After 36–48 hours cervical assessment is done and induction/ augmentation are decided depending on cervical status.

Contraindication

Concurrent long-term corticosteroid therapy, chronic adrenal failure, history of allergy to mifepristone, misoprostol or other prostaglandin, concurrent anticoagulant therapy, hemorrhagic disorders and inherited porphyrias are some of the contraindications.

Adverse Effects

Abdominal cramps, allergic reactions, diarrhea, dizziness, vomiting are some of the adverse effects of mifepristone. It should be used with caution as it has serious drug interactions with some drugs like atorvastatin, mefloquin, triptorelin to name a few.

Cochrane review suggests that there is inadequate clinical trial evidence to support the use of mifepristone to induce labour. However, the studies imply that mifepristone is superior to placebo in lowering the risk of caesarean sections for unsuccessful induction of labour; hence, further trials comparing mifepristone with the standard cervical ripening drugs now in use may be justified. There is little information available on the impact on the baby. There is insufficient data on fetal outcomes and maternal adverse effects to advocate mifepristone for cervical ripening.

Other Drugs

The following methods for induction of labour are not presently recommended—oral or intravenous or intracervical PGE2, relaxin, hyaluronidase, oestrogen, corticosteroids, and vaginal nitric oxide donors.

Suggested Reading

1. Alfirevic Z, Kelly AJ, Dowswell T. Intravenous oxytocin alone for cervical ripening and induction of labour. Cochrane Database Syst Rev. 2009:CD003246. DOI: 10.1002/14651858. CD003246.pub2.
2. Alfirevic Z, Weeks A. Oral misoprostol for induction of labour. Cochrane Database Syst

Rev. 2006:CD001338. DOI: 10.1002/14651858. CD001338.pub2.

3. Hapangama D, Neilson JP. Mifepristone for induction of labour. Cochrane Database Syst Rev. 2009;(3):CD002865.

4. Hofmeyr GJ, Gu¨lmezoglu AM, Pileggi C. Vaginal misoprostol for cervical ripening and induction of labour. Cochrane Database Syst Rev. 2010:CD000941.

5. Induction of labour, GCPR, ICOG-FOGSI 2018.

6. Jerry Kruse, Oxytocin: Clinical Pharmacology and Clinical Applications. The journal of family practice, 1986;vol. 23, no. 5:473–9.

7. Jessica L Morris, Beverly Winikoff, Rasha Dabash, Andrew Weeks, Anibal Faundes, Kristina Gemzell-Danielsson, et al. FIGO's updated recommendations for misoprostol used alone in gynecology and obstetrics. Int J Gynecol Obstet 2017;138:363–6.

8. Kelly AJ, Malik S, Smith L, et al. Vaginal prostaglandin (PGE2 and PGF2) for induction of labour at term. Cochrane Database Syst Rev. 2009:CD003101.

9. Marconi AM. Recent advances in the induction of labour [version 1; peer review: 2 approved] 2019, (F1000 Faculty Rev):1829.

10. Textbook of Essential of Medical Pharmacology, 8th edition by KD Tripathi.

11. Textbook of Williams Obstetrics, 24th edition.

12. Ronan Bakker Stephanie, Pierce Dean Myers. The role of prostaglandins E1 and E2, dinoprostone, and misoprostol in cervical ripening and the induction of labour: A mechanistic approach, Arch Gynecol Obstet, DOI 10.1007/s00404-017-4418–5.

Bronchial Asthma during Pregnancy

• Rashmi Kahar

Introduction

Asthma is one of the most common chronic disease condition occurring during pregnancy.

It is a chronic inflammatory disease which is characterised by increased responsiveness of tracheobronchial tree to multiple stimuli.

This is an episodic disease, the episodes of which lasts from minutes to hours. Patients though appear to recover clinically, may develop chronic airway limitations.

ASTHMA IN PREGNANCY

When the patient is pregnant, the respiratory rate and vital capacity of lung remain unaffected. There is increase in tidal volume, minute ventilation increases by 40% and minute oxygen uptake increase by 20%.

The elevation of diaphragm results in decreased functional residual capacity. Residual volume of air also decreases. This causes a hyperventilatory picture in late trimester of pregnancy.

This results into chronic respiratory alkalosis, decrease in partial pressure of CO_2 and decreased bicarbonates with increase in pH.

Asthma is characterised by inflammation in airways with increase in eosinophils, mast cells and lymphocytes.

This causes increase in secretions and constricts airway diameter by causing bronchial wall edema. The asthma during pregnancy may remain stable or worsen or even improve in equal proportion.

The relative risk of exacerbation is high postpartum. Circulating progesterone and changed beta2 adrenoreceptor response are possible causative factors in asthma in pregnancy.

Can gastroesophageal reflex trigger acute attack of asthma due to aspiration? It is a query till date.

Prevalence of asthma in pregnancy ranges from 1 to 4% worldwide (**Fig. 10.1**).

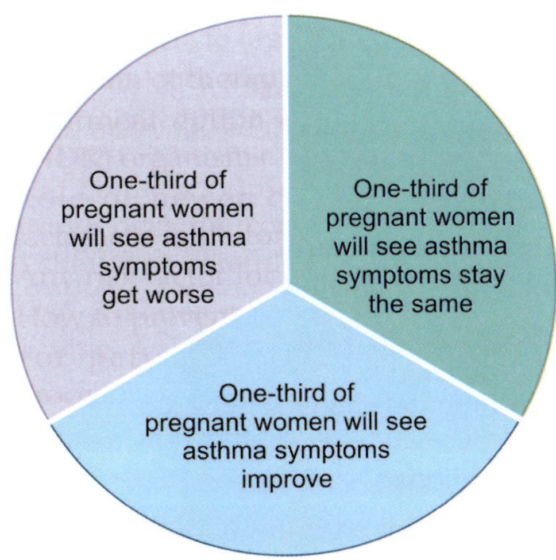

Fig. 10.1: Changes in asthmatic conditions during pregnancy

Symptoms and Signs of Asthma in Pregnancy

- Cough
- Noisy breathing
- Nocturnal awakenings
- Acute exacerbations of attacks
- Shortness of breath.

Features on Examination

- Tachypnoea
- Diffuse wheezes and rhonchi on respiratory system examination
- Bronchovesicular sounds
- Signs of fatigue, lethargy and abnormal breathing.
- Signs of hypoxia and fatigue due to respiratory acidosis.

Factors which Trigger Asthma during Pregnancy

Group 1

Allergens like house dust, mites, cockroach antigens, pollen grains, etc.

Group 2

Irritants like perfumes, deodorants, smoke, chemicals, strong odours.

Group 3

Existing medical conditions like upper respiratory tract infections, sinusitis, etc.

Group 4

Drugs like non-steroidal anti-inflamatory drug (NSAID), betablockers and aspirin.

Group 5

Environmental changes like cold air.

Investigations

- Complete blood count (CBC)
- Chest radiography
- Pulmonary function test.

ANTIASTHMA DRUGS IN PREGNANCY

Principles of Management of Asthma in Pregnancy

- Selection of appropriate treatment should be done based on control level and severity of condition
- The Global Initiative for Asthma (GINA) guidelines suggest that the poor asthma control and acute exacerbations during pregnancy are more risky than taking medicine.
- There should be a written asthma treatment plan for each patient.

The plan should include follow-up details and titrated doses.

LONG-TERM GOALS OF ASTHMA MANAGEMENT

The major goal of long-term management should be maintaining the normal activity levels.

The risk of acute attacks should be decreased and there should be no permanent damage of lung function.

The management should include drugs which have very little side effects and practically should have no effect on fetus in a pregnant patient.

Difference between Pharmacological Therapy in Pregnant and Nonpregnant Asthmatic Patient

- In nonpregnant asthmatic patient, a step-down or step-up treatment approach is appropriate after 3 months of treatment.
- In pregnant patients, the response to treatment should be assessed every month.

Priority should be given to avoid acute exacerbations of attacks.

- So, there is no role of step-up or step-down regimen in pregnant asthmatic patients.
- Some therapies, like IgG monoclonal antibodies and specific immunotherapies should be withheld during pregnancies.

Glucocorticoids

- Budesonide is the most commonly used and the safest glucocorticoid during pregnancy.
- It very effectively inhibits airway inflammation without systemic effect.
- Inhaled glucocorticoids do not alter glucocorticoid regulated pathways in the fetus and thus, do not have any effect on fetal growth and development.
- Inhalational glucocorticoid preparation in a dose of 800 µg/day is apt for first and second trimesters of pregnancy.
- For the third trimester, the dose should be 900 µg/day.

Among oral corticosteroid, prednisone, prednisolone and methylprednisolone can cross placenta even at very low concentration.

Betamethasone reaches fetus at higher concentration by crossing placenta.

Prednisone, before entering fetal blood circulation through placenta gets inactivated by 11-beta hydoxysteroid dehydrogenase-2 (11-beta-HSD-2), thereby has no effect on fetus.

Some studies say that there is increased risk of cleft lip and cleft palate, low birth weight (LBW), preterm delivery, pre-eclampsia with use of oral corticosteroid.

The mechanism postulated for this is corticosteroid when used in early phase of placentation, inhibits trophoblastic proliferation, migration and invasion.

But the general agreement is on the fact that inadequate treatment of asthma during pregnancy has more complications than treatment with glucocorticoids.

Beta-2 Agonists

SABA, *i.e.* short-acting beta-2 agonists including salbutamol, terbutaline, pirbuterol can be used safely in all trimesters in a pregnant patient to treat asthma.

Salbutamol is considered safest of all.

There is no risk of any congenital anomalies with use of SABA.

Studies show that there is risk of cardiac malformations in foetuses when exposed in early trimester.

Maternal asthma itself is closely associated with autistic disorder in offspring, but it does not have any correlation to any medication use per se.

Anticholinergics

- This group includes short-acting muscarine antagonist (SAMA), ipratropium bromide long-acting muscarine antagonist (LAMA).
- SABA plus ipratropium bromide is used in management of severe asthma control.
- There is not much research on the effects of anticholinergics on foetus when used in pregnant patient.

Theophylline

- If the asthma during pregnancy is of mild degree but persistent, low-dose theophylline can be considered as alternative treatment.
- It can be used in conjunction with other agents.
- If the liver function of pregnant patient is compromised, its use should be avoided as it tends to cross the placenta.
- The safest levels of drug in pregnant patient is 5–12 µg/ml and should be maintained. Levels higher than that can cause theophylline adverse reactions. It has no teratogenic effect on fetus.
- Thus, controlled release theophylline preparation is administered in pregnancy.
- It helps by dilating bronchi for 10–12 hours and has proved effective in managing nocturnal attacks of asthma in pregnant patients.

Leucotrine Receptor Antagonists (LTRAs)

- LTRAs include zafirlukast and montelukast and zileuton which is 5-lipoxygenase pathway inhibitor.
- Zikeuton is not recommended in pregnancy.
- The use of LTRAs with inhalational corticosteroids, poses no additional risk of any major congenital birth defect in fetus.

- Some studies show, very little risk of prematurity, gestational diabetes, low Apgar score in neonate and low maternal weight gain in such patients.
- If the patient was asthmatic before conception, and had good control of disease with LTRAs, then it can be continued instead of inhalational corticosteroids. But it is not, per se, preferred drug for mild persistent asthma during pregnancy.

Ornalizumab

- This is IgE monoclonal antibody. It is an add on therapy mainly used in pregnant patients, with moderate disease.
- It reduces frequency of acute attacks and prevents exacerbations.
- The drug can cause serious anaphylaxis reactions and has to be titrated carefully before administration.
- The dose of titration depends upon body weight of patient.
- In a pregnant patient, the weight changes are frequent. This poses a problem in calculating dose and titrating it in pregnant patients.
- The monoclonal antibodies can cross placenta in third trimester but there are no reports of any adverse effects of their use in pregnant asthmatic patients.
- Interleukin contributes to eosinophilic inflammation of airways. Two anti interleukin monoclonal antibodies, mepolizumab and restizumab are used in maintenance therapy in persistent eosinophilic asthma. But there is no substantial data of effect of these drugs in pregnant asthmatic patients.

Allergen Immunotherapy

- This is the exact treatment option for asthma.
- It involves regular subcutaneous injections, oral administration or sublingual administration of a known allergen.
- It should not be used in pregnant patient as it may cause anaphylaxis. But it can be continued in a patient who has already received allergy vaccine and is on a stable dose.
- This modality of treatment is in experimental stage.
- The sublingual and subcutaneous allergy vaccine appear safe during pregnancy.

Acute Attack of Asthma in Pregnancy

- The situation needs urgent hospitalisation. It needs urgent intervention. The acute attacks during pregnancy mainly occur in third trimester. Viral infections act as the major triggers if acute attacks.
- Gaps in regular treatment or under treatment can also lead to acute attacks.
- Can hormonal changes in pregnancy precipitate acute attacks of asthma? It is still a mystery to be solved.
- The patient needs to be hospitalised and continuously monitored for oxygen saturation. It is important to avoid maternal and fetal hypoxaemia and for the same, continuous oxygen inhalation is needed. The patient needs active treatment with SABA, ICS and oral corticosteroids.

Intrapartum Management

Points to remember

- 90% of pregnant patients will not have acute attack during parturition.
- Mother who was on chronic corticosteroid therapy, has risk of adrenal insufficiency during delivery.
- This can be taken care by administering 100 mg hydrocortisone every 8 hours on day 1 and day 2 of delivery.
- Mothers who are on SABA, their newborns should be tested for blood glucose levels.
- Oxytocin is safe for inducing labour in pregnant asthmatic patients.
- Vaginal PGE_2 can be used for induction of labour.
- Narcotics should be avoided for analgesia as they release histamine and cause bronchospasm.

- Central neuraxial anaesthesia is the best choice as it prevents pulmonary infections and atelectasis.

Patient Education

- Patient should be counselled that a good control of asthma during pregnancy is important for fetal wellbeing.
- The woman who smokes, should be encouraged to quit smoking.
- The pregnant patient should have a knowledge of basics of self-care regimen. That consists of correct use of inhalers, adherence to treatment protocol, etc.
- She should avoid triggers.
- It is a good practice to train a pregnant patient to know, how to identity exacerbations and how and when to use prednisone.
- She should avoid allergens, climate changes, drugs, sports, specific environments which can trigger acute attack.

- She can try air filtration as specific control.
- She should avoid viral infections.
- Comorbidities like obesity, gastroesophageal reflux, allergic sinusitis, COPD, should be taken care of.

Conclusion

Structural physical changes, hormones, changes in immunity determines course of disease in pregnant patient.

Pregnancy aggravates bronchial asthma.

Early identification, monitoring signs and symptoms of asthma, monitoring fetal activity, patient education, avoiding triggers, and managing complications actively are important in treatment of asthma in pregnancy.

All pregnant patients should receive symptom-based daily inhaled anti-inflammatory controlled treatment to reduce risk of serious exacerbations.

NATIONAL INSTITUTE FOR HEALTH AND CARE EXCELLENCE (NICE) GUIDELINES ON INTRAPARTUM DRUG USE IN ASTHMATIC PREGNANT PATIENT

Administer 10 units of oxytocin by intramuscular injection at birth at anterior shoulder, before the cord is clamped and cut. Oxytocin, as it is associated with fewer side effects than oxytocin plus ergometrine, is recommended.

Drugs that are not recommended for induction of labour.

- Oral prostaglandin E_2 (PGE_2)
- Intravenous PGE_2
- Extra-amniotic PGE_2
- Intracervical PGE_2
- Intravenous oxytocin.

Suggested Reading

1. Australian Bureau of Statistics: National Health Survey, "First results, 2014-15," 2015, http://www.abs.gov.au/AUSSTATS/abs@.nsf/Lookup/ 4364.0.55.001 Explanatory%20 Notes 12014–15? Open Document.

Flowchart 10.1: Asthma in pregnancy

Types		Managements
Mild • Symptoms less than 2 per week • Night symptoms less than 2 per month	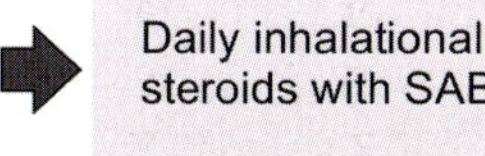	Management SABA
Mild Persistent Type • Symptoms more than 2 per week • Night symptoms 3–4 per month	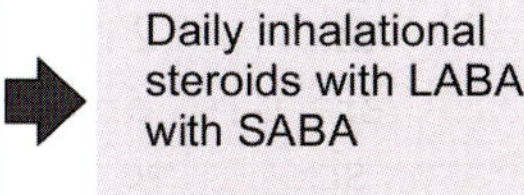	Daily inhalational steroids with SABA
Moderate Attack • Symptoms at night • Symptoms 8–10 per month	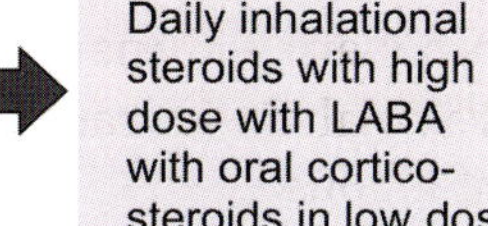	Daily inhalational steroids with LABA, with SABA
Severe Attack Continuous symptoms with pregnant night symptoms		Daily inhalational steroids with high dose with LABA with oral corticosteroids in low dose

SABA: Short-acting beta-2 antagonist
LABA: Long-acting beta-2 antagonist

2. C Nelson-Piercy, "Asthma in pregnancy," Thorax, vol. 56, no. 4, pp 325–328, 2001.

3. C Pitsios, P Demoly, MB Bilò, et al. "Clinical contraindications to allergen immunotherapy: An EAACI position paper," Allergy, vol. 70, no. 8, pp. 897–909, 2015.

4. C Sattler, G Garcia and M Humbert. "Novel targets of omalizumab in asthma," Current Opinion in Pulmonary Medicine, vol. 23, no. 1, pp. 56–61, 2017.

5. E Ellegard, M Hellgren, K Toren, and G Karlsson. "The incidence of pregnancy rhinitis," Gynecologic and Obstetric Investigation, vol. 49, no. 2, pp. 98–101, 2000.

6. EH Bel, SE Wenzel, PJ Thompson, et al. "Oral gluco- corticoid-sparing effect of mepolizumab in eosinophilic asthma," New England Journal of Medicine, vol 371, no. 13, pp. 1189–1197, 2014.

7. Grosso F, Locatelli E, Gini, et al. "The course of asthma during pregnancy in a recent, multicase-control study on respiratory health," Allergy, Asthma and Clinical Immunology, vol. 14, no. 1, p. 16, 2018.

8. HL Kwon, K Belanger, and MB Bracken, "Asthma prevalence among pregnant and childbearing-aged women in the United States: estimates from national health surveys," Annals of Epidemiology, vol. 13, no. 5, pp 317–324, 2003.

9. JM Clark, E Hulme, V Devendrakumar, et al. "Effect of maternal asthma on birthweight and neonatal outcome in a British inner-city population," Paediatric and Perinatal Epidemiology, vol. 21, no. 2, pp. 154–162, 2007.

10. KL Weis. "Asthma management across the life span: the childbearing woman with asthma,"Nursing Clinics of North America, vol. 38, no. 4, pp. 665–673, 2003.

11. M Abramowicz, G Zuccotti, and JM Pflomm, "Benra1: zumab (Fasenra) for severe eosinophilic asthma," JAMA Journal of the American Medical Association, vol. 319, no pp. 1501–1502, 2018.

12. M Castro, S Mathur, F Hargreave, et al. "Reslizumab for poorly controlled, eosinophilic asthma," American Journal of Respiratory and Critical Care Medicine, vol 184, no. 10, pp 1125–1132, 2011.

13. MP Dombrowski, M Schatz, R Wise, et al. "Randomized trial of inhaled beclomethasone dipropionate versus theophylline for moderate asthma during pregnancy," American Journal of Obstetrics and Gynecology, vol 190, no 3, pp. 737–744, 2004.

14. R Majithia and DA Johnson. "Are proton pump inhibitors safe during pregnancy and lactation? Evidence to date," Drugs, vol. 72, no. 2, pp. 171–179, 2012.

15. T Tamada and M Ichinose. "Leukotriene receptor antago- nists and antiallergy drugs," in Handbook of Experimental Pharmacology, vol. 237, pp. 153–169, Springer, Cham, Switzerland, 2017.

16. VE Murphy, H Powell, PAB. Wark, and PG Gibson. "A prospective study of respiratory viral infection in pregnant women with and without asthma," Chest, vol. 144, no. 2, pp. 420–427, 2013.

17. VE Murphy and M. Schatz, "Asthma in pregnancy: a hit for two," European Respiratory Review, vol. 23, no. 131, pp. 64–68, 2014.

18. VE Murphy, ME Jensen, and PG Gibson. "Asthma during pregnancy: exacerbations, management, and health outcomes for mother and infant," Seminars in Respiratory and Critical Care Medicine, vol. 38, no. 2, pp. 160–173, 2017.

19. WH Ibrahim, F Rasul, M Ahmad, et al. "Asthma knowledge, care, and outcome during pregnancy: the QAKCOP study," Chronic Respiratory Disease, vol. 16, 2018.

20. W Kelly, A Massoumi, and A Lazarus. "Asthma in pregnancy: physiology, diagnosis, and management," Postgraduate Medicine, vol. 127, no. 4, pp. 349–358, 2015.

21. Z Ali, L Nilas, and CS Ulrik. "Determinants of low risk of asthma exacerbation during pregnancy," Clinical and Experimental Allergy, vol. 48, no. 1, pp. 23–28, 2018.

Lactation Suppression

• Shreedevi Tanksale • Vidya Thobi

Introduction

Lactation is a process of making and secreting milk from mammary glands. For successful lactation, breasts have to undergo changes in composition, size and shape during various stages of breast development. Breast changes start during pregnancy in order to prepare for lactation post delivery. Every mother has the right to decide whether she wants to breastfeed or give top feeds to her baby. As a part of providing holistic treatment to the new mother, it is our duty to provide her with information about benefits of breast milk.

Breast milk provides most appropriate nutrition needed for a newborn baby. It contains proteins, fats, vitamins and immunoglobulins needed for a newborn. Other anti-infective factors it provides include immunoglobulin-IgA, whey protein (lysozyme and lactoferrin), and oligosaccharides. It protects the baby from risk of asthma, allergies, ear infections, respiratory illnesses, bouts of diarrhea, and the risk of diabetes and obesity.

Although, we are aware of the benefits of breastfeeding, sometimes breastfeeding needs to be avoided. These include stillborn baby, neonatal death, maternal infection, such as HIV, which may be transmitted to the baby via breastmilk, and maternal illness that requires toxic therapy that may be excreted in the breastmilk.[1]

If mothers do not breastfeed, the accumulation of breast milk can lead to breast engorgement and pain in women when no treatment is given. Women may not want to breastfeed for social or personal reasons. If the baby does not suckle at the breast, lactation will stop in the span of days to weeks.[2] This physical pain adds on the emotional trauma in women who experienced fetal loss and inability to breastfeed. The use of breast binding, ice packs, avoiding of tactile breast stimulation have been tried to help relieve physical symptoms.[1] The efficacy of these methods is inconclusive.

Various pharmacological and non-pharmacological methods are used to inhibit lactation after childbirth and relieve associated symptoms.

Indications: Women cannot or may not want to breastfeed due to various reasons including:

1. Stillbirth,

2. HIV-positive mothers,

3. Baby is surrendered for adoption/surrogacy

4. Mother is on certain drugs which can cross over to the baby through breast milk—antineoplastic drugs, chemotherapy agents, benzodiapines, lithium, amiodarone, and retinoids.

5. Mother taking recreational drugs or alcohol should not breastfeed.
6. Mother has an active herpes simplex virus (HSV) infection with lesions present on the breast.
7. Galactosemia—infants with galactosemia should not be breastfed. Galactosemia is detected by newborn screening, allowing proper treatment and diet to begin immediately. If infant is breastfed, it can lead to liver problems, intellectual and developmental disabilities, and shock.
8. Breast surgery—mothers with history of breast surgery or implants may find it difficult to brestfeed and may need lactation suppression.
9. Mother is depressed or critically ill to breastfeed the baby.
10. Social reason—mother can choose not to breastfeed the baby.

Important points to discuss with the patient[3]

○ Do not stimulate breast
○ Express milk to reduce discomfort
○ Wear a firm supportive bra
○ Have a good fluid intake
○ Advise the woman regarding painkillers
○ Do not restart breastfeed/give baby any expressed breastmilk once treatment initiated

PHARMACOLOGICAL METHODS FOR LACTATION SUPPRESSION

Overview of drugs used for lactation suppression

Drug category	Drug
Ergot derivatives	Cabergoline and bromocriptine-cabergoline is the most commonly used drug
Estrogen compounds	Estrogen compounds were used alone or in combination with androgens to suppress the milk Less efficacy Serious side effects like thrombosis and pulmonary thromboembolism
Sympathomimetic drugs	Pseudoephedrine is an adrenergic sympathomimetic Side effects: Stomach pain, irritability, insomnia, tachycardia, cardiac arrhythmias, increased blood pressure and tachycardia

CABERGOLINE

Cabergoline is a long-acting oral dopamine agonist. It is a dopaminergic ergoline derivative that directly stimulates D2-dopamine receptors on pituitary lactotrophs.

Mechanism of Action

- Cabergoline is a long-acting ergot derivative with a high affinity with dopamine D2 receptors.
- It directly stimulates D2-dopamine receptors on pituitary lactotrophs.
- It exerts a central dopaminergic effect via D2-receptor stimulation at oral doses that are higher than those effective in lowering serum prolactin levels.
- Cabergoline has low affinity for D1-, alpha-1, alpha-2 adrenergic and serotonin receptors. Cabergoline has no effect on the basal secretion of other anterior pituitary hormones (GH, FSH, LH, corticotrophin, TSH) or cortisol.

Pharmacokinetics and Pharmodynamics

- Cabergoline is well-absorbed with peak concentrations achieved within 0.5–4 hours and can be administered with or without food.
- Cabergoline is moderately bound to plasma proteins (41%) and has a long elimination half-life (63–69 hours).
- It is extensively metabolized via hydrolysis into inactive metabolites. It is not metabolized by the CYP450 enzyme system and does not cause CYP450 enzyme inhibition or induction.

- No known dose reductions are required for mild or moderate hepatic dysfunction however there are limited data in individuals with severe hepatic insufficiency. No dose reductions are required in renal insufficiency.

Dose

Cabergoline is given as a single 1 mg dose (2 × 0.5 mg tab) during the first day postpartum (preferably within 12 hours postpartum).[4]

Onset of effect occurs within 3 hours of administration and the duration of effect lasts up to at least 14–21 days in puerperal women.

Another regimen followed is to give Cabergoline as a divided dose over 2 days–4 doses of 0.25 mg every 12 hours.

But the 1 mg dose appears to be the most effective for long-term suppression of lactation.

Side Effects[3,4]

- Headache
- Dizziness
- Fatigue
- Orthostatic hypotension
- Acne and pruritis

Contraindications

- Hypersensitivity to the drug, other ergot alkaloids
- Pre-eclampsia or postpartum hypertension.

Drug Interactions

Interaction is more common with antiemetics commonly used in the postpartum period.

Do not use with other dopamine antagonists such as metoclopramide, phenothiazines, butyrophenones and thioxanthines as these may reduce the prolactin lowering effects.

Precautions

- Renal disease
- Gastrointestinal bleeding
- Liver disease
- Raynaud syndrome

- Pulmonary or cardiac fibrotic disorders
- History of psychosis, hypotension.

Rebound lactation (resumption of milk supply) has been documented within one to two weeks after initial pharmacological suppression treatment.[5]

BROMOCRIPTINE

Bromocriptine is an ergoline derivative and dopamine agonist. Currently, it is not used to suppress lactation. It has been withdrawn in the United States and other countries because it increases the risk of maternal stroke, seizures, cardiovascular disorders, death and possibly psychosis.

Dose of 2.5 mg once daily was been used for 3–7 days.

Tips for making suppression more comfortable[6]

- Gentle handling of breasts. As breast milk is expressed less often the supply of milk will also gradually reduce
- Ice packs in bra or cold compresses after a shower or bath can relieve pain and swelling.
- Mild analgesics can help reduce discomfort.
- Advise to wear comfortable bra.

Things to watch out for: If the mother is not breastfeeding the baby, it is necessary to do proper lactation suppression. If not done then it can lead to following complications:

Breast engorgement	*Blocked duct and mastitis*
Breasts become very swollen, tender and hard.	A lump starts forming and the breast begins to feel sore.
Wear a firm bra.	Express more milk than usual to clear the blockage.
Express only for comfort.	If not treated, a breast abscess may develop.

Important Points

- Woman may not be allowed to breastfeed in special situations including:
  - Stillborn baby/intrauterine fetal demise (IUFD),
  - Neonatal death,

- Maternal infection, such as HIV and maternal illness,
- Baby surrendered for surrogacy or adoption, and
- Social reason—mother may choose not to breastfeed
- Cabergoline is a potent long-acting oral dopamine agonist that directly stimulates D2-dopamine receptors.
- Cabergoline is given as a single 1 mg dose (2 × 0.5 mg tab) during the first day postpartum.
- Cabergoline is a relatively safe drug for suppression of lactation with minimal contraindications.

References

1. Spitz AM, Lee NC, Peterson HB. Treatment for lactation suppression Little progress in one hundred years. Am J Obstet Gynecol. 1998;179(6):1485–1490. doi: 10.1016/S0002-9378(98)70013-4.

2. Schanler RJ, Potak DC. Physiology of lactation. UpToDate.

3. LactMed US Library of Medicine. Cabergoline [Internet] Bethesda (MD): US National Library of Medicine, National Institutes of Health; 2015 [updated 2015 cited 2016 Jan12].

4. Briggs GG and Freeman, RK. Freeman, Yaffe, SJ. Drugs in Pregnancy and Lactation: A Reference Guide to Fetal and Neonatal Risk Cabergoline (9th edn).Philadelphia: Wolters Kluwer Health, Lippincott Williams Wilkins.

5. Oladapo OT, Fawole B. Treatments for suppression of lactation. Cochrane Database Syst Rev. 2012 Sep 12;2012(9):CD005937. doi: 10.1002/14651858.CD005937.pub3. PMID: 22972088; PMCID: PMC6599849.

6. Adapted from Supressing Lactation factsheet by Lactation Service, Queensland Children's Hospital.

Malaria in Pregnancy

• Ameya Medhekar • Ameya Purandare

Introduction

Malaria is a common infectious illness in tropical countries. The prevalence of malaria is generally more in pregnant women as compared to non-pregnant women in any given geographic area. The occurrence of malaria in pregnancy is associated with multiple adverse outcomes for both mother and fetus. Pregnant women affected with malaria are at increased risk of maternal death and maternal anemia; while adverse pregnancy outcomes include spontaneous abortion, preterm delivery, intrauterine growth restriction (IUGR) and low birth weight (LBW), stillbirth, congenital infection, and neonatal mortality.

MICROBIOLOGY OF MALARIA

Malarial species that affect humans include *Plasmodium falciparum*, *P. vivax*, *P. ovale*, *P. malariae*, and *P. knowlesi*. Effects in pregnancy are dependent on the infecting parasite species.

P. falciparum can invade red blood cells of all ages, achieve very high parasite burden, sequester in the placental circulation and is consequently responsible for adverse maternal–fetal outcomes.

P. vivax invades young red cells, has lower parasitemia and placental sequestration. It is less likely to cause adverse pregnancy outcomes.

P. ovale, *P. malariae* and *P. knowlesi* are generally uncommon in pregnancy and not associated with poor outcomes. However, a few cases of severe malaria in pregnancy due to *P. knowlesi* have been reported.

LIFE CYCLE (Fig. 12.1)

The malarial sporozoites are transmitted to humans by the bite of an infected female *Anopheles* mosquito. The sporozoites make their way through the blood to the liver and invade the hepatocytes. In the hepatocytes, each sporozoite undergoes a period of asexual reproduction (intrahepatic or pre-erythrocytic schizogony) producing 10,000–30,000 daughter merozoites. The invaded hepatocytes eventually rupture releasing the merozoites into the circulation. These merozoites invade red blood cells (RBC) as trophozoites. The trophozoites multiply 8–20 times every 48 hours (*P. malariae*—72 hrs; *P. knowlesi*—24 hrs). As the trophozoites enlarge, they occupy a major portion of the RBC and consume the hemoglobin. These large forms are called schizonts. The schizonts rupture, ending the intraerythrocytic replication phase, releases 6–30 daughter merozoites that are capable of infecting other RBCs and continuing the cycle.

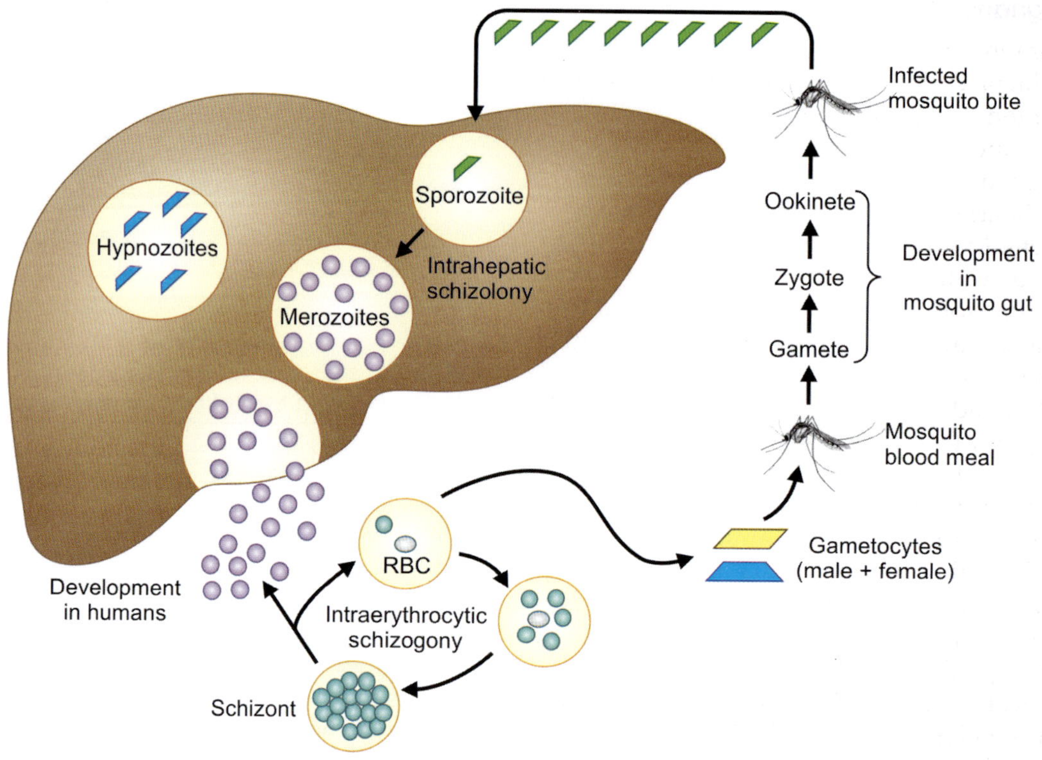

Fig. 12.1: Life cycle of *Plasmodium* species

In *P. vivax* and *P. ovale*, a small number of sporozoites remain quiescent in the hepatocytes and are known as hypnozoites. These dormant forms can multiply later and produce a malarial relapse.

During the intraerythrocytic stage, some trophozoites go on to form specialized forms called gametocytes. The gametocytes are essential for continuation of the malarial life cycle within the biting mosquito, wherein they will undergo sexual reproduction and produce sporozoites that can spread malaria to a susceptible host.

Clinical Features

Malaria is a febrile illness accompanied by other nonspecific features including chills, sweats, fatigue, headache, muscle pains and abdominal discomfort. The malarial paroxysms of regularly occurring fever, chills, rigors and sweats, described in earlier times, are unusual in most cases. Temperatures reaching 104°F (40°C) are often seen and can be accompanied by febrile delirium. Uncomplicated malaria has few clinical signs other than fever, mild anemia and a palpable spleen.

Severe malaria entails vital organ dysfunction. It is most often seen with *P. falciparum* but occasional cases with *P. vivax* and *P. knowlesi* do occur. Major manifestations of severe *falciparum* malaria include unarousable coma and seizures, acidosis, severe anemia, pulmonary edema and acute respiratory distress, renal failure, hypoglycemia, hypotension, disseminated intravascular coagulation, hemoglobinuria and jaundice.

Pregnant women are more likely to have higher parasitemia as compared to non-pregnant women. They consequently experience more severe disease including the occurrence of hypoglycemia and respiratory complaints (pulmonary edema and acute respiratory distress).

Pregnancy Outcome

Women residing in areas with unstable malaria transmission and non-immune women are more likely to have adverse outcomes if they contract malaria during pregnancy.

Malaria is an important cause of maternal mortality during pregnancy. Maternal death is as a result of cerebral malaria, severe organ dysfunction (lungs, liver or renal), acidosis or anemia. Maternal anemia is a common outcome of malaria in pregnancy.

Fetal adverse outcomes include low birth weight (LBW) babies. Low birth weight is as a result of both preterm delivery as well as intrauterine growth restriction (IUGR).

Spontaneous abortions, intrauterine fetal death and neonatal mortality are all devastating outcomes of malaria during pregnancy.

Congenital malaria occurs as a result of vertical transmission of the malarial parasite. All species of malarial parasites can be transmitted *in utero*. Transplacental malaria transmission risk is about 7–10% in non-immune pregnant women.

Diagnosis

Malaria is not a clinical diagnosis. The demonstration of the parasite or parasite antigen/genetic material is essential for diagnosis.

Examination of the peripheral blood smear (thick and thin) is the primary method for malaria diagnosis. In areas where access to microscopy is limited, rapid antigen tests can be used. Polymerase chain reaction (PCR) is an emerging and promising technique for early diagnosis of malaria.

Treatment

Antimalarial drugs are used for the prevention and treatment of malaria. Drugs that are used for treatment essentially target the intraerythrocytic parasite forms which are responsible for symptomatic disease. Additionally, certain antimalarials act on the hypnozoites or dormant intrahepatic parasite forms (*P. vivax* and *P. ovale*) and are used to prevent relapses of malaria that can occur weeks to years after the initial episode.

The role of antimalarials against pre-erythrocytic parasite stages is uncertain. Gametocidal agents are important tools in the interruption of malaria transmission.

DRUGS USED IN THE TREATMENT OF MALARIA

Refer Tables 12.1–12.3 for individual drug dosage.

Table 12.1: Recommended dosages for artemisinin-based combination therapies (ACTs)

Name of drug	Dosage (mg) as per body weight (kg)			
Artemether+Lumefantrine (mg) twice daily for 3 days	5 to <15 kg 20 + 120	15 to 25 kg 40 + 240	25 to 35 kg 60 + 360	>35 kg 80 + 480
Artesunate + Amodiaquine (mg) once daily for 3 days	4.5 to 9 kg 25 + 67.5	9 to 18 kg 50 + 135	18 to 36 kg 100 + 270	>36 kg 200 + 540
Artesunate + Mefloquine (mg) once daily for 3 days	5 to 9 kg 25 + 55	9 to 18 kg 50 + 110	18 to 30 kg 100 + 220	>30 kg 200 + 440
Dihydroartemisinin + Piperaquine (mg) once daily for 3 days (Paediatric dosing)	5 to 8 kg 20 + 160	8 to 11 kg 30 + 240	11 to 17 kg 40 + 320	17 to 25 kg 60 + 480
Dihydroartemisinin + Piperaquine (mg) once daily for 3 days (adult dosing)	25–36 kg 80 + 480	36 to 60 kg 120 + 960	60 to 80 kg 160 + 1280	>80 kg 200 + 1600

Table 12.2: Recommended dosing for Artesunate + Sulfadoxine-pyrimethamine

Name of drug	Dosage (mg) as per body weight (kg)			
Artesunate (mg) once daily for 3 days	5 to 10 kg 25	10 to 25 kg 50	25 to 50 kg 100	>50 kg 200
Sulfadoxine/Pyrimethamine (mg) as single dose on day 1	5 to 10 kg 250/12.5	10 to 25 kg 500/25	25 to 50 kg 1000/50	>50 kg 1500/75

Table 12.3: Dosing schedules for other antimalarial agents

Name of drug	Dosage
Chloroquine	25 mg/kg total dose administered as 10 mg/kg on day 1, 10 mg/kg on day 2, and 5 mg/kg on day 3.
Mefloquine	1250 mg total dose administered as 750 mg initial dose followed 6 to 12 hours later by 500 mg dose.
Atovaquone-proguanil	4 adult tablets orally once daily for 3 days (each adult tablet contains 250 mg atovaquone/100 mg proguanil)
Doxycycline	100 mg twice daily for 7 days
Clindamycin	20 mg/kg per day divided into 3 equal doses (maximum dose 1.8 g/day) for 7 days
Quinine (oral)	650 mg three times a day for 7 days
Arterolane–piperaquine (150 mg/750 mg per tablet)	One tablet at diagnosis, followed by one tablet at 24 hours and 48 hours.

1. Artemisinin Derivatives

The artemisinin derivatives have been used for many centuries in Chinese medicine and are derived from the leaves of *qing hao* (*Artemisia annua* or Chinese sweet wormwood plant). The artemisinin derivatives include artemether, artesunate, dihydroartemisinin and arteether.

Mechanism of action: The drugs bind iron, break down peroxide bridges and generate free radicals that damage parasite proteins. Dihydroartemisinin is the active compound.

These drugs act rapidly against the blood forms of all malarial parasite species and swiftly reduce the parasite burden. They produce the fastest parasite clearance amongst all the available antimalarial agents.

Absorption, fate and excretion: Limited information is available on the pharmacokinetics of artemisinin compounds. Artemether and artesunate are converted to dihydroartemisinin, which is the active agent and has a short half-life of about 45 minutes. Minimal amount of dihydroartemisinin is recovered from urine. Artemether, artesunate and dihydroartemisinin are available as oral formulations. Artesunate and artemether are also available for parenteral use.

Adverse effects: Artemisinin compounds are generally well-tolerated. Type-I hypersensitivity reactions, transient neurologic abnormalities–nystagmus and imbalance, transient neutropenia and elevated aminotransferases have been reported. They are self-limited with unclear clinical significance.

Post-treatment hemolysis following use of intravenous artesunate for treatment of severe malaria with high parasite index can occur.

Safety in pregnancy: There are some concerns about the use of artemisinin derivatives in the first trimester of pregnancy owing to potential for teratogenicity (suggested by animal studies). However, observational reports from use in the first trimester of pregnancy have not shown any adverse pregnancy outcomes in humans. Parenteral artesunate is recommended as first-line therapy for treatment of severe malaria in pregnancy (all trimesters). However, for uncomplicated malaria, artemisinin derivatives should not be used in the first trimester of pregnancy.

Therapeutic uses: Artemisinin compounds are combined with longer-acting agents of another antimalarial group of drugs and formulated as artemisinin-based combination therapy (ACT). ACT provides rapid reduction of the parasite burden, produces durable treatment response, and protects against development of drug resistance. ACTs are oral formulations, typically having fixed doses and 3-day treatment duration.

ACTs are the primary treatment for uncomplicated malaria (any species).

Intravenous artesunate is first-line therapy for severe malaria. Intravenous therapy is given till patients are stable and tolerating orals, after which an ACT is used to complete treatment.

Resistance: Reduced susceptibility to artemisinin compounds as evidenced by delayed parasite clearance has been reported from Southeast Asia. A point mutation in the kelch protein (K13) is associated with this phenomenon. The decreased susceptibility to artemisinin drugs is likely to promote development of resistance to the partner drug used in the ACT.

As ACT is the cornerstone of all current treatment regimens, WHO has banned the use and sale of artemisinin monotherapy.

2. Quinoline Derivatives

The drugs belonging to this group include chloroquine, amodiaquine, quinine, quinidine, mefloquine, lumefantrine, halofantrine and primaquine.

Mechanism of action: These drugs accumulate in the parasite food vacuole. They complex with heme and prevent peroxidation, and inhibit the non-enzymatic polymerization to hemazoin (the inactive malarial pigment). Failure to inactivate heme kills the parasites via oxidative damage to membranes, and digestive proteases.

Chloroquine: Chloroquine was the first drug to be mass produced as an antimalarial agent. It acts against the erythrocytic stages of *P. ovale, P. malariae,* and susceptible stains of *P. vivax.* Most *P. falciparum* strains are resistant to chloroquine.

Absorption, fate and excretion: Chloroquine is well-absorbed after oral administration and has a large volume of distribution being deposited to most tissues. About half of the drug is renally cleared. It has a long half-life and maintains serum concentration for up to 2 months after treatment.

Adverse effects: For doses used in the treatment or prevention of malaria, the drug is extremely well-tolerated and extraordinarily safe. Nausea, vomiting, abdominal discomfort, and diarrhea are common. Headaches and dizziness are also reported. Pruritus may be seen, especially in dark skinned individuals and is not responsive to antihistamines.

Safety in pregnancy: Chloroquine is safe for use in pregnancy in all trimesters.

Therapeutic uses: Chloroquine can be used for the treatment of uncomplicated *P. ovale, P. malariae* and susceptible *P. vivax* malaria. It is also used for chemoprophylaxis in travel to geographic areas that have chloroquine susceptible malarial strains.

Resistance: Resistance to chloroquine is attributed to decreased accumulation of the drug in the parasite food vacuole. *P. falciparum* resistance is widespread. *P. vivax* resistance is also seen in certain parts of the world. *P. malariae* and *P. ovale* remain sensitive to chloroquine.

Amodiaquine: It is structurally similar to chloroquine but retains some activity against chloroquine resistant strains. It is never used as monotherapy and is available as an ACT with artesunate.

Adverse effects include neutropenia and hepatotoxicity, especially with longer duration of therapy. Hence, it is no longer recommended for chemoprophylaxis against malaria.

Piperaquine: It is closely related to chloroquine and amodiaquine. Like amodiaquine, it is not used as monotherapy but combined as ACT with dihydroartemisinin. It is also available in combination with arterolane. It has one of the longest half-lives among antimalarial agents and provides prolonged post-treatment prophylaxis.

Mefloquine: It is an orally-administered agent, effective against the erythrocytic stages of *P. ovale, P. malariae, P. vivax* (including chloroquine-resistant strains) and susceptible strains of *P. falciparum.*

Absorption, fate and excretion: Mefloquine is well-absorbed after oral administration, especially in the presence of food. It is widely distribution and has a half-life of about 20 days. In humans, it undergoes extensive enterohepatic circulation and biliary excretion and is primarily excreted in feces.

Adverse effects: Nausea, vomiting, abdominal discomfort and diarrhea are frequently noted. Dizziness, ataxia, visual and auditory disturbances, and headache can occur but are mild and self-limited. Neuropsychiatric symptoms including disorientation, seizures, psychosis, and encephalopathy are rare.

Safety in pregnancy: Mefloquine is safe for use in pregnancy in the second and third trimesters.

Therapeutic uses: Mefloquine is available as ACT with artesunate and used in the treatment of uncomplicated *P. falciparum* and non-*falciparum* malaria. It is also used for chemoprophylaxis. However, due to the possibility of neuropsychiatric side effects, it is not used in patients with a history of seizures, psychiatric and neurologic illnesses particularly as weekly prophylaxis.

Resistance: Resistance to mefloquine is especially found in Southeast Asia and is due to the increased expression of pfmdr1 which regulates traffic across the digestive vacuolar membrane.

Quinine: Quinine has been used for over 350 years for the treatment of fevers. It is an alkaloid of cinchona, the bark of the South American cinchona tree (Peruvian, Jesuit's, or Cardinal's bark). It remains a mainstay in the treatment of drug-resistant *falciparum* malaria.

Absorption, fate and excretion: Quinine is readily absorbed orally or after intramuscular administration. It has a half-life of about 11 hours and needs to be administered three times per day. The cinchona alkaloids are extensively metabolized in the liver. There is no accumulation of the drug in the body on continued administration as the metabolites are excreted in urine.

Adverse effects: 'Cinchonism' is the characteristic side effect of quinine. Mild forms present with tinnitus, high-tone hearing loss, visual disturbances, headache, nausea, vomiting and orthostasis.

Hypoglycemia due to hyperinsulinemia can occur at therapeutic doses of quinine and should be promptly identified and treated. This is especially problematic in pregnant women and in severe illness.

Quinine rarely causes cardiovascular complications that can be fatal. These are mostly seen after excessively rapid intravenous infusion of quinine. Hypotension accompanied by arrhythmias such as sinus arrest, junctional rhythm, AV blocks and ventricular tachycardia and fibrillation are typical.

'Black water fever' is a severe hypersensitivity reaction to quinine that is seen in treatment of malaria in pregnancy. There is massive hemolysis, hemoglobinemia and hemoglobinuria leading to anuria, renal failure and even death.

Safety in pregnancy: Quinine is safe for use in pregnancy in all trimesters.

Therapeutic uses: Quinine is primarily used for the treatment of complicated and drug resistant *P. falciparum* and non-*falciparum* malaria. It is the drug of choice for treatment of uncomplicated falciparum malaria in the first trimester of pregnancy. It is combined with clindamycin (in pregnancy) or doxycycline for a duration of 7 days.

Resistance: Reduced efficacy to quinine is documented in Southeast Asia. However, when combined with a second agent, efficacy appears to be maintained.

Primaquine: It is an orally-administered agent effective against the late hepatic stages and latent tissue forms of *P. ovale* and *P. vivax*. It is a potent gametocidal agent against all malarial parasite species including *P. falciparum*.

Absorption, fate and excretion: Primaquine has near complete absorption after oral administration, especially in the presence of food. It has wide volume of distribution and is rapidly metabolized. Half-life of primaquine is about 6 hours.

Adverse effects: Nausea, vomiting, and abdominal discomfort are common but are alleviated if the drug is administered after a meal. Its most significant toxicity is acute hemolysis in persons who are glucose-6-phosphate dehydrogenase (G6PD) deficient. It is mandatory to perform testing for G6PD activity prior to administering primaquine.

Safety in pregnancy: Primaquine cannot be used in pregnancy or lactation.

Therapeutic uses: Primaquine is primarily used for the prevention of relapse following infection with *P. vivax* or *P. ovale* (radical cure). It is also used as a gametocidal agent for interruption of malaria transmission.

Tafenoquine: Tafenoquine has a long half life of 17 days and can be used as a single dose therapy for prevention of malaria relapse following *P. vivax* infection. This has significant advantage over the longer and highly dose-dependent primaquine regimen for successful eradication of hypnozoites. It is also used for chemoprophylaxis.

Unfortunately, tafenoquine also causes acute hemolysis in G6PD deficient individuals and hence testing for G6PD activity is mandatory prior to administration. It cannot be used in pregnancy and lactation.

Lumefantrine: It is used with artemether as ACT. The exact mechanism of action is not known. Absorption after oral administration is enhanced by fatty food. It is extensively metabolized in the liver and excreted in bile. It has a half-life of 3–6 days.

3. Arterolane

A rapidly-acting, non-artemisinin, synthetic agent that can be considered an alternative to ACT for treatment of uncomplicated malaria. The advantage of arterolane stems from the production process that is not dependent on the supply of leaves from the *qing hao* plant.

The mechanism of action is similar to the artemisinin derivatives. Arterolane gets concentrated in the parasite food vacuole and cytosol. The free radicals produced as a result of reductive cleavage of the peroxide bond of arterolane causes inhibition of heme detoxification as well as alkylation of essential proteins.

Following oral administration, arterolane has good absorption which is enhanced if taken with food. It has a short half-life of 2–4 hours and a wide volume of distribution. It is combined with piperaquine (longer-acting agent) and thereby provides rapid parasite clearance and prevents recrudescence. The combination is dosed once a day for three days.

Arterolane–piperaquine combination (Synriam) is approved for use by the Drugs Controller General of India (DCGI) for the treatment of uncomplicated *P. falciparum* and *P. vivax* malaria. It is under review for WHO approval. It is not used for preventative therapy or radical cure.

4. Antifolates

This group includes sulfadoxine-pyrimethamine, and proguanil. These drugs inhibit enzymes in folate synthesis, an essential step in parasite DNA production. They primarily target the blood stages of *P. falciparum* and *P. vivax*.

Sulfadoxine-pyrimethamine: This is an orally-administered synergistic antifolate combination that targets two different enzymes in the folate synthesis pathway, namely dihydropteroate synthase (DHPS) and dihyrofolate reductase (DHFR). This is a slow-acting agent with low efficacy and must be combined with a rapid-acting, potent antimalarial drug.

Absorption, fate and excretion: It is administered as a fixed dose tablet with good absorption through the gastrointestinal tract. Sulfadoxine is a sulfonamide with a particularly long half-life of 7–9 days. Pyrimethamine is a diamino-pyrimidine with a half-life of about 4 days.

Adverse effects: Skin rash including the development of Stevens-Johnson syndrome and toxic epidermal necrolysis (SJS-TEN), bone marrow suppression, and hepatitis have been reported.

Safety in pregnancy: It is safe for use in pregnancy.

Therapeutic uses: There is limited role for use of this agent in the treatment of malaria owing to extensive resistance.

Resistance: P. falciparum and *P. vivax* resistance to sulfadoxine-pyrimethamine is widespread in most malaria endemic regions and is due to mutations in the target enzymes, DHPS and DHFR.

Atovaquone–proguanil: This antimalarial drug combination targets the malarial parasite by two different mechanisms essential for nucleic acid replication. Atovaquone blocks the parasite mitochondrial electron transport system. Proguanil, through its active metabolite cycloguanil, inhibits malarial DHFR in the folate synthesis pathway. Proguanil also has intrinsic antimalarial activity that complements atovaquone.

Absorption, fate and excretion: Proguanil is slowly and incompletely absorbed from the gastrointestinal tract. However, adequate drug levels are achieved. It is metabolized to active cycloguanil and an inactive biguanide. The half-life is about 20 hours and about 50% of the drug and metabolites are renally excreted. Proguanil accumulates in erythrocytes and achieves levels that are three times of plasma levels.

Atovaquone absorption is slow, erratic and variable, being enhanced by fatty food. It has a half-life of 1.5–3 days and is not metabolized in the body. It is excreted unchanged almost entirely through the biliary system. There is negligible renal clearance.

Adverse effects: Both drugs are remarkably well-tolerated. Nausea, vomiting, abdominal pain, and diarrhea are the most common side effects. A maculopapular rash can occur but is mild and non-progressive.

Safety in pregnancy: It is not recommended for use in pregnancy.

Therapeutic uses: This combination can be used as an alternative to ACT when these are not available. The main factor limiting the widespread use of these agents is the cost and availability. However, in overweight and obese individuals they may have better efficacy than artemether–lumefantrine combination.

Resistance: Resistance to atovaquone is mediated through cytochrome β-gene mutation. DHFR target mutations induce resistance to proguanil.

5. Antimicrobials

Tetracycline, doxycycline and clindamycin are antimicrobials that have activity against malarial parasites. They target the malarial parasite apicoplast and interfere with protein synthesis. Due to their slow onset of action, they are always combined with a rapidly-acting antimalarial (quinine or artemisinin derivative).

Resistance to these antimicrobials has not yet been documented.

Doxycycline has a longer half-life than tetracycline and is the preferred agent. However, doxycycline cannot be used in pregnant and lactating women and children below 8 years due to deposition in bones and teeth. Clindamycin is the preferred alternative and is safe for use in these individuals.

Side effects of doxycycline include photosensitivity, abdominal discomfort, esophageal irritation and ulceration. Diarrhea and skin rash are the most common adverse effects with clindamycin.

Doxycycline can be used as prophylaxis against malaria. Clindamycin has no role in chemoprophylaxis.

Treatment Regimens for Malaria

The choice of treatment depends on the clinical condition of the patient, severity of malaria, species of malaria parasite and presumed resistance patterns in the geographic area.

Severe or complicated malaria refers to inability of the patient to sit or stand unaided and tolerate oral intake reliably, or evidence of end-organ dysfunction, or high parasite burden on blood smear (>10%).

While definitions for severe malaria exist, if the treating clinician feels uncertain regarding the severity of malaria, it is prudent to use regimens for severe disease.

SEVERE MALARIA
(ANY SPECIES OF MALARIAL PARASITE)

Parenteral therapy is recommended for treatment of severe malaria.

Artesunate is the drug of choice for all patients including pregnant women (any trimester), in lactation and infants.

Dosage for intravenous artesunate is 2.4 mg/kg body weight administered as a bolus. Followed by 2.4 mg/kg body weight at 12, 24 hours and then every 24 hours till the patient can tolerate oral intake reliably. Treatment must be completed with a 3-day ACT regimen once oral intake is established.

If parenteral artesunate is not available, artemether is the alternative. Artemether is administered as an intramuscular injection in the anterior thigh. A loading dose of 3.2 mg/kg body weight followed by 1.6 mg/kg body weight once daily. Patients should be given a 3-day course of ACT as soon as they can tolerate oral treatment.

If parenteral artemisinin derivatives are not available, quinine is the next option. Quinine is given in a loading dose of 20 mg/kg body weight followed by 10 mg/kg body weight every 8 hours. Quinine is usually diluted in 5% dextrose and should be administered slowly over 4 hours to prevent severe hypotension and cardiac arrythmias. A 3-day ACT regimen should be administered, once orals are tolerated for completion of treatment. If an ACT is not available then oral quinine with doxycycline or clindamycin can be used.

Uncomplicated *P. falciparum* Malaria

Patients with symptoms of malaria with a positive diagnostic test for *P. falciparum* malaria and without any features of severe malaria are deemed to have uncomplicated *P. falciparum* malaria.

The recommended treatment for uncomplicated malaria in all individuals (except pregnant women in the first trimester) is ACT. The treatment duration must be 3 days to cover 2 asexual reproduction cycles of the malarial parasite.

The ACTs approved by WHO for treatment include artemether–lumefantrine, artesunate–amodiaquine, artesunate–mefloquine, dihydroartemisinin–piperaquine, artesunate–pyronaridine and artesunate–sulfadoxine–pyrimethamine.

Pregnant women in the first trimester should be treated with quinine in combination with clindamycin.

Uncomplicated *P. vivax*, *P. ovale*, *P. malariae* or *P. knowlesi* Malaria

In areas with chloroquine-susceptible infections, adults and children with uncomplicated *P. vivax*, *P. ovale*, *P. malariae* or *P. knowlesi* malaria should be treated with either ACT (except pregnant women in their first trimester) or chloroquine.

In areas with chloroquine-resistant infections, adults and children with uncomplicated *P. vivax*, *P. ovale*, *P. malariae* or *P. knowlesi* malaria (except pregnant women in their first trimester) should be treated with ACT.

When ACT is considered as the therapeutic option, ACTs containing piperaquine, mefloquine or lumefantrine are recommended. Resistance to sulfadoxine-pyrimethamine among *P. vivax* is more rampant compared to *P. falciparum* and will compromise efficacy of the regimen.

In areas with chloroquine resistant malaria, pregnant women in the first trimester should be treated with quinine in combination with clindamycin.

Radical Cure

Treatment for the clearance of hypnozoites is recommended following *P. vivax* and *P. ovale* malaria. To prevent relapse of *P. vivax* or *P. ovale* malaria in children and adults (except pregnant women, infants aged <6 months, women breastfeeding infants, and people with G6PD deficiency), treatment with a 14-day course of primaquine is recommended in all transmission settings.

The dose of primaquine to be used is 0.25–0.5 mg/kg body weight per day in a single dose for 14 days. A higher dose has been found to be more effective in high transmission settings.

In pregnant and breastfeeding women, weekly chloroquine chemoprophylaxis may be considered to prevent relapse till such time that primaquine can be administered based on maternal G6PD status.

Chemoprophylaxis

Travelers to malaria endemic areas are often prescribed malaria chemoprophylaxis. Malaria is the most common identifiable cause of fever in a returning traveler. Chemoprophylaxis is effective and most failures are due to non-adherence to prescribed regimens.

Agents used for chemoprophylaxis include mefloquine, doxycycline, atovaquone–proguanil and tafenoquine.

Suggested Reading

1. Chamma-Siqueira N; Higher-Dose Primaquine to Prevent Relapse of Plasmodium vivax Malaria; N Engl J Med 2022; 386:1244–53.
2. Goodman and Gilman's The Pharmacological Basis of Therapeutics; 13th edition; Brunton, et al.
3. Harrison's Principles of Internal Medicine, 21st edition; Loscalzo, et al.
4. Llanos-Cuentas A, et al; Tafenoquine versus Primaquine to Prevent Relapse of Plasmodium vivax Malaria; N Engl J Med 2019; 380:229–241.
5. WHO Guidelines for malaria, 18 February 2022. Geneva: World Health Organization; 2022 (WHO/UCN/GMP/2022.01).

Toxoplasmosis in Pregnancy

• Arundhati Tilve • Niraj Mahajan

Introduction

Toxoplasmosis is a disease that affects many hosts, including about one-third of humans. Toxoplasmosis is caused by the sporozoite parasite *Toxoplasma gondii* (*T. gondii*). It has acute and chronic effects in humans. Most healthy people recover from toxoplasmosis without treatment. Toxoplasmosis presents with a variety of symptoms ranging from congenital neurotoxoplasmosis to eye symptoms.

Congenital toxoplasmosis occurs due to acquisition of toxoplasma as the primary infection in a pregnant woman. Toxoplasmosis can cause serious health problems in fetuses, newborns and immunocompromised patients. The parasite crosses the blood–placental barrier to reach the fetus.

The rate and severity of congenital toxoplasmosis infection depend on the gestational age at which the infection is transmitted.[1,2]

Although rare, congenital toxoplasmosis can cause brain or eye disease (causing blindness) and anomalies of the heart and brain.[3]

Fetal infection in the first trimester often causes miscarriages. However, it can cause stillbirths or develop neonatal brain abnormalities (hydrocephalus, intracranial calcifications, deafness, mental retardation, convulsions) and eyes (retinochoroiditis causes blindness).

Infection in the second trimester or later is unlikely to cause miscarriage.

Retinochoroiditis and learning difficulties may occur after birth. Retinochoroiditis is the most common symptom of ocular toxoplasmosis, usually caused by a congenital toxoplasmosis infection.

It manifests as posterior uveitis, vitritis, focal necrotizing granulomatous retinitis, and reactive granulomatous choroiditis.[4]

Treatment for toxoplasmosis is still varied, including antibiotics and antiparasitic agents. The effectiveness of the drug is affected by intolerance, side effects, and parasite resistance. Unfortunately, all drugs currently used, target acute toxoplasmosis and have little or no effect on chronic disease.

Therefore, toxoplasmosis prevention education should be included in antenatal.

TREATMENT

The mainstay of treatment for toxoplasmosis is antibiotics and antiparasitic agents.[5]

Treatment strategies for this disease vary according to the condition of the disease and the immune system.

The Centers for Disease Control and Prevention (CDC) recommends a combination of drugs such as pyrimethamine and sulfadiazine, as well as folinic acid. Drugs currently approved for the treatment of toxoplasmosis target the tachyzoite stage of the parasite.

These drugs do not remove the encysted toxoplasma from the tissues. Pyrimethamine is a part of the standard treatment and is considered the best medicine against toxoplasmosis.

Trimethoprim and sulfamethoxazole available as a fixed drug combination is also available as an alternative. Other combinations such as atovaquone and pyrimethamine plus azithromycin have not been studied.[6,7]

Lymphadenopathic toxoplasmosis is usually selflimited and does not require treatment in healthy adults.

In obvious visceral disease or when symptoms are severe or persistent, treatment should be continued for 2 to 4 weeks.[6]

CONGENITAL TOXOPLASMOSIS

In congenital toxoplasmosis, the combination of pyrimethamine and sulfadiazine is the recommended first-line therapy.[8]

For the treatment of congenital toxoplasmosis, the infected newborns are usually given pyrimethamine and folinic acid for 12 months.[9] The recommendations of the National Toxoplasmosis Reference Laboratory (PAMF-TSL) and the University of Chicago Toxoplasmosis Center for the treatment of infected infants are: Pyrimethamine: 2 mg/kg, orally, twice daily for the first 2 days; then 1 mg/kg daily from third day to second month (or sixth month if symptoms are present); then 1 mg/kg per day orally for 3 times a week. Sulfadiazine: 100 mg/kg, orally, daily in two divided doses and folinic acid (leucovorin): 10 mg three times a week.[6]

OCULAR DISEASE

Blindness should be treated after a complete evaluation of the eye. The decision to treat an ocular toxoplasmosis depends on many variables, including the severity and degree of inflammation, visual impairment, and the location, size, and persistence of the lesion. Treatment should not be initiated for a healed lesion. The 'classic treatment' for ocular toxoplasmosis includes: Adults—100 mg pyrimethamine daily for 1 day, followed by 25 to 50 mg daily, 2 to 4 grams of sulfadiazine daily for 2 days, followed by 500 mg to 1 g four times daily plus folinic acid 5–25 mg with every pyrimethamine dose.

Pediatric dose: Pyrimethamine 2 mg/kg, day 1, followed by 1 mg/kg/day, plus sulfadiazine 50 mg/kg, twice daily, plus leucovorin 7.5 mg per day.

Treatment should be continued for 4 to 6 weeks, after which the patient should be reassessed.[6,10] Corticosteroids may be prescribed in addition to antiparasitic medication.

TREATMENT OF ACQUIRED IMMUNODEFICIENCY SYNDROME (AIDS)

Pyrimethamine 200 mg orally initially and 50–75 mg daily along with leucovirin 10 mg daily with sulfadiazine 4–8 g daily for 6 weeks, then treatment of life or until immunocompetent.

The antibiotics used in AIDS patients (CD4 <100) were oral pyrimethamine 50 mg/day and oral sulfadiazine 1–1.5 g/day plus leucovorin 10 mg/day for life or until immunocompetence is restored. Steroid therapy may be beneficial in patients with AIDS, CNS toxoplasmosis, and evidence of increased intracranial pressure or midline shift.

Diagnosis of toxoplasmosis in the absence of tissue or culture evidence can be dangerous because serology can be misleading and false-positive IgM results are relatively common. Empirical treatment should be avoided.[6]

Pyrimethamine

Pyrimethamine is a dihydrofolate reductase (DHFR) inhibitor, and acts by blocking the synthesis of purines and pyrimidines.

It falls into pregnancy category C. Information on the use of pyrimethamine in pregnant women is limited. By allowing the use of pyrimethamine and sulfadoxine during the second and third months of pregnancy, the World Health Organization (WHO) decided that the benefits of the treatment outweigh the risks of preventing malaria. Evidence suggests that pregnant women in the first trimester should avoid using pyrimethamine and supplement pyrimethamine with folinic acid during the second and third trimesters of pregnancy. Pyrimethamine also passes into breast milk.

Both the American Academy of Pediatrics and the World Health Organization classify pyrimethamine as suitable for breastfeeding. Breastfeeding women should be cautious when using pyrimethamine with other medications.[6]

Sulfadiazine

Sulfadiazine is a dihydrofolate synthase (DHPS) inhibitor. *T. gondii* synthesizes folic acid *de novo*, and this combination produces its antiparasitic effect by blocking the parasitic folic acid biosynthesis, thereby inhibiting the nucleic acid synthesis and parasite replication.

It falls into pregnancy category C. Information on the use of sulfadiazine during pregnancy is limited. Evidence suggests that sulfonamides should be avoided after 32 weeks of pregnancy. The use of sulfadiazine during pregnancy is only necessary if the benefit outweighs the risk to the fetus. Sulfadiazine also passes into breast milk.

The World Health Organization recommendation is to avoid breastfeeding with sulfadiazine therapy. Sulfadiazine is contraindicated during breastfeeding.[6]

To reduce side effects of pyrimethamine/ sulfadiazine, of which the most important is myelosuppression if used together with folinic acid, an active metabolite of folic acid and an important coenzyme for the synthesis of nucleic acids.[5]

A combination of medications containing pyrimethamine, sulfadiazine, and folinic acid should be used to treat women with confirmed or suspected fetal infection at or after 18 weeks of pregnancy (usually positive by amniotic fluid polymerase chain reaction.[3]

CDC-Recommended dose for adults: Add 100 mg of pyrimethamine loading dose on day 1, followed by 25 to 50 mg per day and 2 to 4 grams of sulfadiazine 2 times a day, followed by 500 mg to 1 gram four times a day, folinic acid 5–25 mg per pyrimethamine.[6]

This treatment has many side effects and causes 44% of patients to stop treatment. In patients allergic to sulfonamides, clindamycin should be used instead of sulfadiazine. However, pyrimethamine–clindamycin is less effective in preventing relapse and has similar toxicity.[11]

Clindamycin

Clindamycin falls in pregnancy category B. Data on the use of clindamycin in pregnant women are limited, but there are no reported congenital anomalies.

Clindamycin can be used in pregnant women, who will definitely benefit from the drug. Clindamycin passes into breast milk. The American Academy of Pediatrics classifies clindamycin as compatible with breastfeeding.[6]

Trimethoprim–Sulfamethoxazole (TMP-SMX)

This fixed drug combination falls in category C during pregnancy. It should be used in pregnancy.

TMP–SMX should be avoided in the last trimester because of the risk of neonatal hyperbilirubinemia and kernicterus. TMP-SMX passes into breast milk. TMP-SMX is generally suitable for breastfeeding healthy, term infants, after the newborn period. Breastfeeding of premature, jaundiced, sick, or stressed infants or infants with glucose-6-phosphate dehydrogenase deficiency should avoided when being treated TMP-SMX.[6]

TMP–SMX can be used instead of pyrimethamine-sulfadiazine if the patient is not allergic to sulfa and has pyrimethamine intolerance or is not available.[12]

Pyrimethamine, sulfadiazine, and trimethoprim-sulfamethoxazole are all class C drugs and all are secreted in breast milk. These medicines should only be given after careful consideration of the potential benefit to the fetus.

Spiramycin

Spiramycin is a 16-ring macrolide (antibiotic). It was discovered in 1952 as a product of *Streptomyces ambofaciens*. For oral administration, the drug has been used since 1955, and in 1987 the parenteral form was introduced into therapy.

The antibiotic activity of spiramycin includes inhibition of protein synthesis in bacterial cells during translocation.[13]

If the mother is infected before 18 weeks of pregnancy but the fetus no documented or suspected infection, spiramycin should be given for fetal prophylaxis to prevent maternal-to-fetus by blocking transplacental transmission. Polymerase chain reaction (PCR) is done on the amniotic fluid, usually around 18 weeks of pregnancy to determine if the baby has the disease.[6]

The drug is concentrated in the placenta and has been shown to reduce transmission by 60%. Spiramycin is given orally at a dose of 1 gram every 8 hours or 1–2 grams twice a day on an empty stomach. Oral spiramycin therapy is generally well-tolerated; abdominal side effects are the most common.

If the fetus is not infected (toxoplasma is confirmed by amniotic fluid polymerase chain reaction), continue spiramycin until the baby is born. However, since spiramycin does not cross the placenta well, it cannot be used to treat fetal toxoplasmosis; in this setting, pyrimethamine and sulfadiazine are recommended.

If the amniotic fluid test is positive for *Toxoplasma gondii*: 3 weeks of pyrimethamine (50 mg/day, PO) and sulfadiazine (3 g/day in 2–3 divided doses) alternating with 3 weeks of spiramycin 1 g, thrice a day for maternal therapy.

Alternatively, pyrimethamine (25 mg/day, PO) and two/four doses of sulfadiazine (4 g/day, PO) until delivery (this may be associated with myelosuppression and pancytopenia) and oral 10–25 mg/day folinic acid therapy to prevent myelosuppression.

CDC RECOMMENDATIONS FOR PREVENTION OF TOXOPLASMOSIS[6]

To avoid toxoplasmosis, food must be cooked to safe temperatures. Red meat should be cooked to at least 145°F, and pork, ground meat, and wild game meat cooked to 180°F in the thigh to guarantee thorough cooking.

Fruits and vegetables should be peeled or thoroughly washed before consumption.

Cutting boards, dishes, counters, utensils, and hands should always be meticulously washed with hot water and soap after they have come in contact with raw meat, poultry, seafood, or unwashed fruits or vegetables.

It is recommended that pregnant women should wear gloves when gardening and during any contact with soil or sand because it may be contaminated with cat waste. After gardening or contact with soil or sand, hands need to be thoroughly washed with soap and water.

Pregnant women should avoid changing cat litter if possible. However, if no one else is available, the use of gloves and then thorough and meticulous handwash is recommended. Also, the litter box needs to be changed daily because *Toxoplasma* oocysts require several days to become infectious. Pregnant women should be encouraged to keep their cats inside and not adopt or handle stray cats. Cats should be fed only canned or dried commercial food or well-cooked table food. Raw or undercooked meats are to be avoided.

Health education and information for women of reproductive age should also include information about meat-related and soilborne toxoplasmosis prevention.

References

1. Robbins JR; Zeldovich VB; Poukchanski A; Boothroyd JC; Bakardjiev AI. Tissue barriers of the human placenta to infection with *Toxoplasma gondii*. Infect. Immun. 2012, 80, 418–428.

2. Singh S. Congenital toxoplasmosis: Clinical features, outcomes, treatment, and prevention. Trop. Parasitol. 2016, 6, 113–122.

3. Paquet C, Yudin MH; Society of Obstetricians and Gynaecologists of Canada. Toxoplasmosis in pregnancy: prevention, screening, and treatment. J Obstet Gynaecol Can. 2013 Jan;35(1):78–81. English, French. doi: 10.1016/s1701-2163(15)31053-7. PMID: 23343802.

4. Vasconcelos-Santos DV; Dodds EM; Orefice, F. Review for disease of the year: Differential diagnosis of ocular toxoplasmosis. Ocul. Immunol. Inflamm. 2011, 19, 171–179.

5. Dunay IR; Gajurel K; Dhakal R; Liesenfeld O; Montoya JG. Treatment of Toxoplasmosis: Historical Perspective, Animal Models, and Current Clinical Practice. Clin. Microbiol. Rev. 2018, 31, e00057-17.

6. https://www.cdc.gov/parasites/toxoplasmosis/treatment.html Page last reviewed: July 13, 2022. Content source: Global Health, Division of Parasitic Diseases and Malaria. Accessed on 12th August 2022.

7. Montoya JG, Boothroyd JC, Kovacs JA. *Toxoplasma gondii* in Mandell, Douglas, and Bennett's Principles and Practice of Infectious Diseases, 8th, Edition, 2017 Mandell GL, Bennett JE, Dolin R, Eds. Churchill Livingstone Elsevier, Philadelphia, PA).

8. Blume M; Seeber F. Metabolic interactions between *Toxoplasma gondii* and its host. F1000 Research 2018;7:1719.

9. Maldonado YA, Read JS. AAP Committee on Infectious Diseases. Diagnosis, treatment, and prevention of congenital toxoplasmosis in the United States. Pediatrics. 2017;139(2):e20163860.

10. de-la-Torre A, Stanford M, Curi A, Jaffe GJ, Gomez-Marin JE. Therapy for ocular toxoplasmosis. Ocul Immunol Inflamm. 2011;19:314–20.

11. PH Alday, et al. Drugs in development for toxoplasmosis: Advances, challenges, and current status Drug Des. Dev. Ther (2017).

12. Hagras NA, Allam AF, Farag HF, Osman MM, Shalaby TI, Fawzy Hussein Mogahed NM, Tolba MM, Shehab AY. Successful treatment of acute experimental toxoplasmosis by spiramycin-loaded chitosan nanoparticles. Exp Parasitol. 2019 Sep;204:107717. doi: 10.1016/j.exppara.2019.107717. Epub 2019 Jun 20. PMID: 31228418.

13. Vacek V. Spiramycin [Spiramycin]. Cas Lek Cesk. 1994 Jan 17;133(2):56–60. Czech. PMID: 8131182.

Drugs in Urinary Tract Infection

• Geeta Agrawal

Introduction

The doctor should be well-acquainted with the chapter of drugs used in urinary tract infection (UTI) because:

- Urinary tract infections are among the number 1 infections that lead to the prescription of antibiotics after a visit to the doctor.
- The top most urinary tract infections reported by National Healthcare Safety Network are catheter induced.

Collateral damage can be prevented by the appropriate use of antibiotics. Collateral damages refer to adverse environmental effects due to organism which become drug resistant by inappropriate use of antibiotics, for example use of broad-spectrum cephalosporins and fluoroquinolones in UTIs.

Judicious Use of Antibiotics

Reduce

1. Inappropriate use of antibiotics
2. Broad spectrum use of antibiotics

It helps to adjust the necessary treatment for the shortest effective time.

Pathophysiology

Cystitis is lower urinary tract infection which is more common in women due to short urethra and moist periurethral environment. Pyelonephritis is infection of upper urinary tract which develops when the pathogens ascend to the kidneys. This infection occurs due to catheter, stones in urinary tract and due to trapping of pathogens in any physical obstruction in the tract.

Epidemiology

Three-fifths of women have at least single episode of urinary tract infection in their lifetime. Sexually active women are more prone to it.

Age group: Reproductive age group

Risk factors

- Diabetes
- Barrier method of contraception of low quality, specially having spermicides
- Past history of urinary tract infections
- Urinary tract infections in mother or sisters
- Coitus
- Poor hygiene

Age group: Postmenopausal women

Risk factors

- Lack of estrogen
- Physical or mental disability
- History of urinary tract infections in reproductive age group
- Urinary catheter
- Urinary incontinence
- Sanitization

Structural Abnormalities in Urinary Tract

- Extrarenal obstruction associated with ureteric or urethral anomalies or calculi, extrinsic ureteral compression.
- Intrarenal obstruction due to stone and uric acid nephropathy.
- Polycystic kidney disease, renal lesion associated with hypokalemia or analgesic use and sickle cell disease.

TYPES OF UTIs

1. Uncomplicated UTI occurs when a healthy nonpregnant woman suffers from dysuria, frequency, urinary urgency.
2. Complicated UTI occurs in pregnancy, stones, immunocompromised patient, in renal shutdown and transplantation, retention of urine from neurological disease, *in situ* catheters and sling surgery.
3. Catheter-induced UTI: It is the presence of $\geq 10^2$ colony-forming unit per ml (CFU/ml) bacteria from single catheter urine sample or midstream sample from a patient in whom catheter has been removed in the previous 48 hours.
4. Asymptomatic bacteriuria is defined as when the patient has no symptoms and on 2 consecutive midstream samples there is isolation of $\geq 10^5$ CFU/ml bacteria. The sample should be obtain form full retracted labia or if $\geq 10^5$ CFU/ml bacteria are isolated from single catheterized urine sample.
5. Recurrent UTI is said to occur when a patient suffers from 2 episodes of infection in 6 months or 3 such episodes in a year.

Typical Causative Organism

It is primarily caused by Gram-negative bacteria. More than 95% of uncomplicated UTIs are monobacterial.

Causative Agents in Type of UTIs

1. Uncomplicated UTI is most common caused by *E. coli*, *S. saprophyticus*, *Enterococcus* spp., *K. pneumoniae*, *P. mirabilis*.

S. saprophyticus is mostly involved in sexually active women.

2. In complicated UTI, same organisms are involved as of uncomplicated UTI and antibiotic-resistant *E. coli*, *P. aeruginosa*, *Acinetobacter baumannii*.

Enterococcus spp. and *Staphylococcus* spp. cause kidney abscess by bloodborne spread.

3. Catheter-induced UTI is mostly caused by *P. mirabilis*, *Morganella morganii*, *Providencia stuartii*, *C. urealyticum*.
4. Recurrent UTI is caused by *P. mirabilis*, *K. pneumonia*, *Enterobacter* spp., antibiotic-resistant *E. coli*, *Enterococcus* spp. and *Staphylococcus* spp.

Infectious window period (IWP) is defined as a period of 7 days, during which all the infection-specific criteria must be met. It includes the collection of first positive diagnostic test that is used as an element to meet site-specific infection criterion that is 3 calendar days before and 3 calendar days after the test.

Asymptomatic Bacteriuria

Definition: Asymptomatic bacteriuria (ABU) is defined as when the patient has no symptoms and on 2 consecutive midstream samples, there is isolation of $\geq 10^5$ CFU/ml bacteria. The sample should be obtained form full retracted labia or if $\geq 10^5$ CFU/ml bacteria are isolated from single catheterized urine sample.

*ABU is a blessing in disguise if found, it is protective against symptomatic UTI.

ABU in pregnancy: It occurs in 2–10% of all pregnant women and may lead to symptomatic infection.

It preferably occurs at 12 to 16 weeks of gestation.

Management of ABU

The current recommendations for the management of ABU are:

Flowchart 14.1: How to differentiate between symptomatic urinary tract infection (SUTI) and asymptomatic bacteremic UTI (ABUTI)

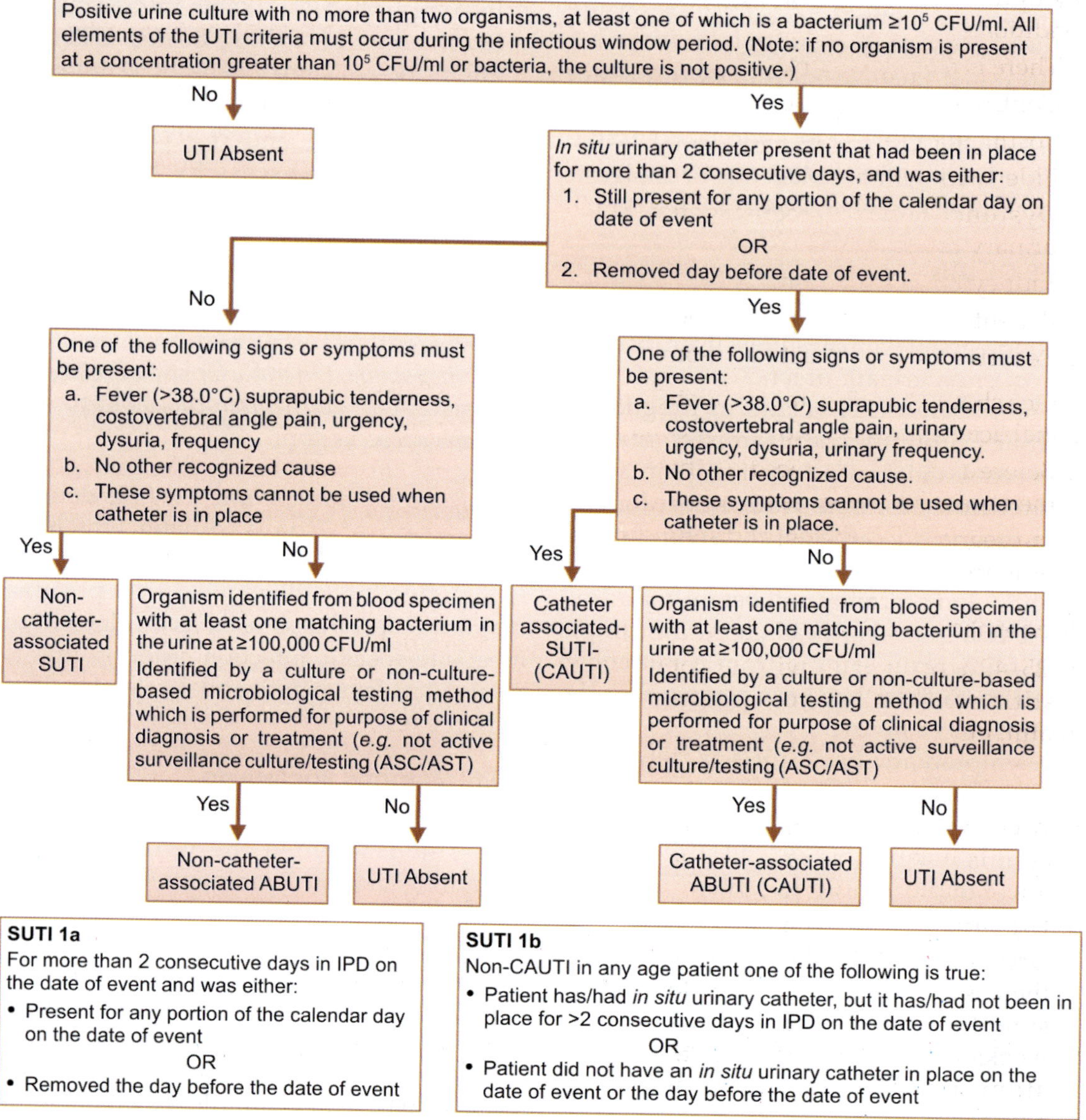

CFU: Colony-forming unit, IPD: Indoor patient department; IPD: Individual patient data

Note: This classification is given by Centers for Disease Control and Prevention (CDC) in Jan 2021. It does not affect the treatment.

One should not investigate or treat asymptomatic bacteriuria in the following conditions:

1. There is no risk factors.
2. Controlled diabetes mellitus.
3. Postmenopause.
4. Elderly indoor patients.
5. Dysfunctional or reconstructed lower urinary tracts.
6. Kidney transplantation.
7. Patients before arthroplasty operations.
8. Recurrent urinary tract infections.

One should investigate and treat asymptomatic bacteriuria done in following conditions:

1. Before a urological procedure that violates the mucous membrane.
2. In pregnant women with standard short-term treatment.

Uncomplicated Cystitis

In 25–42% of women with uncomplicated cystitis resolves without any antibiotic treatment.

How to Diagnose Uncomplicated Cystitis

a. A woman is said to have uncomplicated cystitis if she has no risk factors and has lower urinary tract symptoms.
b. Use urinalysis to diagnose.
c. Urine cultures should be done only when there is suspicion of acute pyelonephritis, symptoms do not subside within four weeks of stopping treatment, there are atypical symptoms or the woman is pregnant.

Treatment of Uncomplicated Cystitis

1. Fosfomycin trometamol, pivmecillinam or nitrofurantoin to be used as first line of treatment.
2. Do not use aminopenicillins or fluoro-quinolones **(Tables 14.1 and 14.2)**.

Recurrent UTI

Recurrent UTI (rUTI) is said to occur when a patient suffers from 2 episodes of infection in 6 months or 3 such episodes in a year.

Risk Factors for rUTI Related to Age

1. *Reproductive age group:* The most common risk factors in this age group are coitus, multiple sexual partner, spermicidal use, mother with history of UTI and past history of UTI.
2. *Post-menopausal women:* The risk factors are past history of UTI, urinary incontinence, atrophic vaginitis, cystocele and increased post-void urine volume.

A patient who has a relative having a history of UTI has some genetic risk and behavioral patterns which make them more prone to UTI.

Secretary status: It is set to be positive when there is presence of water soluble ABO blood group antigen in person's body fluids. These people are more susceptible to cross infections.

Antibiotic prophylaxis: Women with recurrent cystitis can be educated to self-administer short-term therapy lasting for 3 to 5 days at symptom onset after assessing patient compliance. Refer to the table for the

Table 14.1: First-line therapy for the treatment of uncomplicated symptomatic UTIs

Treatment effects	Nitrofurantoin	TMP-SMX	Fosfomycin
Cure rate	88–93%	90–100%	83–91%
Antimicrobial spectrum	Narrow: *E. coli, S. saprophyticus*	Typical uropathogens	Covers VRE and ESBL
Collateral damage	No	Minimum	No
Resistance	Low	Increasing	Currently low

Table 14.2: Antibiotic recommendations by type of UTIs

Antibiotics	Dose	Duration	Comments
Acute uncomplicated cystitis			
Nitrofurantoin monohydrate macrocrystal	100 mg PO BD	5 days	Dosage listed assumes normal renal function (>60 ml/ min/per 1.73 m²). Avoid in cases of early pyelonephritis.
Trimethoprim/ Sulfamethoxazole	160/800 mg PO BD	3 days	Use empirically if *E. coli* resistance to trimethoprim/sulfamethoxazole is <20%
Trimethoprim	100 mg PO BD	3 days	In sulpha-sensitive patients
Fosfomycin	3 g PO	Once	
Alternative agents			
Amoxicillin/Clavulanate	500/125 mg PO q8hr	5–7 days	
Cefodoxime proxetil	100 mg PO BD	5–7 days	
Cefdinir	300 mg PO BD	5–7 days	
Cephalexin	500 mg PO BD	5–7 days	Widely used, but limited data.
Ciprofloxacin	250 mg PO BD	3 days	Use empirically if FQ resistance in *E. coli* is <10%
Levofloxacin	250–500 mg PO daily	3 days	

drugs used in recurrent UTI **(Table 14.5)**. Use of cranberry juice, D-mannose, topical oestrogen therapy, probiotics show weak evidence in preventive strategies of recurrent UTI.

Recommendations for Diagnostic Evaluation and Treatment of Recurrent UTIs

- Diagnosed by urine culture examination.
- Do not do ultrasound or cystoscopy in women under 40 years with low risk factors.
- Do behavioral modification in active patients to reduce the risk of rUTI.
- Use vaginal estrogen therapy in post-menopausal women.
- Use of immunoactive prophylaxis with OM-89 reduces rUTI.
- Continuous use or prophylactic postcoital use reduces the risk of rUTI.
- For patients who are willing to comply, can be given self-administered short-term therapy.

Uncomplicated Pyelonephritis

Diagnosis of Uncomplicated Pyelonephritis

1. Perform urine dipstick to assess white blood cell (WBC), red blood cell (RBC) and nitrite.

2. In patients with pyelonephritis, do urine culture and sensitivity.

3. Do a urinary tract imaging if the fever persists for >72 hours or in case any complication arises, *e.g.* sepsis.

Treatment of Uncomplicated Pyelonephritis

1. Use short course fluoroquinolone (FQ) as first-line treatment in OPD.
2. Indoor patients treat with IV antibiotics initially.
3. Change from IV to oral therapy, if there is clinical improvement.
4. Avoid using nitrofurantoin, oral fosfomycin, and pivmecillinam **(Table 14.3)**.

Complicated UTIs

Risk factors

- Obstruction at any location
- Foreign body
- Pregnancy
- Incomplete voiding
- Vesicoureteral reflex—immune suppression
- Recent history of instrumentation
- Healthcare-associated infections
- Diabetes mellitus.

Table 14.3: Treatment of acute uncomplicated pyelonephritis

Antibiotics	Dose	Duration	Comments
Recommended antibioties for outpatient (OP) management			
Ciprofloxacin	500 mg, PO, BD	7 days	If local fluoroquinolone resistance is >10%, give ceftriaxone 1 g IV once or a dose of an aminoglycoside culture results
Ciprofloxacin	1 g ER, PO, daily	7 days	
Levofloxacin	250–500 mg, PO, daily	3 days	
Alternative or definitive therapy if susceptibility is confirmed			
Trimethoprim/ Sulphamethoxazole	160/800 mg, PO, BD	14 days	Give ceftriaxone 1g IV once or amino-glycoside pending culture results
Cefpodoxime axetil	200 mg, PO, BD	10–14 days	
Amoxillin clavulanate	500 mg, PO, BD	10–14 days	
Inpatient management or in those unable to take oral medication			
Ciprofloxacin	400 mg, IV, q12hr	7 days	May add aminoglycoside pending culture results. Complete the course with PO antibiotics after afebrile for 48 hrs
Levofloxin	500 mg, IV, q24hr	7 days	
Ceftriaxone	1 g, IV, q24hr	7 days	
Cefepime	1–2 g, IV, q12hr	14 days	
Piperacillin/tazobactum	3.375 g, IV, q6hr		

Treatment of Complicated UTI

a. Use amoxicillin + aminoglycoside combination or second generation cephalosporin + aminoglycoside. Use IV third-generation cephalosporins as empiric treatment of complicated UTI with systemic symptoms.

b. Use ciprofloxacin only if the percentage of local resistance is <10% when the patient can take oral medicines, can be treated on OPD basis and the patient is sensitive to beta-lactam antimicrobial agents.

c. Ciprofloxacin and other FQs should not be used, empirically in the urology-ward patients and patients who have received FQs in the past 6 months.

d. Treat any neurologic issue or any complicating factors **(Table 14.4)**.

Catheter Associated UTI (CA-UTI)

Diagnosis of CA-UTI

1. In asymptomatic catheterized patient do not do urine culture.

2. Pyuria is not a soul indicator for catheter-associated UTI.

3. Only presence or absence of cloudy or odorous urine does not differentiate between symptomatic and asymptomatic Catheter-associated UTI.

Management and Prevention of CA-UTI

1. Symptomatic CA-UTI is considered as a complicated UTI.

2. Collect a culture of urine from which the catheter has been removed before starting therapy. An existing catheter may make culture results less useful due to bacterial biofilms.

3. Do not treat asymptomatic bacteriuria in a catheterized patient.

4. Treat asymptomatic bacteriuria before traumatic interventions in the urinary tract.

5. Remove or replace a catheter *in situ* that was in place >7 days prior to treatment initiation.

Table 14.4: Treatment of acute complicated pyelonephritis or urosepsis or patients with CA-UTI, who are seriously ill

Recommended empiric therapy for hospitalized, not seriously ill	See inpatient management of acute uncomplicated pyelonephritis		
Recommended empiric therapy for hospitalized, seriously ill patients including urosepsis			
Ceftriaxone	1g, IV, q24hr	Add aminoglycoside initially (gentamycin 5–7 mg/kg, once daily)	
Ceftazidime	1–2 g, IV, q8hr		
Cefepime	1 g, IV, q24hr		Direct antibiotic therapy according to susceptibility results and treat for total of 14 days
Piperacillin/Tazobactum	3.375–4.5 g, IV, q6hr		
Aztreonam	1–2 g, IV, q8hr		
Metropenam	1 g, IV, q8hr		The decision to use carbepenam for empiric therapy should be individualized based on local resistance data followed by timely de-escalation to ensure judicious use
Doripenam	500 mg, IV, q8hr		
Definitive therapy if susceptible to			
Trimethoprim/sulphamethoxazole	160/800 mg, PO, BD	14 days	
Ciprofloxacin	500 mg, PO, BD	5 days	
Levofloxacin	700 mg, PO, BD	5 days	
CA-UTI (see acute complicated cystitis for stable patients)			

6. Topical antiseptics or antimicrobials should not be applied to the catheter or urethral meatus.
7. Prophylactic antimicrobials use should be avoided to prevent CA-UTI.
8. The number of days a patient should be catheterized should be minimal.
9. Prophylactic use of antibiotic should be avoided after catheter removal.

The Infectious Diseases Society of America (IDSA), European Association of Urology (EAU) recommends treating CA-UTI for 7 days, if symptoms resolve in time and for 10 to 14 days, if the response is delayed, bacteremia, hypotension or severe sepsis occurs. In the absence of symptoms indicating pyelonephritis, women under the age of 65 years can be treated for 3 days after removal of the *in situ* catheter. CA-UTI patients who are not very sick can be treated with levofloxacin for 5 days.

In short-term catheterization, the infection is caused by a single organism, while in long-term catheterization of >30 days, multiple organisms are involved. Asymptomatic candiduria is common in nosocomial infections. Changing and removing the catheter clears it up, and in 20–40% of cases no treatment is needed. Fluconazole is highly recommended in these cases due to the high

Table 14.5: Prevention of recurrent UTI

Prevention of recurrent UTI	Dose	Duration	Comment
Nitrofurantoin	50 mg qHS		
Trimethoprim/ sulphamethoxazole	40/200 mg PO daily		
UTIs and asymptomatic bacteriuria in pregnant women			
Nitrofurantoin monohydrate/macro crystals	100 mg PO BD	5 to 7 days	Except during first trimester or near term
Amoxacillin	500 mg PO TDS	3 to 7 days	
Amoxicllin/clavulanate	500 mg PO TDS	3 to 7 days	
Cefalexin	500 mgPO QID	3 to 7 days	Drug of choice in first trimester
Cefpodoxime	100 mg PO BD	3 to 7 days	
Fosfomysin	3 g PO once	Once	
Trimethoprim/ sulphamethoxazole	160/800 mg PO BD	3 days	Except during first trimester or near term

BD: Twice daily; CBA: Colistin base activity; CRE: Carbepenam-resistant Enterobacteracae; ER: Extended release; ESBL: Extended spectrum beta-lactase; FQ: Fluoroquinolone; IV: Intravenously; PO: Orally; Q: Every; QD: Daily; QHS: Night; QID: 4 times daily; TDS = Three times daily. VRE: Vancomycin-resistant *E.coli*

concentration in the urine. Flucytosine is used in cases resistant to fluconazole.

Sepsis

Sepsis is a potentially fatal organ failure caused by a uncontrolled host reaction to infection. A rapid sequential organ failure assessment (SOFA) score was developed for rapid identification which includes respiratory rate of 22/min or greater, altered thinking, or systolic blood pressure of 100 mmHg or less.

Septic Shock

Septic shock is a type of sepsis in which extreme circulatory, cellular, and metabolic failures are associated with a increased mortality. These patients need for a vasopressor to maintain a mean arterial pressure of 65 mmHg or greater and a serum lactate level greater than 2 mmol/litre (>18 mg/dl) without hypervolemia.

GOALS OF THERAPY OF UTI

a. We need to identify the type of UTI.

b. Empirical regimen with low potential for collateral damage should be chosen.

c. We must know the most appropriate definitive treatment.

d. Drugs compatible with breastfeeding and pregnancy.

e. Duration of therapy.

f. Treatment option in multidrug-resistant (MDR) organisms.

g. Role of newer cephalosporin/beta-lactamase inhibitor combinations.

h. Any risk factor for recurrence for patient.

i. How to prevent rUTI?

j. For patient undergoing urological procedure, what is the strategy to minimise urosepsis postoperatively.

A patient with cystitis responds within 24 hours and with pyelonephritis response within 48–72 hours with proper antibiotic usage. Imaging studies should be done if the patient does not respond within 72 hours.

Hydration

There is not enough evidence to prove that hydration improves the outcome of UTIs.

Nitrofurantoin

Mode of action has a broad mechanism of action. It works by damaging bacterial DNA, which attacks ribosomal proteins, DNA respiration, and the metabolism of pyruvate. Therefore, when nitrofurantoin is used, the development of resistance is low. It is recommended in cystitis especially caused by *E. coli*. It reaches a high concentration in the urine, but poorly penetrates into the renal parenchyma; therefore, not to be used in pyelonephritis. Common side effects are diarrhea, headaches, and numbness.

Contraindication: It should not be used in a patient with creatinine clearance CrCL of 60 ml/min/1.73 m^2 or less because of lack of efficacy and toxicity which will lead to peripheral neuropathy and pulmonary side effects. It causes hemolytic anemia in newborns, so it should be avoided at term and during delivery. It should also be avoided in patients with glucose-6-phosphate dehydrogenase (G6PD) deficiency.

Trimethoprim/Sulphamethoxazole

It is also known as cotrimoxazole. The two drugs are present in a ratio of 1:5.

Mode of action: Bacterial production of dihydrofolic acid is blocked by sulphamethoxazole by competing with para-aminobenzoic acid (PABA). The conversion of tetrahydrofolic acid from dihydrofolate reductase is blocked by trimethoprim. Therefore, it has a broad-spectrum action. It is safe during breastfeeding.

Common side effects are nausea, vomiting and diarrhea.

It is drug of choice is uncomplicated cystitis. It works wonderfully, when the resistance rate in *E. coli* is <20% but works up to cure rate of 85%, even if the resistance rate is 30%.

Fluoroquinolones

It is effective against Gram-positive and Gram-negative bacteria. It disrupts DNA replication. Widespread veterinary use of quinolones has been implicated in resistance.

Levofloxacin or ciprofloxacin can be used in uncomplicated pyelonephritis, complicated urinary tract infections including urosepsis when local resistance is <10%.

Moxifloxacin is 20% excreted unchanged in the urine and is therefore not recommended in UTIs.

Adverse effects: Collateral damage, tendinitis, peripheral neuropathy, and central nervous system (CNS) effects.

Fosfomycin

Fosfomycin has *in vitro* activity against most *Enterobacteria* including extended-spectrum beta-lactomases (ESBL)-producing variants and *Enterococcus* spp. (regardless of vancomycin sensitivity). It has high susceptibility of *E. coli* and low potential for collateral damage, fosfomycin is the recommended agent.

Its routine use is increasing resistance and the price is also high which limits its use.

Aminoglycoside

Mode of action: Works by inhibiting protein synthesis. It is effective in gram-negative infection and aerobic infection. Gentamycin is used together with cephalosporins for complicated UTIs.

Side effects: Causes sensorineural hearing loss. It causes oscillopia in some patients.

Contraindications: It is contraindicated in myasthenia gravis because it worsens weakness.

Oral Vaccine-89 (OM-89)

It is a bacterial lysate with anti-inflammatory and immunomodulating effects. It is used for recurrent UTIs.

Oral β-Lactam Agents

They are considered alternative agents in management of uncomplicated UTIs because of there lower efficacy than FQs and trimethoprim/sulphamethoxazole.

It is commonly used in on an OPD basis and is an acceptable alternative for the treatment of uncomplicated cystitis and ASB. It is used to treat ASB or UTIs only when culture and sensitivity shows susceptibility.

Beta-lactamase Inhibitor

They are used in combination with beta-lactam antibiotics to increase its effectiveness. Ceftazidime/avibactam and ceftozolone/tazobactum are newer agents that have a promising result in treating complicated urinary tract infections caused by multidrug-resistant (MDR) *P. aeruginosa* or Enterobacteriaceae, especially carbapenem-resistant enterobacteriaceae (CRE) strains that are or are not New Delhi metallo-beta-lactamase (NDM) producers.

CONCLUSION

Urinary tract infection is the top most infection leading to the prescription of antibiotics. However, not all bacteriurias require therapy. One should be judicious in the use of antibiotics to avoid collateral damage.

Suggested Reading

1. American urological association (AUA) guidelines on UTI.
2. Antimicrobial guidelines for urinary tract infections - ICMR.
3. A study on recurrence of UTI in Indian women- international journal of science and research (IJSR).
4. Delia Scholes, Thomas R.Hawn ,Thomas M Hotoon: family history and risk of Recurrent cystitis and pyelonephritis in pregnancy.
5. Helen S Lee, Pharma D, BCPS-AQ, ID; and Jennifer Lee, pharma D, MAS, FIDSA, FCCP, FCSHP, BCPS-AQID Urinary tract infection: American College of pharmacy.
6. J Curtis Nickel, MD, FRCSC.
7. Urinary tract infection - CDC.
8. Urological infections - European association of urology 2020 edition.

Drugs in Gestational Diabetes Mellitus

• Pratima Verma • Ruchika Garg

Introduction

Diabetes in pregnancy is a commonly encountered complication worldwide. Epidemic of obesity and type-2 diabetes mellitus may be possible reasons. The International Diabetes Federation (IDF) estimates that one in six live births (16.8%) are as prevalence of hyperglycemia in pregnancy. While 16% of these cases may be due to diabetes in pregnancy (either pre-existing diabetes—type-1 or type-2—which antedates pregnancy or is first identified during testing in the index pregnancy), the majority (84%) is due to gestational diabetes mellitus (GDM).

In India, incidence of GDM is about 10–14.3%.[5] As of 2010, there were approximately 22 million women aged 20 to 39 with diabetes, and an additional 54 million women in the same age group had impaired glucose tolerance (IGT) or pre-diabetes, putting them at risk of developing GDM, if they become pregnant. It is expected that the incidence of GDM will increase to 20%, meaning that one in every five pregnant women is likely to experience GDM. The prevalence of GDM was 17.8% in urban areas, 13.8% in semi-urban areas, and 9.9% in rural areas.

Women diagnosed with GDM, face a higher risk of experiencing several adverse maternal outcomes, such as pre-eclampsia, cesarean section, and operative vaginal delivery. Additionally, there is a significant concern that they may be more susceptible to developing type-2 diabetes later in life, with a risk as high as 70%.

Furthermore, GDM also poses potential fetal complications, including macrosomia (large birth weight), congenital anomalies, growth restriction, neonatal hypoglycemia (low blood sugar), hyperbilirubinemia (elevated bilirubin levels), polycythemia (high red blood cell count), respiratory complications, shoulder dystocia (difficulties during delivery), stillbirth, and birth trauma. These risks highlight the importance of early detection and appropriate management of GDM to safeguard the health and well-being of both the mother and the baby.[1] It is utmost important to screen all pregnant women, diagnose them, and initiate appropriate management. These women will need glucose monitoring, so that blood glucose control can be achieved and we can prevent adverse fetomaternal outcome owing to uncontrolled blood sugar levels.

Topic of discussion of this chapter is drugs, so diagnosis criteria of GDM and lifestyle management will not be discussed and obstetric care pertaining to drugs will be discussed.

Most women can be managed with lifestyle modification (nutrition counseling, diet modification and exercise), approximately 25–30% will ultimately require pharmacologic therapy.[1]

Drugs for glycemic control are:
1. Insulin
2. Oral hypoglycemic agents:
   a. Metformin
   b. Glyburide
   c. Novel drugs

Insulin has always been incorporated in standard care of diabetes in pregnancy but in recent past use of oral antidiabetic medications like metformin and glyburide for treatment of GDM has also gained importance.

INSULIN

Most professional societies recommend insulin as first-line treatment of gestational diabetes after failure of lifestyle modification (**Table 15.1**). Due to its relatively small molecular size, insulin does not pass through the placenta. This characteristic ensures that insulin remains confined to the maternal bloodstream and does not affect the developing fetus.

Mechanism of Action

Insulin initiates its action by binding to a glycoprotein receptor on the surface of the cell. This receptor consists of an alpha-subunit, which binds the hormone, and a beta-subunit, which is an insulin-stimulated, tyrosine-specific protein kinase. These specific receptors are located on practically all cells but liver and fat cells have these receptors in abundance.

Insulin stimulates glucose transport across cell membrane by ATP-dependent translocation of glucose transporters GLUT-4 and GLUT-1 to the plasma membrane and achieves hypogycemia. Exogenous insulin improves insulin availability and acts similar to endogenous insulin. Main actions are illustrated in **Fig. 15.1**.

Flowchart 15.1 and **Table 15.2** are showing different types of insulin. Thorough knowledge of insulin is mandatory to understand its usage.

Pharmacokinetics: Insulin requirements according to gestational age is given in **Table 15.3**.

Salient Points about Commonly Used Insulin

A. Rapidly-acting Insulin

1. Insulin Aspart (NovoLog)
Onset—approximately 15 minutes
Timing—it should be taken at the beginning of a meal, which is different from the timing of regular insulin.

Table 15.1: Indications of insulin in GDM as per different guidelines	
International Federation of Gynecology and Obstetics (FIGO), 2015	Oral therapy failure or One of the risk factors; • Diagnosing diabetes before 20 weeks of gestation • Oral therapy for >30 weeks • Fasting plasma blood glucose above 110 mg/dl • 1-hour postprandial glycemia above 140 mg/dl • Weight gain over 12 kilograms during pregnancy
Canadian Diabetes Association (CDA), 20118	If glycemia control is not achieved in 2 weeks after the initiation of medical, nutritional intervention
American Diabetes Association (ADA), 2018	First-line therapy if glycemic control is not achieved after diet intervention
American College of Obstetricians and Gynecologists (ACOG), 2018	First-line therapy it glycemic control is not achieved after diet intervention

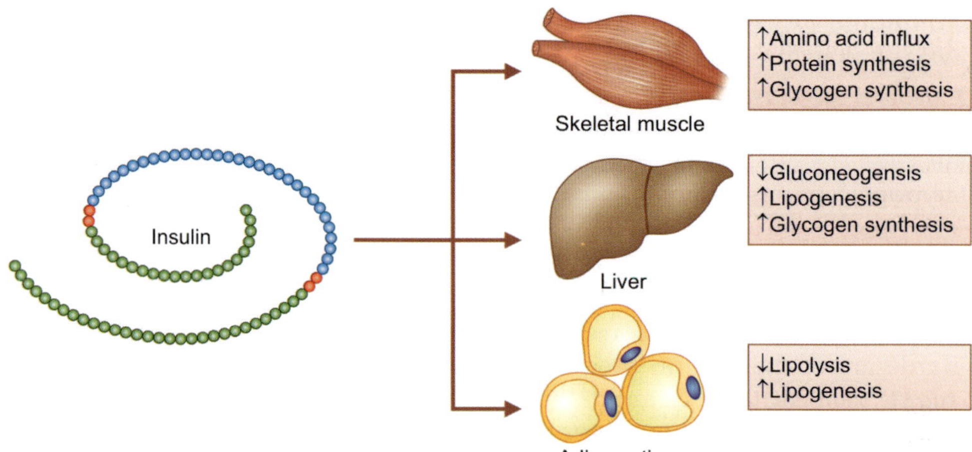

Fig. 15.1: Mechanism of action of insulin. Courtesy: Clinical Diabetes and Endocrinology—Biomed Central

2. Insulin lispro (humalog): Very similar to aspart. Timing—at the start of a meal given.

B. Short-acting Insulin

Regular insulin:

Timing—at least 10 to 15 and up to 30 minutes before a meal. Available in U-100 and U-500 strength, U-500 useful in patients with insulin requirement >200 units per day

Flowchart 15.1: Types of insulin

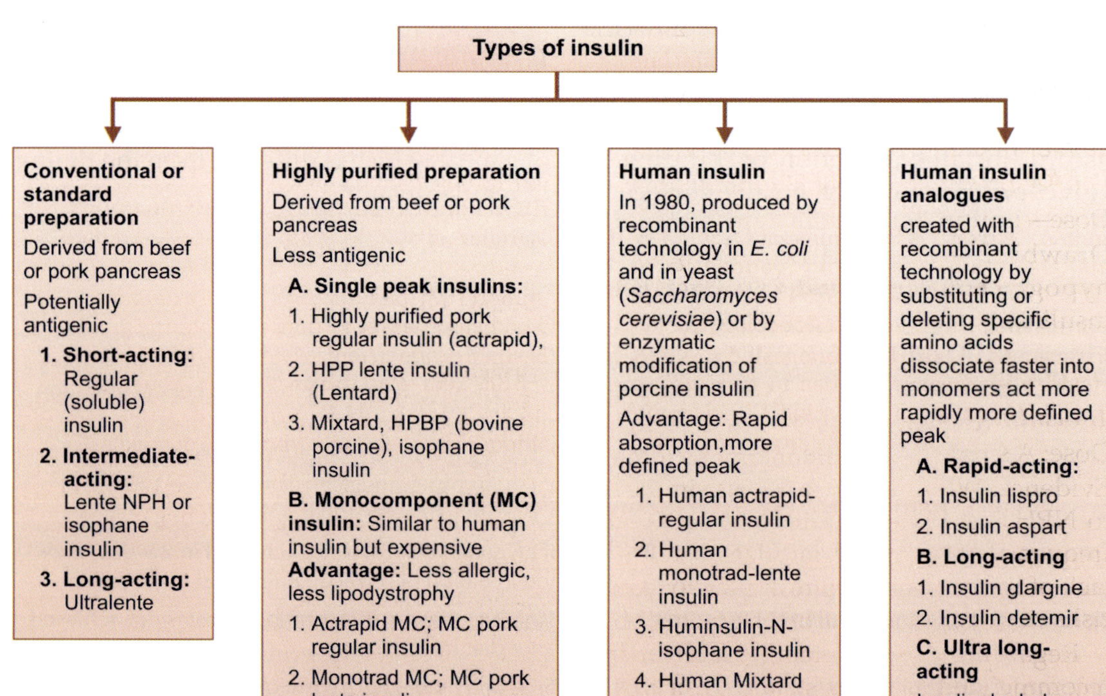

Table 15.2: Different types of insulin

S. No.	Type of insulin	Onset of action	Peak of action (hours)	Duration of action (hours)	Remarks	FDA category
1.	Insulin lispro	1–15 min (rapid-acting)	1–2	4–5	Decreased risk of severe maternal hypoglycemia compared with regular insulin	Category B
2.	Insulin aspart	1–15 min (rapid-acting)	1–2	4–5	Impart better glycemic control higher satisfaction of patients than regular insulin	Category B
3.	Regular insulin	30–60 min (short-acting)	2–4	6–8	Covers insulin needs for mealseaten within 30–60 minutes	Category B
4.	NPH	1–3 hour (intermediate-acting)	5–7	13–18	Covers insulin needs for about half the day or overnight	Category B
5.	Insulin glargine	1–2 hour (long-acting)	No peak	24	Insulin is delivered at a steady level	Category C
6.	Insulin detemir	1–3 hour	Minimal peak at 8–10	18–26	Less incidence of hypo-glycemia compared to NPH	Category B
7.	Premixed 30/70	30 min	2–4 hours	14–24 hours	These are usually taken two or three times a day before mealtime	Safe
	50/50	30 min	2–5 hour	18–24 hours		

FDA: Food and Drug Administration; NPH: Neutral protamine hagedron

C. Intermediate-acting Insulin-NPH-insulin (Novolin H, Humulin N)

Dose—multiple times.

Drawback—increased risk of night-time hypoglycemia (contrast to longer-acting insulins).

D. Long-acting Insulins

1. Insulin glargine (lantus)

Dose: A single daily dose.

Evidence: While glargine shows similarities to NPH insulin and is linked to a reduced frequency of hypoglycemic events, there is a lack of information regarding the long-term risks of glargine use during pregnancy.

Regarding insulin detemir (Levemir), it is recommended to administer the dosing every 12 hours to effectively manage blood glucose levels in pregnant women. Proper monitoring and adherence to medical guidance are essential for optimizing maternal and fetal health during this period.

Special Mention

1. Insulin glulisine

Onset: 10–15 minutes
Peak: 55 minutes
Duration of action: 4–5 hours
Category C drug in pregnancy.

2. Nasal insulin

Onset: 15 minutes
Peak: 50 minutes
Duration of action: 2 hours
Equivalent to Lispro
Disadvantage: Bronchospasm
Category C drug in pregnancy.

3. Insulin degludec

Onset: One hour

Long duration of action, no peak

Dose: Once daily

Category C drug in pregnancy.

Insulin Regimens

The insulin regimen should be based on the blood glucose profile. Commonly used insulin regimens are:

1. Split mix regimen or premix regimen
2. Multiple daily injections (MDI) or basal-bolus regimen
3. Continuous subcutaneous infusion.

When regimens one and two are compared, maternal and fetal outcomes, total insulin doses, and overall glycemic control, both found to be equivalent.

Table 15.3: Insulin requirement according to gestational age
First trimester: 0.7–0.8 U/kg
Second trimester: 0.8–0.9 U/kg
Third trimester: 1 and 1.2 U/kg
Postpartum: 0.55 U/ kg
Type 2 diabetes: 1.2 and 1.6 U/kg (in the second and third trimesters)

Different insulin regimens are given in **Table 15.4.** Maternal and fetal outcomes, the total insulin required, and overall management of blood glucose levels during pregnancy, both found to be equivalent in regimens 1 and 2.

Adjustments

It is necessary to titrate and individualise the regimen. It is utmost important to rapidly

Table 15.4: Different insulin regimen		
1. Split mix regimen or premix regimen Two injections (intermediate + soluble) or premix per day Before breakfast and before bedtime		
Calculate total insulin requirement as per given formula • Two-thirds of the total dose given in morning and one-third in evening If neutral protamine hagedorn (NPH) and regular insulin or rapid-acting insulin is being given ↓ Morning dose: Two-thirds NPH (before breakfast) + One-third regular insulin or insulin lispro or aspart (with breakfast) Evening dose: Half NPH (bed time) + Half regular insulin or insulin lispro or aspart (with dinner)		
2. MDI or basal-bolus regimen Most physiologic and most flexible regimen A multiple daily injection regimen involves administering insulin 4 to 7 times throughout the day. These injections are given before meals and at bedtime to maintain proper blood-glucose control. Insulin glargine/detemir and rapidly-acting insulin is being given Divide total required dose into ↓ Half dose (basal insulin)—insulin glargine (OD, evening) or insulin detemir (BD) Rest half dose—lispro or aspart insulin is divided into three equal doses, and each dose is taken with meals.		
3. Continuous subcutaneous insulin infusion If adequate glycemic control is not achieved by MDI regimen		
4. Special situations • Only fasting glucose levels are high—basal insulin only • Only post-prandial glucose levels are high—mealtime insulin only		

adjust dose to achieve glycemic control for better fetal and maternal outcome.

Target Capillary Blood Glucose Levels

As per International Federation of Gynecology and Obstetrics, FIGO (2015); American Diabetes Association, ADA (2018); American College of Obstetricians and Gynecologists, ACOG (2018) and Goverment of India guidelines (2018) target capillary blood glucose levels are:

- Capillary pre-prandial glucose <95 mg/dl (5.3 mmol/L)
- Capillary 1 hour post-prandial glucose <140 mg/dl (7.8 mmol/L)
- Capillary 2 hour post-prandial glucose <120 mg/dl (6.7 mmol/L)

There is insufficient evidence to suggest the optimal frequency of blood glucose testing in women with GDM. Based on the data available, recommendation is for daily glucose monitoring four times a day, once after fasting and again after each meal.

Route: Subcutaneous for all preparations. Only regular insulin can be injected IV (in intensive care settings)

Insulin Delivery Device

1. Vials and syringes
2. Pen
3. Insulin pump

This approach proves particularly beneficial for individuals with volatile or unstable diabetes. It offers notable advantages in managing the condition without raising the incidence of diabetic ketoacidosis (DKA) or severe hypoglycemic events.

Injection Sites (Fig. 15.2)

1. Abdomen (most common)
2. Front of thigh
3. Side of upper arm
4. Buttocks.

Storage of Insulin

Insulin vials should be stored in a refrigerator between 4°C to 8°C (usually in the door of the

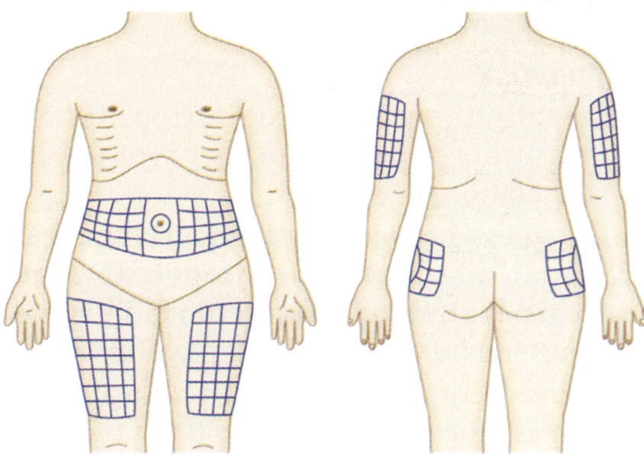

Fig. 15.2: Insulin injection sites

refrigerator), and in areas with inconsistent electricity supply, it is essential to have a battery backup to maintain the appropriate temperature.

Never store insulin vials in the freezer compartment of the refrigerator. If mistakenly placed in the freezer and frozen, the vials should not be used and must be discarded.

Insulin vials should be shielded from direct heat or sunlight. They remain stable within a temperature range of 2°C to 30°C.

Open insulin vials currently in use should be stored in the refrigerator or in a cool and dark place. Once opened, they should be used within a month. If not used within a month, they should be discarded, and the date of opening must be marked on the vial.

Syringes can be stored at room temperature, avoiding direct exposure to sunlight or heat.

Unopened insulin pens should be stored in the refrigerator. After opening, they can be kept at room temperature away from direct sunlight.

Adverse Effects

Hypoglycemia

Most frequent and potentially the most serious reaction.

Causes

1. Inadvertant injection of large doses of insulin
2. Missing a meal
3. Vigorous exercise

Diagnosis of Hypoglycemia

1. Symptoms

a. Sweating, anxiety, palpitation, tremor (because of counter regulatory sympathetic stimulation)

b. Dizziness, headache, behavioural changes, visual disturbances, hunger, fatigue, weakness, muscular incoordination, sometimes fall (neuroglucopenic symptoms)

c. Mental confusion, seizures and coma (blood glucose levels than 40 mg/dl).

Treatment: Glucose must be given orally or IV (for severe cases). It reverses the symptoms rapidly. Pregnant women using insulin therapy should be advised to keep a readily accessible source of fast-acting carbohydrates, such as sugar, jaggery, or glucose powder, at home. This precautionary measure will help them promptly treat any episodes of hypoglycemia that may arise.

2. Local reactions

Swelling, erythema and stinging

Lipodystrophy–not seen with newer preparations

3. *Allergy:* Very rare with human insulin

4. *Edema:* In some patients develop short lived dependent edema.

Drug Interactions

1. Beta adrenergic blockers prolong hypoglycaemia

2. Thiazides, Furosemide, corticosteroids, oral contraceptives, salbutamol,nifedepine tend to raise blood sugar and reduce effectiveness of insulin

3. Acute ingestion of alcohol can precipitate hypoglycaemia

4. Salicylates, Lithium and theophylline may also accentuate hypoglycaemia.

Barriers to insulin Use

1. Compliance of patients

2. Fear of many injections in a day and scarring

3. Difficulty in administration and pain

4. Risk of hypoglycaemia

B. Oral Hypoglycaemic Agents

Insulin has always been incorporated in standard care of Diabetes in pregnancy but in recent past use of oral antidiabetic medications like metformin and glyburide for treatment of GDM has also gained importance. Table 15.5 shows comparison of oral hypogycemic agents and insulin.

Table 15.5: Comparison of oral hypogycemic agents and insulin

Studies	*Outcome*
Nicholson, et al.—4RCT (n = 1229), 5 observational studies (n = 831) 1 RCT of metformin versus insulin 3 RCT of glibenclamide versus insulin 1 RCT of acarbose versus insulin 5 observational studies	No difference in maternal and neonatal outcome but higher neonatal hypoglycemia in insulin arm (8.1%) compared to OHA (3.3%), P = 0.008 No difference in maternal and neonatal outcomes
Dhulkotia, et al.—6 RCT (n = 1388) 2 RCT of metformin versus insulin 4 RCT of glyburide versus insulin	No difference in glycemic control or of maternal hypoglycemia 0.34 (95% Cl, 0.02–5.82) with OHA, trends of higher hypertensive disorders in insulin arm. No differences in CS rate, preterm birth, neonatal hypoglycemia, BW, LGA, NICU admission, RDS, SGA and IUFD
Nicholson, et al. – 8 RCT – 2 RCT of met formin versus insulin	No difference in any outcome, trends of increased maternal hypoglycemia in insulin arm

METFORMIN

Recently Society for Maternal–Fetal Medicine (SMFM) endorsed metformin as a safe first-line alternative to insulin. In **Table 15.6** Role of metformin as per different guidelines is beautifully depicted.

Mechanism of Action

Metformin, a biguanide analogue, operates through three main mechanisms:

1. It restrains hepatic gluconeogenesis, which helps to reduce the liver's production of glucose.
2. It stimulates glucose uptake in peripheral tissues, leading to improved glucose utilization by the body.
3. It lowers gastrointestinal glucose absorption, resulting in lower glucose levels after meals.

While metformin relies on the presence of insulin to enhance its effectiveness, it

Table 15.6: Role of metformin as per different guidelines

Guide	Country	Year	Requirements
The American Diabetes Association (ADA)	American	2020	Insulin is the first-line treatment for GDM in the United States. Although several randomized controlled trials have supported the limited efficacy of metformin and glyburide in reducing glucose levels in the treatment of GDM, these drugs are not recommended as first-line agents for GDM because they are known to cross the placenta and lack data to demonstrate offspring safety; metformin, when used to treat polycystic ovary syndrome and induce ovulation. should be discontinued by the end of the first trimester
American Congress of Obstetricians and Gynecologists (ACOG)	American	2018	For women refused to use insulin, or obstetrician or obstetric nurses think women cannot safely use insulin, patient with metformin is a reasonable second-line choice, but it is necessary to inform patients the risk of adverse events, such as increasing prematurity, drugs through the placenta, and lack of long-term data on drug exposure assessment of the risks of late fetal growth
International Federation of Gynecology and Obstetrics (FIGO)	—	2015	Insulin, glyburide and metformin are safe and effective treatment options during second and third trimesters of pregnancy if blood glucose cannot be controlled by lifestyle changes alone
The National Institutes of Health and Care Excellence (NICE)	UK	2015	Metformin is used if the blood sugar target is not achieved through lifestyle changes within 1–2 weeks. If the patient is intolerant or cannot accept metfonnin, insulin is used
International Diabetes Federation (IDF)	–	2009	If blood sugar targets are not met within 1–2 weeks of lifestyle changes, blood sugar levels should be lowered. Insulin is a treatment of choice, but there is now sufficient evidence to consider metformin and glyburide in women who are known to be at risk. Combination therapy has not been studied specifically
The Australasian Diabetes in Pregnancy Society (ADIPS) and Ille Australian Electronic Treatment Guidelines (e TG)	Australian	2005	It is recommended to change treatment to insulin and to use metformin only in the following cases: patients are opposed to injections

GDM: Gestational diabetes mellitus

does not prompt insulin secretion itself. Consequently, metformin usage is not linked to hypoglycemia, making it a safer option for diabetes management.

Dose

The initial dose for metformin is 500 mg taken at bedtime during the first week. Afterward, the dosage is raised to 500 mg twice daily.

The maximum daily dose should be between 2500 to 3500 mg, divided into 2 to 3 separate doses throughout the day.

Metformin has a half-life ranging from 2 to 5 hours, indicating the time it takes for half of the medication to be cleared from the body.

Highest plasma concentrations—4 hours

Extended Release Metformin

Half-life—7 to 8 hours
Maximum limit—2000 mg daily.

Advantages

- Lesser gastrointestinal side effects
- An advantage of this medication is that it offers simplified dosing, allowing for once daily administration instead of multiple divided doses.

Side Effects

Common side effect (2.5 to 45.7% of patients)
- GI upset
- It may cause two serious side-effects:
  - Lactic acidosis
  - Hypoglycemia.

Limitations

This medication can pass through the placenta, leading to concentrations in the fetus that are comparable to those found in the mother's bloodstream.

Its indication and contraindications are given in **Table 15.7**.

Pros and cons of using metformin are given in **Table 15.8**.

GLYBURIDE

Also known as glibenclamide. It is a second generation sulfonylurea.

Mechanism of Action

It interacts with pancreatic beta-cell adenosine triphosphate—calcium-channel receptors
1. Act to increase insulin secretion
2. Increase sensitivity in peripheral tissues.

Table 15.7: Indications and contraindications of metformin

Relative indications	Contraindications
As monotherapy: • GDM not responding to medical nutrition therapy and exercise, if FPG <110 mg/dl • Poor compliance or refusal to use insulin • Lack of skills and /or resources for self-management of diabetes with insulin	**Medical status:** • Diagnosis in early gestation • Elevated BMI with significant hyperglycemia • Gastrointestinal intolerance • Previous adverse reaction or allergy to metformin • Renal or hepatic dysfunction
Add-on to insulin therapy: • High insulin dose requirements • Excessive maternal weight gain	**Metabolic status:** • Significant hyperglycemia (FPG:2:110 mg/dl) • Ketosis or ketonuria
	Obstetric status: • History of major congenital anomaly in previous pregnancy • Presence of hydramnios • Maternal distress • Fetal distress

Table 15.8: Pros and cons of metformin

	Pros	Cons
Mechanism of action	Reduces insulin resistance, the main pathophysiology in GDM	May fail to achieve adequate glycemic control in presence of insulinopenia
Pharmacokinetics	Oral route of administration Easy dose titration	Increased renal clearance—need for higher doses Significant placental transfer—exposure of fetus Gastrointestinal intolerance
Efficacy	Glycemic control comparable to insulin or glyburide Low risk of maternal hypoglycemia	Failure rate in 14–16% women, who require suplemental insulin Slow onset of action—time lag in presence of significant hyperglycemia
Social and other considerations	Better patient acceptability Less cost Less need for self-monitoring of blood glucose	Not approved for use in pregnancy—category B, use is off-label Discordant views among leading guidelines
Maternal outcomes	No adverse maternal outcomes Less risk of hypoglycemia Lower maternal weight gain Less risk of pregnancy-induced hypertension	Slightly lower gestational age at delivery
Short-term fetal outcomes	No increased risk of teratogenicity in fetuses exposed in first trimester No increased risk of perinatal complications Reduced neonatal hypoglycemia Reduced NICU admissions Lower birth weight, reduced risk of LGA and macrosomia	Increased risk of preterm birth (inconsistent results)
Long-term effects of exposure of fetus	No evidence of growth or motor–social development abnormalities may result in more favorable distribution of adipose tissue	Insufficient data of long-term effects of exposure *in utero*

Dose

The recommended daily dosage of this medication ranges from 2.5 to 20 mg, which can be taken as a single morning dose or divided into two separate doses throughout the day. For optimal effectiveness, it is advised to take the medication 30 minutes to 1 hour before meals.

The peak concentration of the drug occurs within 2 to 3 hours after administration, with insulin secretion being directly linked to the level of glyburide in the body. Drug concentrations return to baseline levels after approximately 8 hours, suggesting that three times daily dosing may be more suitable for some individuals. It is crucial not to exceed a daily dose greater than 20 mg, as this may elevate the risk of hypoglycemic events, including neonatal hypoglycemia, and is not recommended. Regarding its use during pregnancy, although glyburide appears to cross the placenta, the levels are sufficiently low to be considered safe for the developing fetus **(Table 15.9)**.

Pregnant women diagnosed with gestational diabetes mellitus (GDM) require specialized obstetric care during their antenatal period.

Table 15.9: Comparison of insulin, metformin and glyburide

S. No.	Features	Insulin	Metformin	Glyburide
1.	History	Standard of care—first-line therapy by most guidelines	Approved recently as alternative to insulin	As second choice after metformin
2.	Placental transfer	Not known to cross the placenta	Crosses placenta	Crosses placenta
3.	Fetomaternal outcome	Safe	Similar to insulin, superior to glyburide	Safer in pregnancy but with more longstanding data required
4.	Advantages	Long-term safety data	Satisfacton of patient, Less cost, reduces several common short-term adverse outcomes related to GDM	Suitable, economical, and more convenient administration and storage options compared to insulin
5.	Drawbacks	Decreased compliance, costly substantial education of patient	No long-term safety data, potential detrimental effect of metformin on fat mass, fetal programming	Meta-analyses suggest that glyburide may increase the risk for LGA infants and neonatal hypoglycemia

Only salient points pertaining to GDM in pregnancy will be discussed in this section.

- Many guidelines worldwide, including the American and Canadian guidelines, recommend universal screening using a two-step approach. However, in India, the government has recently endorsed the 'single-step procedure' for screening and diagnosing GDM using a 2-hour 75 g post-blood sugar level of ≥140 mg/dl **(Flowchart 15.2)**.
- Evidences specific to India indicate that pregnant women in our country face a significantly higher risk of developing glucose intolerance during pregnancy when compared to white women. Moreover, adherence to recommended screening and treatment protocols can be a genuine challenge in some cases.

Maternal and Fetal Risk

After confirming a diagnosis of GDM, the initial management approach entails medical nutrition therapy (MNT) and engaging in regular physical exercise for a period of 2 weeks. Following these 2 weeks of MNT and physical activity, a 2-hour post-meal blood sugar test (PPBS) should be conducted to evaluate the effectiveness of the management plan. If it is not controlled with MNT (lifestyle changes), metformin or insulin therapy is added.

If 2-hour PPBS is >200 mg/dl at diagnosis, insulin has to be started straightaway.

During follow-up visits, the dosage of the medication will be adjusted as needed. Simultaneously, it is crucial to continue adhering to the MNT and maintaining regular physical exercise as prescribed. Consistency in both medication management and lifestyle modifications is an essential component of the overall treatment plan for GDM **(Flowchart 15.3)**.

- For cases diagnosed with GDM before 20 weeks of pregnancy, a fetal anatomical survey using ultrasonography (USG) should be conducted at 18–20 weeks.
- For all pregnancies with GDM, a fetal growth scan is recommended at 28–30 weeks of gestation and repeated at 34–36 weeks of gestation.

Flowchart 15.2: Universal Screening GDM, Guidelines for the Diagnosis and Management of Gestational Diabetes Mellitus—Technical and Operational Recommendations, GOI 2018.

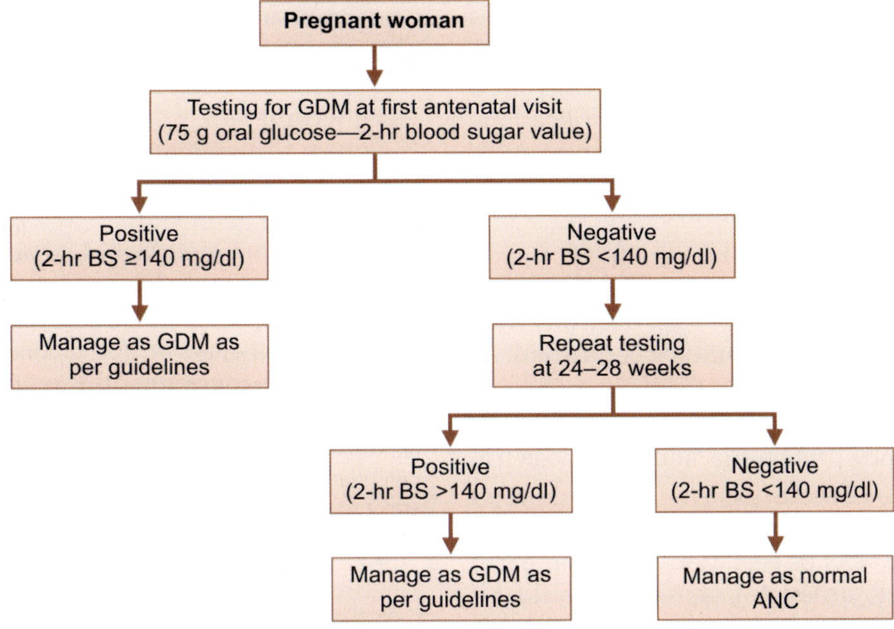

Flowchart 15.3: Management of GDM in pregnancy. Diagnosis and management of Gestational Diabetes Mellitus. Technical and Operational Guidelines, GOI 2018.

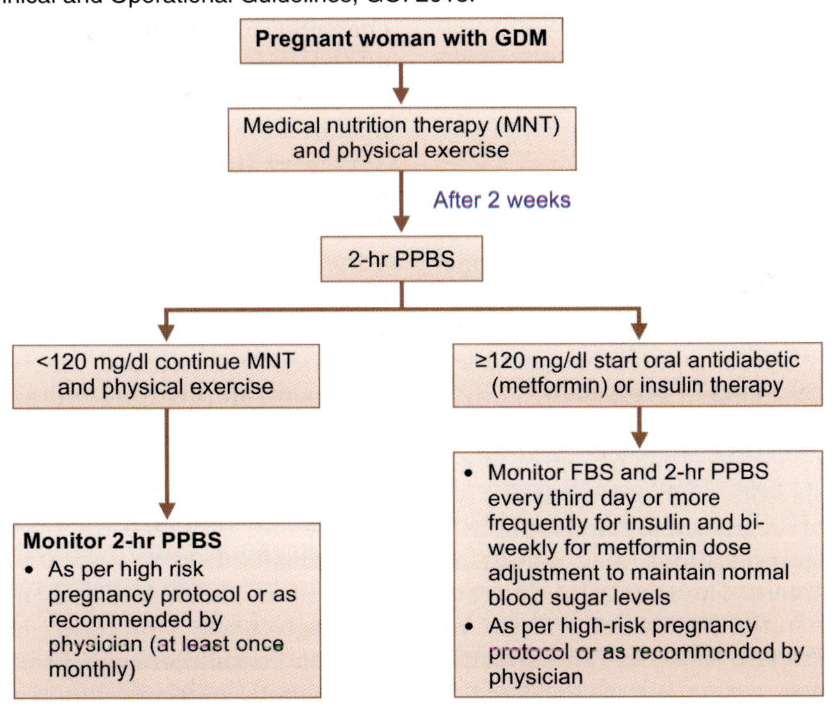

- Pregnant women should be educated about daily fetal activity assessment to ensure regular monitoring of the baby's movements.
- Pregnant women with well-controlled blood sugar levels and no complications related to GDM should continue with regular antenatal visits following the high-risk pregnancy protocol.
- During each antenatal care (ANC) visit, monitoring for abnormal fetal growth (macrosomia/growth restriction) and polyhydramnios should be conducted.
- Diligent monitoring of pregnant women with GDM is necessary for hypertension in pregnancy, proteinuria, and other obstetric complications.
- In pregnant women with GDM between 24–34 weeks of gestation requiring early delivery, antenatal steroids should be administered according to the guidelines issued by the Government of India (GoI). This involves administering Inj. Dexamethasone 6 mg, IM, every 12 hours for 2 days. Following the injection, blood sugar levels should be closely monitored for the next 72 hours, and insulin doses should be adjusted if necessary in case of raised blood sugar levels during this period **(Flowchart 15.4)**.

Labour and Delivery

- If a pregnant woman with GDM maintains well-controlled blood sugar levels and has not undergone spontaneous delivery, induction of labour should be scheduled at or after 39 weeks of pregnancy.
- Pregnant women with GDM, who experience poor blood sugar control, along with risk factors such as hypertensive disorders of pregnancy, previous stillbirth, and other complications, may require an earlier delivery. The timing of delivery should be individually determined by the obstetrician based on the specific circumstances.

- Vaginal delivery is preferable for pregnant women with GDM, and a lower segment cesarean section (LSCS) should only be performed for obstetric indications.
- If fetal macrosomia is detected (estimated fetal weight >4 kg), consideration should be given to a primary cesarean section at 39 weeks to reduce the risk of shoulder dystocia.
- It is important to note that GDM pregnancies are associated with delayed lung maturity in the fetus. As a result, routine delivery prior to 39 weeks is not recommended. Careful consideration and evaluation of the fetus' lung maturity are essential before planning the delivery timing.

Special precautions during labour for pregnant women with GDM:
- Pregnant women with GDM who are on medical management (using metformin or insulin) need regular blood sugar monitoring during labour, which can be done using a glucometer.
- On the day of induction of labour, the morning dose of insulin/metformin should be withheld, and the pregnant women should begin 2-hourly blood sugar monitoring.
- An intravenous (IV) infusion with normal saline (NS) should be started, and regular insulin should be added based on blood sugar levels, as indicated in the table below **(Table 15.10)**.

Immediate neonatal care for babies born to mothers with gestational diabetes mellitus:
- All neonates should receive essential newborn care promptly, with a focus on early breastfeeding to prevent hypoglycemia.
- If necessary, sick neonates should be immediately resuscitated following the guidelines provided by the Government of India (GoI).
- Newborns should be closely monitored for hypoglycemia. Monitoring should begin within 1 hour after birth. In all babies born to diabetic mothers, blood sugar levels

Flowchart 15.4: Insulin therapy in GDM. Diagnosis and management of Gestational Diabetes Mellitus Technical and Operational Guidelines, GOI 2018

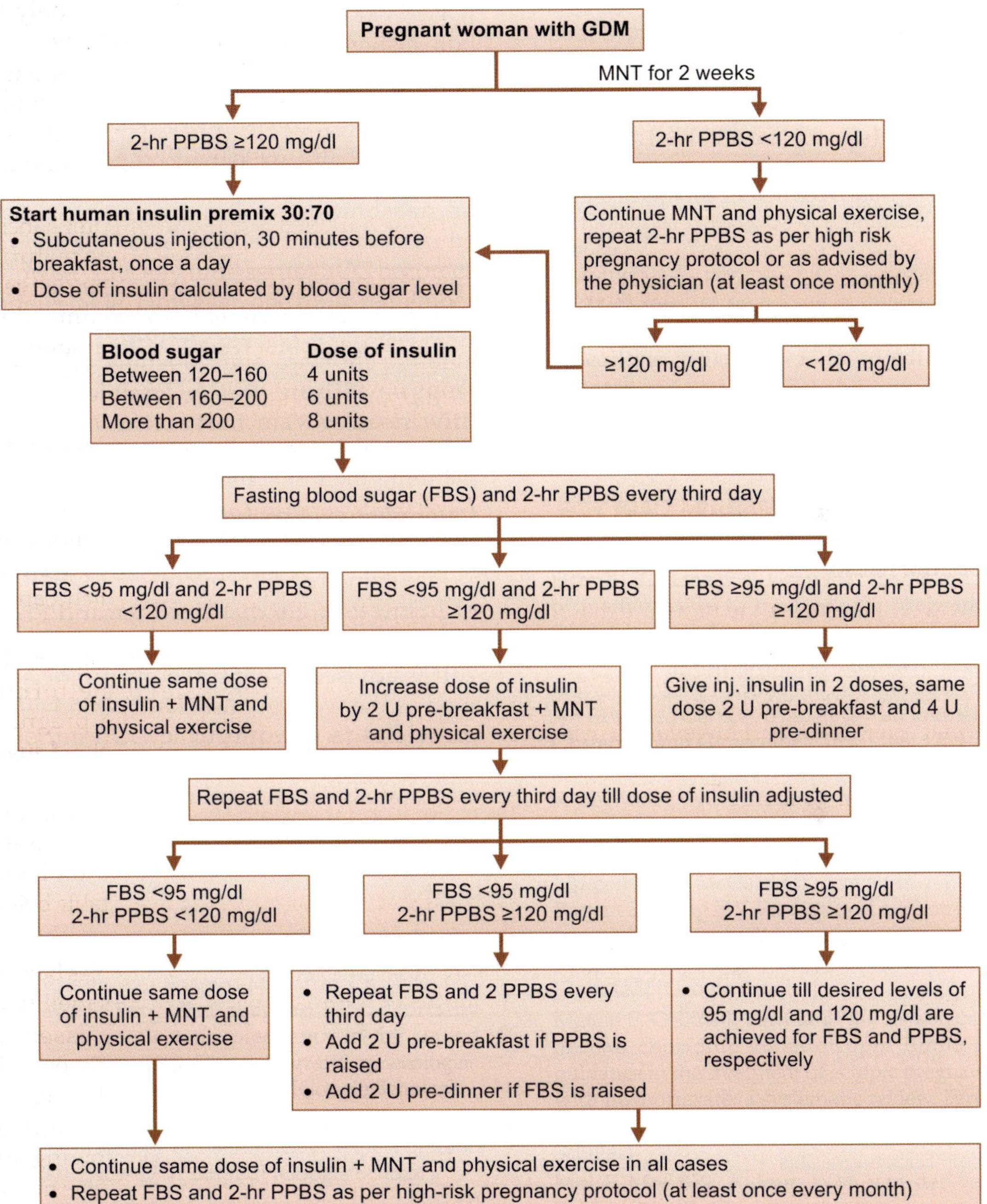

Table 15.10: Insulin on sliding scale

Blood sugar level	Amount of insulin added in 500 ml NS	Rate of NS infusion
90–120 mg/dl	0	100 mVhr (16 drops/min)
120–140 mg/dl	4U	100 mVhr (16 drops/min)
140–180 mg/dl	6U	100 mVhr (16 drops/min)
>180 mg/dl	8U	100 mVhr (16 drops/min)

should be checked using a glucometer between 1–2 hours after birth to detect and manage any potential hypoglycemic episodes effectively.

THE IMMEDIATE POSTPARTUM CARE FOR WOMEN WITH GESTATIONAL DIABETES MELLITUS (GDM)

However, it is essential to be aware that these women are at a higher risk of developing type-2 diabetes mellitus in the future.

Typically, maternal glucose levels return to normal after delivery. However, to evaluate the woman's glycemic status, it is crucial to conduct a 75 g oral glucose tolerance test (OGTT) at 6 weeks postpartum, measuring both fasting and 2-hour postprandial glucose levels. Regular monitoring and maintaining a healthy lifestyle are essential for women with a history of GDM to reduce the risk of developing type-2 diabetes mellitus in the long term.

Flowchart 15.5 is showing this algorithm.

PRE-CONCEPTION CARE AND COUNSELING FOR WOMEN WITH A HISTORY OF GESTATIONAL DIABETES MELLITUS (GDM)

Women with a history of GDM should receive counseling regarding their body mass index (BMI) and blood sugar estimation before planning their next pregnancy.

Desired blood sugar levels for pre-conception:
- Fasting blood sugar (FBS) should be maintained at <100 mg/dl.
- 2-hour Postprandial Blood Sugar (PPBS) - should be kept at <140 mg/dL.

It is advised to consult a gynecologist as soon as the woman misses her period when considering a new pregnancy.

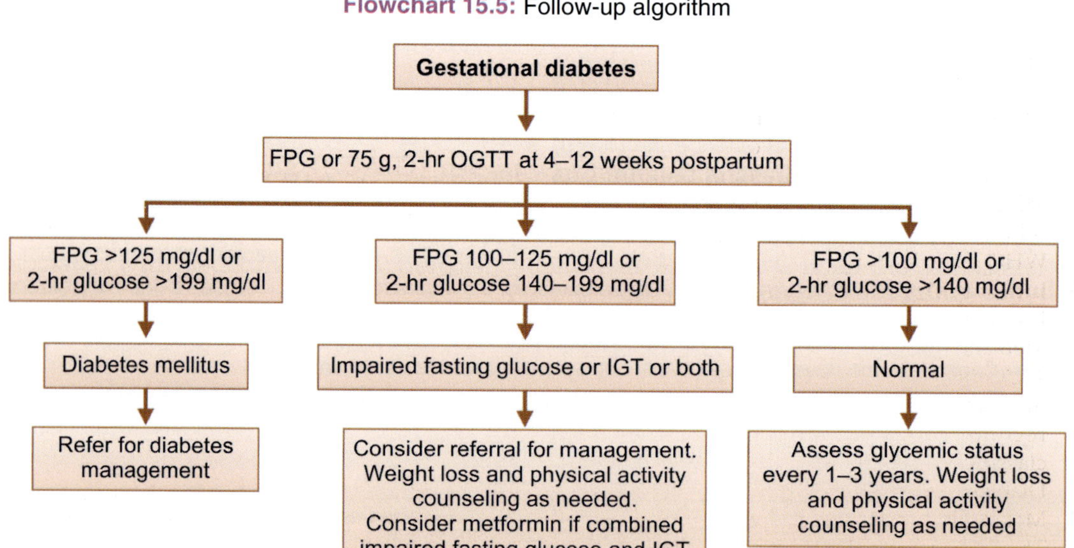

Flowchart 15.5: Follow-up algorithm

SUMMARY (Table 15.11)

Table 15.11: Summary of delivery protocol in GDM. Diagnosis and Management of gestational diabetes mellitus—technical and operational guidelines step 1

Intra-delivery protocol and method of delivery

Elective cesarean section

- Women with type-1 diabetes should be placed first on the operating list and admitted either the previous day or early on the morning of surgery
- Long-acting insulin is taken as normal before a light supper
- The mother should fast from 22:00 hrs in the evening before surgery and should be first on the operating list the next day; rapid-acting insulin should be withheld
- 1 to 2 hours surgery, hourly monitoring of blood glucose begins; and a glucose–insulin infusion is commenced, if necessary, to maintain blood glucose between 4 and 7 mmol/L
- The insulin dose and/or rate is adjusted in response to maternal/capillary glucose

Induction of labor

- Women should continue their current insulin regimen until labor is confirmed
- Often, an early morning breakfast is consumed with their normal morning insulin dose
- Once labor is confirmed and mother is fasting, glucose–insulin infusion is commenced as per protocol, unless delivery is imminent
- Maternal blood glucose levels should be monitored hourly
- Blood glucose levels should be maintained between 4 and 7 mmol/L
- The insulin dose and/or rate is adjusted in response to maternal blood glucose

Spontaneous labor

- Following admission in spontaneous labor, the patient is fasted
- A blood glucose level should be taken on admission and hourly thereafter
- Once labor is confirmed, a glucose–insulin infusion is commenced as per protocol
- Capillary glucose levels should be maintained between 4 and 7 mmol/L
- The insulin dose and/or rate Is adjusted according to the local protocol in response to maternal blood glucose

References

1. Gestational diabetes mellitus. ACOG Practice Bulletin No.190. American College of Obstetricians and Gynecologists. Obstet Gynecol. 2018;131:e49–e64.

2. World Health Organization. Diagnostic criteria and classification of hyperglycaemia first detected in pregnancy.WHO/NMH/MND/13.2. Geneva: WHO;2013.http://apps.who.int/iris/bitstream/10665/85975/1/WHO_NMH MND_13.2_eng.pdf

3. International Association of Diabetes and Pregnancy Study Groups Consensus Panel, Metzger BE, Gabbe SG, Persson B, Buchanan TA, Catalano PA, et al. International association of diabetes and pregnancy study groups recommendations on the diagnosis and classification of hyperglycemia in pregnancy. Diabetes Care 2010;33(3):676–82.

4. Moshe Hod, Anil Kapur, David A. Sacks, et al. The International Federation of Gynecology and Obstetrics (FIGO) Initiative on gestational diabetes mellitus: A pragmatic guide for diagnosis, management, and care#International Journal of Gynecology and Obstetrics 131,S3 (2015) S173–S211.

5. Government of India. Maternal and Health Division, National Guidelines for Diagnosis and Management of Gestational Diabetes Mellitus. New Delhi, India: Ministry of Health & Family Welfare, New Concept Information Systems; 2014.

6. Mishra S, Bhadoria AS, Kishore S, Kumar R. Gestational diabetes mellitus 2018 guidelines: An update. J Family Med Prim Care 2018;7:1169–72.

7. Kelley KW, Carroll DG, Meyer A. A review of current treatment strategies for gestational diabetes mellitus. Drugs Context. 2015;4: 212–282.

8. KDT, Essentials of Medical Pharmacology, Fifth edition, chapter 18, page 235–253.

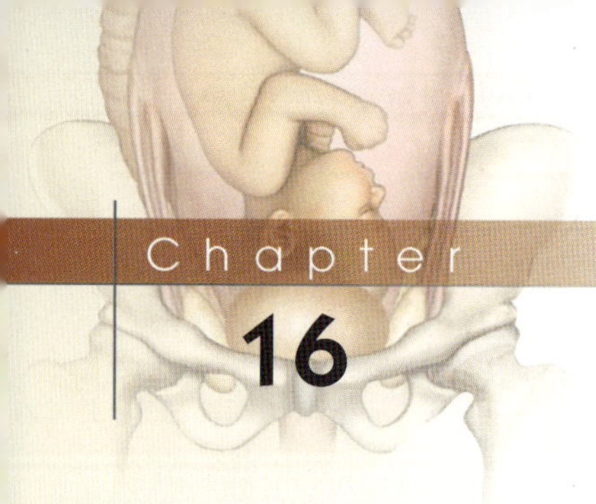

Induction of Abortion

• Punit Bhojani • Bhumika Kotecha Mundhe

Introduction

Induced abortion in first trimester of pregnancy is an option available for women with an unplanned and unwanted pregnancy. It includes sequential use of two drugs, namely mifepristone and misoprostol. This induced abortion can be done under MTP Act to ensure that every pregnant individual has an access to legally eligible safe abortion care with adequate protection of health and human rights.

MIFEPRISTONE

Mifepristone also known as RU-486 and typically derives its name from an abbreviation for the pharmaceutical company Roussel-Uclaf plus a serial number.[2] It is a synthetic steroid which has antiprogesterone, antiglucorticoid and a weak antiandrogen properties.

Indications

It has been approved by FDA for two indications.

1. For termination of intrauterine pregnancy along with misoprostol.
2. Control of blood sugars in patients with Cushing syndrome.

Additionally, its off-label uses are as follows—for postcoital emergency contraception, cervical softening and as an adjunct to treatment for uterine fibroids.[3]

Mechanism of Action

When administered in lower doses, it has high-binding affinity to progesterone receptor and thus acts as a competitive progesterone receptor antagonist. If administered in higher doses, it binds to the glucocorticoid receptors and blocks cortisol. This in turn has an effect on hypothalamic–pituitary-adrenal axis

WHO recommendations of medical management of induced abortion at <12 weeks of gestation[1]

Recommendations	Combination regime (recommended) Mifepristone >1–2 days >misoprostol	Misoprostol-only (alternate)
Induced abortion <12 weeks	Mifepristone—200 mg, PO, once followed by 1–2 days interval Misoprostol—800 µg, B, PV or SL	800 µg, B, PV or SL

However, in India, it is approved up to 9 weeks of gestation or up to 63 days of early pregnancy.

which leads to higher circulating cortisol levels and thus controls hyperglycemia in a few patients.[4]

Being a progesterone antagonist, in medical abortion, it typically affects endometrial decidua and causes cervical priming. In addition, it increases the production of prostaglandins and also the sensitivity of myometrium to the prostaglandin activity leading to myometrial contractions.[2] This ultimately leads to disruption of the endometrium and thus the bleeding gets initiated.

Pharmacokinetics

It has been observed that the half-life of the drug is a complex. The drug label mentions that the elimination at first is slow, $t_{1/2}$ being 12–72 hours and then the elimination is quite fast. The elimination half-life being 18 hours. However, the radiolabelled assay has observed that the terminal half-life is 90 hours. Metapristone is one of the major metabolites of mifepristone.[2]

Side Effects[4]

- Nausea, vomiting
- Abdominal pain, diarrhea, gastroesophageal reflex disease (GERD), constipation
- Headache, dizziness, sinusitis, pharyngitis
- Hypertension, hypokalemia, peripheral edema, hypertension, dyspnea, hypoglycemia
- Maculopapular rash, pruritis
- Anaphylactic reactions, toxic epidermal necrolysis, angioedema, and
- Teratogenesis, fetal death.

Contraindications[4]

1. Hypersensitivity
2. Cushing syndrome patients taking simvastatin, lovastatin, and CYP3A substrates (*i.e.* cyclosporine, dihydroergotamine, ergotamine, fentanyl, sirolimus, and tacrolimus).
3. In pregnant patients for control of hyperglycemia.

MISOPROSTOL

Misoprostol belongs to prostaglandin E_1 group of drugs and is a synthetic analogue.

Chemical formula: $C_{22}H_{38}O_5$

Indications

1. The key role of misoprostol is dose-dependent protection of gastrointestinal mucosa and is used for prevention and treatment of gastric and duodenal ulcers.
2. It also widely used in medical abortions and to treat postpartum bleeding due to atonic uterus.
3. In women with previous event of failure of intrauterine device insertion or those with previous cesarean section, misoprost may be used to avoid failure of insertion of intrauterine device. However, its routine use for the same is not recommended.[5]
4. Another use is in patients aspiring myomectomy for uterine fibroids is to reduce intraoperative blood loss and may be blood transfusion.[6]

FDA Approval Status

In current scenario, the only FDA approved indication is to prevent and treat stomach and duodenal ulcers when administered concurrently with NSAIDs. The other parallel indication is for treatment of active duodenal or gastric ulcers which have been formed due to other causes and can be continued transiently. However, this indication has not been approved by FDA.

In obstetric and gynecological practice, it is used for the following indications:

a. Induction of medical abortion in combination with other chemotherapeutic drug, namely mifepristone. Mifepristone along with misoprostol is approved as an abortion regime. The approved mifepristone dosing regimen is:
   - *On day one:* 200 mg of mifepristone, orally.
   - *24 to 48 hours later:* 800 µg of misoprostol, buccally.

The clinicians use the same regime in the management of missed and incomplete abortion.

b. It also been used as an uterotonic agent alone or in combination with other medications for prophylaxis and treatment of postpartum hemorrhage. However, this indication of misoprost is not FDA approved. This is more commonly preferred in low resource settings of remote areas where other uterotonic agents are not readily available and/or the efficacy of oxytocin is questionable due to its cold chain maintenance.[7]

c. Other off-label use is in induction and ripening of cervix in full-term pregnancies and those with an intrauterine fetal demise in minimal doses.[8]

Pharmacokinetics

Misoprostol once absorbed is converted to its free acid form by the process of de-esterification. This acid form is detectable in plasma. The final form prostaglanding-F_1 analog is achieved by beta-oxidation of alpha side chain and omega-oxidation of alpha-side chain followed by reduction of ketones. The active form of misoprostol is 81–89% protein bound. The T_{max} of misoprostol acid by oral route is 12 ± 3 minutes and a terminal half-life of 20–40 minutes. The mean values attained after single dose show a linear relationship with the dose range of 200–400 µg.

Mean ±SD	C_{max} (pg/ml)	AUC (0–4) (pg·hr/ml)	T_{max} (min)
Fasting	811 ± 317	417 ± 135	14 ± 8
With antacid	689 ± 315	349 ± 108*	20 ± 14
With high fat breakfast	303 ± 176*	373 ± 111	64 ± 79**

SD: Standard deviation of the mean; AUC: Area under the curve; C_{max}: Peak concentration; T_{max}: Time to peak concentration

Comparisons with fasting results statistically significant, p <0.059.

The radiolabelled oral dose of misoprostol of $73.2 \pm 4.6\%$ was recovered in urine.[10]

Within 1 hour of single dose 200 µg and 600 µg of misoprost the concentration achieved was 7.6 pg/ml (CV 37%) and 20.9 pg/ml (CV 62%), respectively and this was at its maximum. However, the breast milk concentrations of misoprostoic acid declined to <1 pg/ml at 5 hours post-dose.[9]

Pharmacodynamics

Misoprostol inhibits gastric acid secretion via stimulation of prostaglandin-E_1 receptors on parietal cells in the stomach. Misoprostol also facilitates mucus and bicarbonate secretion which leads to thickened mucosal bilayer. This protection of mucosal bilayer in turn results in reduced backflow of hydrogen ions and improved blood flow of this mucosal layer. Thus its ability to regenerate new mucosal cells is preserved.[11] However, this action of misoprostol is dose-dependent and has been shown at doses of ≥ 200 µg.[12]

With non-steroidal anti-inflammatory drugs (NSAIDs) ingestion, there is inhibition of prostaglandin synthesis which in turn leads to decreased bicarbonate and mucus secretion and thus may damage the gastric mucosa. Hence, administration of misoprostol in patients with NSAID-induced gastric ulcer would be of help.

Studies conducted using isolated canine parietal cells and misoprostol in its acid form have shown that there is stereo-specific binding of misoprost with specific prostaglandin receptors. This receptor binding is also saturable and reversible. It is also seen that the receptors have affinity for acid metabolite of misoprostol which is E type prostaglandin. However, this affinity is not for other F or I prostglandin type or other compounds like cimetidine or histamine. This receptor-specific action of misoprostol also allows it to be effective even if it is taken with food even if the serum concentration of the drug is low.[9]

Effects on gastric acid secretion: Misoprostol inhibits basal and nocturnal gastric acid secretion via activation of prostaglandin-E_1

receptors which are present on the gastric parietal cells. This inhibition is seen after food, alcohol, NSAIDs, histamine, caffeine, etc. This action is dose-dependent with effects being moderate and short term at 50 µg dosage and significant effects are noted with dosage of 200 µg dose.

Uterine effects: Misoprostol binds to the prostaglandin receptors present within the smooth muscle of the uterus and this leads to its uterotonic effect and its abortifacient action as well. This uterotonic effect is used for prevention of postpartum hemorrhage. However, misoprostol may cause excessive contractions of pregnant uterus, thus leading to uteirne tachysystole and non-reassuring fetal heart status.

With increased intensity and frequency of uterine contractions, there is degradation of collagen within the cervical stroma and thus reduction in its tone. This leads to cervical ripening and dilation.

Other pharmacologic effects: It found that misoprostol has no significant effect on other systems of the body.

Drug Interactions

It has been found in the pharmacokinetcis of aspirin that the AUC decreases by 20%. Although this is not found to be a significant decrease.

Mode of Administration

This drug is available in the tablet form and the possible modes of administration are oral, sublingual, buccal, vaginal, or rectal. There has been extensive research about the preferred mode of administration in terms of its efficacy and safety with minimalistic adverse effects. However, no conclusive evidence could be drawn from the available data.[13] The only FDA-approved route of administration is orally.

Also the available studies show that the patient may witness misoprost-induced diarrhea if there is concomitant intake of magnesium-containing antacids.

Monitoring

This drug has no monitoring guidelines since it is generally a well-tolerated drug with an acceptable safety profile. This is true in case of its obstetric and gynecological indications as well. However, monitoring of maternal vital signs, fetal heart rate (FHR), signs of fetal distress, and uterine contractions should be done when used for induction of labour. A recent Cochrane review supports its use in outpatient settings in a low-risk pregnancy for induction of labour.[14]

Adverse Effects

The most common ones are:
- Mild and include shivers/chills
- Diarrhea
- Abdominal pain
- Hyperthermia
- Nausea, vomiting
- Flatulence
- Constipation
- Dyspepsia
- Headache
- Breakthrough bleeding, and irregular menstrual cycles.

Relatively severe and not very frequent ones are:
- Hypotension
- Sinus tachycardia
- Fetal bradycardia
- Uterine contractions and pain
- Vaginal bleeding
- Edema, myocardial infarction
- Uterine rupture
- Cervical laceration
- Fetal death
- Pulmonary embolism
- Anaphylactoid reactions
- Thrombosis and
- Teratogenesis

It has been noted that the misoprostol failure in cases of first trimester-induced abortion may lead to terminal transverse limb reduction defects, Moebius syndrome, cranial nerve palsies, arthrogryposis and brain anomalies like holoprosencephaly and hydrocephalus. The probable explanation for these anomalies is vascular disruption. It is recommended that these anomalies should be counseled to the patient aspiring for such a first trimester medical abortion. Additionally, pregnancies survived after an unsuccessful attempt of induced abortion in the first trimester should be terminated surgically.[12]

Contraindications

1. Suspected ectopic pregnancy
2. Pelvic infections/sepsis
3. Hemodynamically unstable
4. Allergic to misoprostol
5. Previous cesarean section
6. Mitral stenosis
7. Hypertension
8. Glaucoma
9. Brochial asthma[13]
10. Labor induction in term pregnancy— previous uterine surgery, multiple gestation, cord prolapse, active genital Herpes infection, vasa previa, complete placenta previa, or if any unknown vaginal bleeding, any abnormal fetal heart tracings, abnormal fetal positions.[14]

References

1. WHO guidelines on Medical management of abortion, 2018 ISBN 978-92-4-155040-6
2. Wikipedia-Mifepristone.
3. Hcini N, Jolivet A, Pomar L, Mchirgui A, Maamri F, Elcadhi Y, Lambert V, Carles G. Cervical maturation using mifepristone in women with normal pregnancies at or beyond term. Eur J Obstet Gynecol Reprod Biol. 2020 May;248:58-62.
4. Blake M. Autry; Roopma Wadhwa.Mifepristone-stat pearls(internet).Last updated on may 8, 2022.
5. Tassi A, Parisi N, Londero AP (February 2020). "Misoprostol administration prior to intrauterine contraceptive device insertion: a systematic review and meta-analysis of randomised controlled trials". Eur J Contracept Reprod Health Care. 25 (1): 76–86.
6. Wali S, Balfoussia D, Touqmatchi D, Quinn S (February 2021). "Misoprostol for open myomectomy: A systematic review and meta-analysis of randomised control trials". BJOG. 128 (3): 476–483.
7. "Misoprostol". The American Society of Health-System Pharmacists. Archived from the original on 21 February 2015. Retrieved 20 February 2015.
8. Rostom A, Dube C, Wells G, Tugwell P, Welch V, Jolicoeur E, McGowan J (2002). "Prevention of NSAID-induced gastroduodenal ulcers". The Cochrane Database of Systematic Reviews. 2011 (4): CD002296.
9. Cytotec (misoprostol) tablet – drug lable. https://www.accessdata.fda.gov/drugsatfda_docs/label/2018/019268s051lbl.pdf
10. Schoenhard G, Oppermann J, Kohn FE: Metabolism and pharmacokinetic studies of misoprostol. Dig Dis Sci. 1985 Nov;30(11 Suppl):126S-128S. doi: 10.1007/bf01309397.
11. Turner JV, Agatonovic-Kustrn S, Ward H. Off-label use of misoprostol in gynaecology. Facts Views Vis Obgyn. 2015 Dec 28;7(4):261–264.
12. Marissa Krugh; Christopher V. Maani. Misoporostol. NCBI Bookshelf. A service of the National Library of Medicine, National Institutes of Health. StatPearls [Internet]. Treasure Island (FL): StatPearls Publishing; 2022 Jan.
13. Alfirevic Z, Aflaifel N, Weeks A. Oral misoprostol for induction of labour. Cochrane Database Syst Rev. 2014 Jun 13;(6):CD001338.
14. den Hollander WJ, Kuipers EJ. Current pharmacotherapy options for gastritis. Expert Opin Pharmacother. 2012 Dec;13(18):2625–36.
15. Sura Alwan, Jan M. Friedman, in Emery and Rimoin's Principles and Practice of Medical Genetics and Genomics (Seventh Edition), 2019.
16. Wu HL, Marwah S, Wang P, Wang QM, Chen XW (May 2017). "Misoprostol for medical treatment of missed abortion: a systematic review and network meta-analysis". Scientific Reports. 7 (1): 1664.
17. Tang OS, Gemzell-Danielsson K, Ho PC. Misoprostol: pharmacokinetic profiles, effects on the uterus and side-effects. Int J Gynaecol Obstet. 2007 Dec;99 Suppl 2:S160–7.

Magnesium Sulphate

• Amarjeet Kaur Bava • Neha Kamath

Molecule

Magnesium sulphate (formulation $MgSO_4$) is an amalgam having magnesium cation Mg^{2+} (20.19% by mass) and the sulfate anion SO_4^{2-}. A chemical salt marketed as a white crystalline solid soluble in water but insoluble in ethanol. Generally, encountered in the form of a hydrate $MgSO_4 \cdot nH_2O$ with values of n ranging from 1 to 11. Heptahydrate $MgSO_4 \cdot 7H_2O$ is the most common hydrate sold in the market as Epsom salt or bath salt, used as a home remedy with mineral health benefits **(Fig. 17.1).**[1]

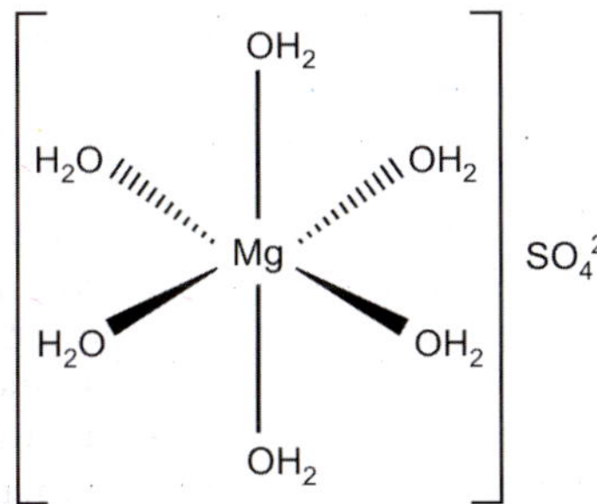

Fig. 17.1: Magnesium sulphate hexahydrate

Source

Magnesium sulphate is directly procured from dry lakes and other natural sources. In the laboratories it is prepared by reacting base magnesite (magnesium carbonate, $MgCO_3$) or magnesia (oxide, MgO) with sulfuric acid (H_2SO_4). One more procuring way is from seawater or magnesium-containing industrial wastes treatment to precipitate magnesium hydroxide and reacting the precipitate with sulfuric acid.

Further, magnesium sulfate heptahydrate (epsomite, $MgSO_4 \cdot 7H_2O$) is prepared by dissolving magnesium sulfate monohydrate (kieserite, $MgSO_4 \cdot H_2O$) in water followed by crystallization of the heptahydrate.

Pharmacokinetics

Using United States Pharmacopeia (USP) standards, magnesium sulfate USP is $MgSO_4 \cdot 7H_2O$ containing 8.12 mEq magnesium per 1 g.

After parenteral administration, approximately 40% of plasma magnesium is protein-bound, while the unbound ionized magnesium increases proportionately to the total serum concentration of magnesium. The free magnesium ions diffuse into the extravascular space, bones, and through the placenta and amniotic membranes to enter the fetus and amniotic fluid. Magnesium is almost completely excreted by the maternal kidneys, and approximately 90% of the dose is excreted in the urine within the first 24 hours after an IV dose. Hence, magnesium toxicity rarely occurs with normal or only slightly-reduced glomerular filtration rate. Adequate urine output usually signifies a preserved glomerular filtration rate. That is, magnesium excretion is independent of urine flow, and urinary volume per unit time does not predict renal function. Therefore, serum creatinine levels should be checked to diagnose a decreased glomerular filtration rate.

Therapeutic range for eclampsia is between 4–7 mEq/L (4.8–8.4 mg/dl), *i.e.* eclamptic convulsions are almost always prevented or controlled by maintaining plasma magnesium levels between 4 to 7 mEq/L, 4.8 to 8.4 mg/dl, or 2.0 to 3.5 mmol/L. Careful monitoring for toxicity is required beyond this recommended concentration. The first warning of occurence or possible occurrence of magnesium toxicity in the mother is the loss of the patellar reflex at concentrations between 3.5 and 5 mmol/L or 10 mEq/L or 12 mg/dl possibly due to the curariform action.

Respiratory paralysis and cardiac arrest may occur at or over a supratherapeutic concentration of 5 mmol/L or 10 mEq/L. When plasma levels rise above 10 mEq/L, respiration becomes weakened. At or beyond 12 mEq/L, respiratory paralysis and respiratory arrest follow (Somjen, 1966). Hence, close monitoring for the loss of deep tendon reflexes, respiratory rate <12 breaths/ minute, urine output <30 ml/hour, and high plasma magnesium concentrations are of paramount importance.

Respiratory depression (mild or moderate) can be reversed by treatment with calcium gluconate or calcium chloride, 1 g, intravenously. Discontinuation of further magnesium sulfate should be mandatory in such conditions. Also availability of either of these agents should be checked whenever magnesium treatment is started.

In cases of steady-state toxic level, the effects of intravenously administered calcium may be short-lived. Endotracheal intubation and mechanical ventilation are life-saving for severe respiratory depression and arrest. Direct toxic effects of high magnesium concentration on the myocardium are rare. Since magnesium is almost completely excreted by renal excretion, the described dosages will become excessive if glomerular filtration is reduced. An initial 4g loading dose of magnesium sulfate can be safely given regardless of renal function. There is no need to reduce the standard loading dose under the mistaken conception that diminished renal function requires it. This is because after distribution, a loading dose achieves the desired therapeutic level, and the infusion maintains the steady-state level. Thus, only the maintenance infusion rate should be altered with diminished glomerular filtration rate. Renal function is estimated by measuring plasma creatinine. Whenever plasma creatinine levels are >1.0 mg/ml, it is essential to determine serum magnesium levels to help guide the infusion rate.

Following a 4 g dose injected intravenously over 15 minutes, there is a slight decrease in mean arterial pressure with a 13% increase in cardiac index. This means, magnesium helps in lowering systemic vascular resistance and mean arterial pressure. During the same time, cardiac output is found to be increased. These findings were accompanied with transient nausea and flushing, and the effects on cardiovascular system last for only 15 minutes despite continued infusion of magnesium.[2]

Pharmacodynamics

Magnesium sulphate action on the central nervous system (CNS) and vascular endothelium helps in explaining its anti-convulsant process, which is intervened via the neuromuscular junction (NMJ). CNS depression is generalized and happens through the voltage-dependent N-methyl-D-aspartate (NMDA) receptor blockade and NMJ blockade by reducing the calcium conductance, acetylcholine release, and motor endplate irritability to acetylcholine release. In addition, it causes vasodilation via synthesis of prostacyclin I_2 (PGI_2) and nitric oxide in vascular endothelial cells. Thus, this effect of $MgSO_4$ upon the small caliber intracranial vessels helps to decrease cerebral ischemia after administration for the prevention and therapy of eclampsia.

Thurnau, et al. (1987) showed that after magnesium administration, there was a noteworthy rise in the total magnesium concentration of the spinal fluid. This rise is reciprocal to the rise in concentration of serum. High serum magnesium concentrations in the uterus suppress contractions of myometrium both *in vitro* and *in vivo*. After following the dosage schedule which has been suggested, no depression of the myometrium was observed, except for a temporary reduction in uterine activity stat after giving the first loading dose given intravenously. The standard magnesium therapy does not cause increased blood loss after delivery.

However, stopping uterine contraction relies on the dose of drug administered, and magnesium levels between 8 to 10 mEq/L is required to prevent uterine activity.[2]

Magnesium has uterine relaxant effect (tocolytic) by competing calcium in the sarcoplasmic reticulum, slowing the inter-action of calcium with the actin–myosin complex and interfering with myometrial repolarization. It also blocks entry of extracellular calcium and inhibits intracellular release of calcium via the inositol triphosphate pathways. Finally, the reduced release of acetylcholine at the neuromuscular junction, results in decreased amplitude of motor endplate potential and thus reduced sensitivity.[11]

Mechanism of Action (Fig. 17.2)

- Presynaptic liberation of glutamate which is a neurotransmitter is reduced.
- Blocks glutamatergic N-methyl-D-aspartate (NMDA) receptors.
- Improves adenosine action.
- Improves buffering of calcium by mitochondria.
- Blocks entry of calcium via voltage-gated channels (Arango, 2008; Wang, 2012).

Effects

- CNS depression, peripheral neuromuscular transmission is blocked, produce anti-convulsant effect; reduced release of acetylcholine amount at the endplate caused by motor nerve impulse.
- It delays the rate impulse generation at the SA node in the heart (myocardium), hence prolongs conduction time.
- Facilitates moving of calcium, potassium, and sodium inside and outside of cells and stabilizes membranes which are excitable.

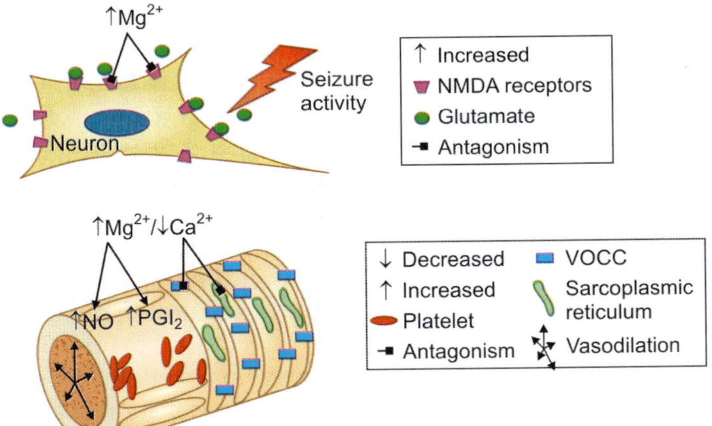

Fig. 17.2: Mechanism of action of $MgSO_4$

- In gastrointestinal (GI) system, it boosts retaining of fluid in colon by its osmotic effect, thus causing increased peristalsis and emptying of bowel.

Uses

$MgSO_4$ is put to use outside (as Epsom salt) as well as inside.

- Anticonvulsant
- Tocolytic
- Neuroprotection in preterm
- Laxative
- Thrombophlebitis dressing
- Arrhythmias
- Bronchodilator in Asthma

Dosage and Administration

Available as 50% w/v and 25% w/v solutions of magnesium sulfate is $MgSO_4 \cdot 7H_2O$ and not $MgSO_4$.

50% w/v, 5 ml ampoule, 2 ml = 1 g $MgSO_4$ used IM/IV 25% w/v, 2 ml ampoule = 0.5 g $MgSO_4$, used only IV **(Fig. 17.3)**.

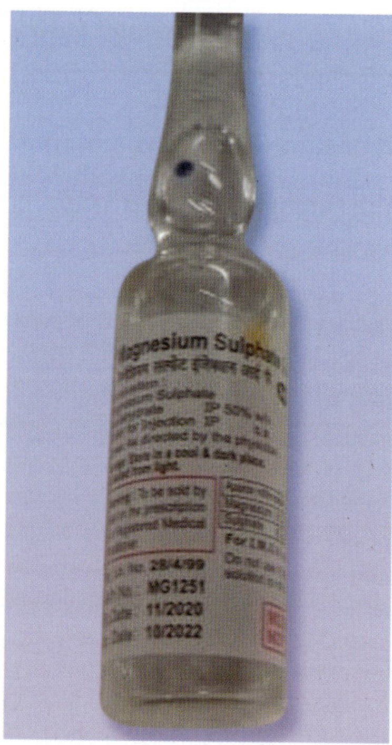

Fig. 17.3: Vial of magnesium sulphate, 50% w/v

4 g IV = 50% w/v = 8 ml = +12 ml normal saline = 20 ml, give 5 ml/1 g over one minute. 4 g IV = 25% w/v = 8 ampules = 16 ml = + 4 ml normal saline = 20 ml give 5 ml/1 g over 1 minute.

5 g IM = 50% w/v = 10 ml given deep IM (with 10 cc syringe and 22 number needle) in buttocks after proper cleaning with betadine to prevent abscess.

ECLAMPSIA

Pritchards regimen

- Loading dose =14 g = 4 g IV (20% solution) + 10 g, deep IM 5 g (50% solution) in both buttocks
- Maintenance/subsequent dose = 5 g deep IM, in alternate buttock, at interval of 4 hours up to 24 hours after last convulsion or delivery.
- Monitor parameters = Respiratory rate >16/min/patellar reflexes present/urine output >30 cc/hour or 100 cc in the last 4 hours.

Zuspan regimen

- Loading dose = 4 g, slow IV as 20 ml 20% solution.
- Maintenance dose = 1 g/hour through infusion pump [5 g, *i.e.* 5 amps of 50% w/v to be added to 500 ml Ringer lactate (RL)]

Note: When magnesium sulphate is administered parenterally to control seizures in eclamptic women, 10 to 15% of them were found to have a repeat seizure. In such a condition, slowly administer an extra 2 g of $MgSO_4$ in a 20% solution, slow IV. This supplementary 2 g $MgSO_4$ in small woman is given once and in larger woman given twice. At Parkland Hospital, only 5 of 245 women with eclampsia required the use of alternative supplementary anticonvulsant drugs to control seizures (Pritchard, 1984). For these, an injectable barbiturate is administered slowly, intravenously. Single small doses of midazolam or lorazepam can also be used, but multiple doses should not be given as there are high chances of maternal mortality from aspiration pneumonia (Royal College of Obstetricians and Gynecologists, 2006).

NEUROPROTECTION

- $MgSO_4$ reduces neuronal damage by 'downregulating' excitatory stimuli.
- Neuroprotection of preterms (between 24+0 and 33+6 weeks of pregnancy) that is pregnant women who are having preterm labour (threatened/established) or having a planned preterm birth or come with preterm premature rupture of membranes (P-PROM) [2015, amended 2019], are given a 4 g, IV bolus of $MgSO_4$ slowly in 15 minutes, subsequently $MgSO_4$, IV infusion at a rate of 1 g per hour till delivery of the patient or 24 hours is given. [2015][9]
- Maintenance = dilute 20 ml (2 ml = 1 g) + 30 ml of NS = 50 ml; infuse 5 ml/hour for 24 hours.

TOCOLYSIS

- For tocolysis, $MgSO_4$ acts as a competitive calcium ion inhibitor and also has direct relaxing action on myometrium.
- The dose is 4–6 g, slow IV bolus over 20 minutes after which $MgSO_4$ at a rate of 1–2 g/hour infusion is continued up to 12 hours after contractions have stopped.
- Contraindications are renal impairment and myasthenia gravis.
- Side effects seen with patients were weakness of muscles and respiratory depression.

Clinical Trials

- $MgSO_4$ decreased the possibility of recurrent seizures in pregnant women with eclampsia by 52% as compared with diazepam and by 67% when compared with phenytoin a Multinational Collaborative Eclampsia Study published in The Lancet in June 1995.[4]
- Magpie study (Magnesium Sulphate for the Prevention of Eclampsia a randomized controlled trial), conducted on 10141 women in 175 hospitals across 33 countries between 1998 and 2001 and published in 2002, the results showed the efficacy of $MgSO_4$ use in severe pre-eclampsia. Treatment with $MgSO_4$ in severe pre-eclampsia prevented progression to eclampsia by more than half without serious consequences on the mother and fetus and also reduced maternal mortality.[3]
- A study on $MgSO_4$ versus lytic cocktail regime showed that $MgSO_4$ was better than diazepam, phenytoin or lytic cocktail when used in eclampsia patients. This was published in july 2000 in a Cochrane review on Magnesium sulphate as the anticonvulsant of choice for pregnant patients with eclampsia. Lytic cocktail should be abandoned.[5]
- Improved perinatal outcomes of neonates born to mothers on $MgSO_4$ as compared to phenytoin. Neuroprotection was observed in preterm babies born between 28 to 31 weeks gestation.
- In a Study from Parkland Hospital by Tudela and colleagues (2013) done on obese women, the observations after administration of $MgSO_4$ showed that >60% of women with body mass index (BMI) greater than 30 kg/m^2 and received the 2 g/hr dose were found to have subtherapeutic levels after 4 hours. Therefore, obese women need 3 g/hr to keep magnesium levels in therapeutic range. Hence, many studies done recently do not suggest regular measurements of magnesium levels. (American College of Obstetricians and Gynecologists, 2013; Royal College of Obstetricians and Gynecologists, 2006).
- The Dhaka regimen follows loading dose of 10 g $MgSO_4$ and 2.5 g every 4 hourly for 24 hours after first dose This is about 50% dose of Pritchard regime and proved to have similar effect in controlling recurrent convulsions/seizures. Multiple such researches have been done, like the Dhaka regimen, Sokoto regimen using

low-dose regime of $MgSO_4$ loading, and maintenance doses proved usage in adequately managing patients of eclampsia. These help in reducing the burden on healthcare resources by helping treat the condition and thereby reducing complications due to toxicity. The Dhaka study summarized effectivity of 50% of standard magnesium sulphate dose appears to be effective to manage seizures and maintain serum levels of magnesium in the therapeutic range.[10]

Fetal and Neonatal Effects

$MgSO_4$ rapidly crosses the placenta, when administered parenterally to maintain balance in fetal serum and to a lesser extent in amniotic fluid. Timing of maternal infusion of $MgSO_4$ is directly proportional to its level in amniotic fluid. The effect is seen on cardiotocograph (CTG), specially the fetal heart beat-to-beat variability. In 2012, Duffy and associates reported that on CTG baseline fetal heartrate was on lower side of the normal range; reduced beat to beat variability; and some prolonged decelerations. No adverse outcomes were noted after delivery. Thus, maternal magnesium therapy appears to be safe for perinatal period.

A study of >1,500 premature babies born to mothers on $MgSO_4$ by the maternal–fetel medicine units (MFMU) network found no association between newborn needing resuscitation and serum magnesium levels of cord blood. However, some side effects in newborns have been seen with $MgSO_4$ therapy in mothers.

A research done at Parkland Hospital showed that 6% out of 6,654 term exposed newborns had hypotonia. In addition, newborns had lower first and fifth minute Apgar scores, needing intubation and admission to specialized care units.

This study demonstrates that neonatal depression only occurs when hypermagnesemia is severe at birth.[2]

Magnesium has a preventative effect in very-low-birthweight newborns from cerebral palsy as per few observational studies. At least five randomized studies have also evaluated $MgSO_4$ neuroprotection effect in premature neonates. Nguyen, et al. (2013) expanded the possibility to include the term neonatal neuroprotection, but the data were insufficient to draw a conclusion.

Finally, $MgSO_4$ when given for several days for tocolysis in patients with respiratory failure has been associated with neonatal osteopenia (American College of Obstetricians and Gynecologists, 2016c).

As per the National Institute for Health and Care Excellence (NICE) guidelines corticosteroids and $MgSO_4$ should be given between 24 weeks and 33.6 weeks of gestational age to women with preterm labour (threatened or established), having a planned preterm birth or have P-PROM.[7]

Maternal Safety and Efficacy

Total 1687 women with eclampsia were part of the multinational Eclampsia Trial Collaborative Group study (1995), they were randomly assigned to one of three different methods of anticonvulsant treatment: magnesium sulfate, diazepam, or phenytoin. This proved that largely $MgSO_4$ therapy in women had lower incidence of recurrent seizures (9.7%) than women who were given phenytoin (28%) or diazepam (17%).

The overall maternal mortality rate, especially for magnesium sulfate was 3.2%, which was <5.2% for the two other methods.[6]

Side Effects

Magnesium toxicity

- Deep tendon reflexes are lost ≥7 mEq/L (9.6–12 mg/dl)
- Respiratory system depression/reduced breathing ≥10 mEq/L (12–18 mg/dl)
- Respiratory paralysis/breathing stops ≥12 mEq/L
- Cardiac arrest ≥25 mEq/L (24–30 mg/dl)

When toxicity is suspected what should be done?

- If absent, deep tendon reflexes stop or omit the next dose of $MgSO_4$.
- Administer oxygen by nasal prongs/mask/intubation depending on respiratory condition
- Antidote = Calcium gluconate = 10 milliliter of 10% Calcium gluconate is given over a period of 10 minutes.
- Calcium gluconate 1 g IV + with holding $MgSO_4$, usually reverses mild-to-moderate respiratory depression.
- Prompt endotracheal intubation and mechanical ventilation are life-saving for severe respiratory depression and arrest.
- As $MgSO_4$ is excreted by renal excretion, give only half of the intramuscular $MgSO_4$ maintenance as long as the RFT is ≥ 1.3 mg/dl. Plasma $MgSO_4$ levels should be checked periodically in patients with renal insufficiency.

Cardiovascular effects

- Acute cardiovascular effects: Parenteral $MgSO_4$ can cause lowering of systemic vascular resistance ($\downarrow$SVR) and mean arterial pressure and increased carbon monoxide ($\uparrow$CO), without myocardial depression, also may lead to nausea and flushing.
- The CVS effect lasts only for 15 minutes even with a drip of $MgSO_4$ at 1.5 g per hour.
- Magnesium-related heart dysfunction is caused by respiratory arrest and hypoxia.
- With proper ventilator support, the heart functions satisfactorily even at high-plasma levels of magnesium.

Uterine effects

- Mg inhibits uterine contractions due to high extracellular concentrations of Mg which inhibits calcium entry into myometrial cells.
- The magnesium levels in serum between 8 to 10 mEq/L are effective to prevent uterine contractions, hence tocolytic effect is dose-dependent.
- Thus, it is evident that there is no uterine effect with $MgSO_4$ dose given in eclampsia or severe pre-eclampsia.

Fetal effects

- The placental barrier is crossed by Mg to bring balance in fetal serum, also in amnionic fluid.
- If severe hypermagnesemia occurs in second stage of labor there are chances of neonatal depression.
- Mg effect is seen on CTG as decrease in heartrate variability, though it has protective effect in very-low-birthweight infants from developing cerebral palsy.[2]

Clinical Approach to Tackle the Disease
Eclampsia

- Resuscitation
- Ensure patent airway
- Give oxygen
- Establish IV access and send blood investigations.
- Restrict IV fluids
- Prevent injuries, tongue bite and aspiration
- Prevent further seizures—start magnesium sulphate and monitor for toxicity.
- *Control of hypertension:* Use antihypertensive agents to lower BP to <160/100 mm Hg. Either labetolol or nifedepin preferred.
- If preterm, give corticosteroids.
- Delivery: Strict monitoring until delivery.

Criteria for Magnesium Sulfate Neuroprophylaxis

In a woman with new-onset proteinuric hypertension, at least one of the following criteria is required:

- Systolic BP 160 or diastolic BP 110 mm Hg
- Proteinuria 2+ by dipstick in a catheterized urine specimen
- Serum creatinine >1.1 mg/dl
- Platelet count <100,000/µl
- Aspartate aminotransferase (AST) elevated twice upper limit of normal

- Laboratory values
- Round-the-clock headache or scotomata
- Continuous midepigastric or right-upper quadrant pain

MgSO$_4$ in Preterm Labour

- Complete bed rest
- Tocolysis
- Corticosteroids for fetal lung maturity
- MgSO$_4$ has been recommended for neuro-protection of the fetus, as it protects the offspring from risk of developing cerebral palsy.

Indications:

- P-PROM
- Preterm labor
- Planned preterm birth for fetal or maternal indication.

References

1. "Quick Cures/Quack Cures: Is Epsom Worth Its Salt?". The Wall Street Journal. 9 April 2012. Archived from the original on 12 April 2012. Retrieved 15 June 2019.
2. Hypertensive disorders In: Cunningham FG, Leveno KJ, Bloom SL, Spong CY, Dashe JS. Williams obstetrics, 25e. New York, NY, USA: Mcgraw-hill; 2018.
3. Group TM. Do women with pre-eclampsia, and their babies, benefit from magnesium sulphate? The Magpie Trial: a randomised placebo-controlled trial. The Lancet. 2002 Jun 1;359(9321):1877–90.
4. Group TE. Which anticonvulsant for women with eclampsia? Evidence from the Collaborative Eclampsia Trial. The Lancet. 1995 Jun 10; 345(8963):1455–63.
5. Duley L, Guelmezoglu AM, Chou D. Magnesium sulphate versus lytic cocktail for eclampsia. Cochrane Database of Systematic Reviews. 2010(9).
6. Bansal V, Damania K, Hypertensive Disorders in Pregnancy In: Arias F, Bhide AG, Arulkumaran S, Damania K, Daftary SN, editors. Arias' Practical Guide to High-Risk Pregnancy and Delivery: A South Asian Perspective. Elsevier Health Sciences; 2019 Oct 16.
7. National Institute for Health and Care Excellence. Preterm labor and Birth[Internet]. [London]: NICE; 2015 [updated 2022 June] (NICE Guideline NG 25). Available from:https://www.nice.org.uk/guidance/ng25/chapter/recommendations
8. Nguyen TM, Crowther CA, Wilkinson D, Bain E. Magnesium sulphate for women at term for neuroprotection of the fetus. Cochrane Database of Systematic Reviews. 2013(2).
9. Crowther CA, Hiller JE, Doyle LW. Magnesium sulphate for preventing preterm birth in threatened preterm labour. Cochrane Database of Systematic Reviews. 2002(4).
10. Begum R, Begum A, Johanson R, Ali MN, Akhter S. A low dose ('Dhaka') magnesium sulphate regime for eclampsia: Clinical findings and serum magnesium levels. Acta obstetricia et gynecologica Scandinavica. 2001 Jan 1;80(11):998–100.
11. Martin RJ, Fanaroff AA, Walsh MC. Fanaroff and Martin's neonatal-perinatal medicine e-book: diseases of the fetus and infant. Elsevier Health Sciences; 2014 Aug 20.

Management of Peripartum Psychiatric Disorders

• Milan Balakrishnan • Bhavini Shah

Introduction

There's a silent crisis that affects women during their most fertile years—a heightened vulnerability to mental health issues—prime culprits. The rollercoaster ride of neuro-hormonal and psychological changes, compounded by social and emotional hurdles, especially prevalent during pregnancy and childbirth.

There is ample evidence of significant structural and functional brain changes, we lack enough longitudinal studies to fully comprehend these complex changes.

Research indicates that significant transformations occur in women's brains during pregnancy, with a decrease in overall grey matter volume across gestation.

Evidence also points to anatomical adjustments in key structures such as the amygdala, hippocampus, and pituitary gland.[1]

Depressive and anxiety disorders stand out as the mental health conditions most commonly encountered by women.[1]

This is particularly true for women who have a previous history of any psychiatric conditions.

Psychiatric illnesses most prominently depression and anxiety are more prone to relapse in the peripartum period. This is more likely if they have had 2 or more such previous episodes.[2]

Woman with a past history of psychiatric disorders should have a thorough pre-pregnancy psychiatric assessment, ideally in the pre-conception period. This interaction should address the safest approach as they plan to conceive, discuss issues during pregnancy and postpartum. For women on psychiatric medications, the consultation should include a review of any previous attempts of trying to stop the medication. If a patient has quickly relapsed after discontinuing, she may need to remain on the medication while pregnant. However, if she has been able to remain well for at least several months while off the medication, she may be able to taper and discontinue the medication prior to attempting to conceive. A risk–benefit approach in collaboration with the couple and including the psychiatrist would be most helpful. This liaison should continue over the course of the pregnancy and should be carefully documented.

The discussion should include the following:

1. Sharing maximum available information on the risks of medication exposure during pregnancy and lactation.
2. The limitations of the data (*e.g.* small sample sizes, limited information on potential sequelae of prenatal medication exposure, naturalistic designs that do not

account for confounding factors, such as maternal use of nicotine, maternal health, habits, etc.)

3. Treatment alternatives
4. The patient's risk of a psychiatric relapse during pregnancy and postpartum.
5. Measures that may reduce the likelihood of relapse (*e.g.* psychotherapy; couples therapy, focus on psychosocial stressors).
6. The general incidence of birth defects (approx. 2–4%) regardless of medication exposure.

GENERAL PRINCIPLES OF TREATMENT OF PERIPARTUM PSYCHIATRIC DISORDERS[3,4]

Non-pharmacological interventions include individual and group psychotherapy, couple and family counseling, relaxation techniques, and a focus on psychosocial stressors.

However, drugs can be required if non-pharmacological strategies have been tried in the past without success or if nonpharmacological interventions are ineffective or inappropriate for the patient's ailment. No matter the method of therapy, the woman should be urged to enlist the help of family and friends to care for the baby, to get as much sleep and rest as she can, and to scale back on her other commitments.

Aim to keep doses at the bare minimum required.

Always prefer monotherapy over polytherapy. Try using the drug with the lowest known risk.

Whenever possible, medication use should be minimized or avoided at least in the first trimester, particularly if pregnancy data on its safety are limited and adjust doses as pregnancy and illness progresses.

DEPRESSION DURING PREGNANCY[5–9]

Approximately, 10% of pregnant women develop or have a pre-existing depressive illness. Around 30% of postpartum depression begins before birth. There is a significant increase in new psychiatric episodes in the first 3 months after delivery. At least 80% are mood disorders, particularly severe depression. Women who have had a previous episode of depressive illness (postpartum or otherwise) are at higher risk of further episodes during peripartum. The risk is highest in women with bipolar illness who are also at risk of mania or mixed affective episodes. There is some evidence that depression increases the risk of spontaneous abortion, having a low-birth weight or small-for-gestational-age baby, or of preterm delivery, though effects are small.

The mental health of the mother influences fetal well-being, obstetric outcome, and child-brain growth and development and has long-term impact on the mental health of the child. The risks of not treating depression include:

Harm to the mother due to poor self-care, lack of pregnancy care, or risk of self-harm. Harm to the fetus or neonate (ranging from neglect to infanticide).

Symptoms of Depression

A depressive episode is characterised by a period of low mood or diminished interest in activities occurring most of the day, nearly everyday during a period lasting at least two weeks accompanied by other symptoms such as difficulty concentrating, feelings of worthlessness or excessive or inappropriate guilt, hopelessness, recurrent thoughts of death or suicide, changes in appetite or sleep, psychomotor agitation or retardation, and reduced energy or fatigue. There have never been any prior episodes of mania, hypomania, or mixed episodes, which would indicate the presence of a bipolar disorder.

Significant anxiety symptoms (*e.g.* feeling nervous, anxious or on the edge, not being able to control worrying thoughts, fear that something bad will happen, having trouble relaxing, muscle tension, autonomic symptoms) have been present for most of the time during the episode. Mental or behavioural disorders associated with pregnancy, childbirth or the puerperium, without psychotic symptoms is an additional diagnostic code used for mood episodes that arise during pregnancy or commencing within about 6 weeks of delivery that include delusions, hallucinations, or other psychotic symptoms.

Assessing patient suspected for having depression involves asking 2 key questions—do you have persistent feelings of sadness and secondly lack of pleasure in previously pleasurable activities. Screening can be done by using Edinburgh postnatal depression scale (EPDS) a 10 question inventory or by using the Becks depression inventory (BDI). The primary care evaluation of mental disorders patient health questionnaire (PRIME-MD, PHQ) is considered an accurate instrument for the detection of recent psychosocial stressors and functional impairment due to mood disorders in pregnant patients.[10–15]

Management

Crafting a treatment plan essentially revolves around the intensity of depression and the associated symptoms. It is crucial that the path to recovery is charted on a case-by-case basis, with the patient at the heart of decision-making, while being guided by their trusted healthcare providers.

Psychotherapeutic Interventions

When it comes to tackling mild-to-moderate depression, cognitive behaviour therapy (CBT) and interpersonal therapy (IPT) have the best evidence in the psychotherapy arena.

CBT includes identifying problems, recognizing cognitive distortions, generating alternative thoughts, problem-solving, activity scheduling, and anxiety management through relaxation techniques.

IPT focuses on losses, role disputes and changes, social isolation, impairment in social skills, and other interpersonal factors that may affect depression.[16,17]

Treatment with Antidepressants

Some data suggest that antidepressants may increase the risk of spontaneous abortion (but note that confounding factors were not controlled for), preterm delivery, low-birth weight, respiratory distress in the neonate, a low Apgar score at birth, and admission to a special care baby unit.[18] Most studies are observational and do not control for maternal depression. In a large cohort study, the presence of depressive symptoms but not antidepressant use[19] was associated with preterm birth and babies small-for-gestational-age. Interestingly, a large Finnish study found selective serotonin reuptake inhibitor (SSRI) use to be associated with a lower risk of preterm birth and cesarean delivery compared with unexposed women diagnosed with a psychiatric illness,[20] and untreated maternal depression itself is associated with an increased risk of both low-birth weight and preterm birth.[60] SSRIs do not appear to increase the risk of stillbirth or neonatal mortality.[21,22]

Discontinuing medication can lead to higher relapse rates in individuals with a history of depression. It is especially relevant for women who have experienced severe or recurrent bouts of depression to continue their treatment and reduce risk.[23]

Sertraline appears to result in the least placental exposure. SSRIs appear not to be major teratogens,[24–27] with most data supporting the safety of fluoxetine.[28–33]

All SSRIs, such as citalopram, escitalopram, sertraline and fluoxetine seem to be safe with the exception of paroxetine. Paroxetine has been specifically associated with cardiac malformations particularly after high dose (>25 mg/day) but other studies have failed to replicate.[34–38]

Tricyclic Antidepressants[39–41]

Foetal exposure to tricyclics is found to be high. Tricyclic antidepressants (TCAs) have been widely used in the past throughout pregnancy without apparent detriment to the foetus.

Use of TCAs in the third trimester is known to produce neonatal withdrawal effects;

agitation, irritability, seizures, respiratory distress and endocrine and metabolic disturbances. These are usually mild and self-limiting.

Use of nortriptyline is recommended over amitriptyline and imipramine because of lower anticholinergic side effects.

TCA use during pregnancy increases the risk of preterm delivery.

Monoamine oxidase inhibitors (MAOIs) should be avoided in pregnancy because of a suspected risk of congenital malformations and because of the risk of hypertensive crisis.[42]

Duloxetine is unlikely to be a major teratogen.

Bupropion exposure *in utero* has been associated with an increased risk of attention deficit hyperactivity disorder (ADHD) in the child.[43,44]

For patients who are already receiving antidepressant treatment and are at high risk of relapse, it is recommended to continue with the same antidepressant during and after pregnancy. In cases, where a moderate-severe or severe depressive illness develops during pregnancy, treatment with antidepressant medication is recommended.

When initiating an antidepressant during pregnancy or for women considering pregnancy, the individual's previous response to treatment should be taken into account. The antidepressant that has previously been effective should be considered as the first choice. For untreated patients, sertraline may be selected as a treatment option.

During pregnancy, it is important to screen for alcohol use and monitor for the development of hypertension and pre-eclampsia. Women taking SSRIs may have an increased risk of postpartum hemorrhage. When SSRIs are taken in late pregnancy, there may be a slight increase in the risk of persistent pulmonary hypertension of the newborn, although the absolute risk is very low.

Newborns may experience discontinuation symptoms if the mother has taken antidepressants during pregnancy. These symptoms are usually mild and can include agitation, irritability, and rarely, respiratory distress and convulsions (particularly with short half-life drugs such as paroxetine and venlafaxine). Continuing to breastfeed and gradually transitioning to mixed feeding (breast and bottle) may help reduce the severity of these reactions.[45–61]

Electroconvulsive therapy (ECT): There is no evidence to suggest that ECT causes harm to either the mother or foetus during pregnancy[62] although general anesthesia risks need to be considered. The National Institute for Health and Care Excellence (NICE) recommends ECT for pregnant women with severe depression, severe mixed affective states or mania, or catatonia, whose physical health or that of the fetus is at serious risk.

POSTPARTUM DEPRESSION (PPD)

The major risk factor for postpartum depression is a past episode of major depressive disorder. Other risk factors include a history of severe premenstrual dysphoria, family history of mood disorder, marital discord, lack of a supportive relationship, family support, and repetitive stressful life events in the last year. In terms of perinatal events, pregnancy loss is associated with post-traumatic symptoms and depression, but, in general, studies of the impact of obstetrical complications on postpartum mood have been mixed.[63–74]

The prevalence of infanticidal thinking in women with PPD, with or without psychosis, is quite high. A study of severely ill and hospitalized women in India found that 43% reported infanticidal ideas, whereas 36% reported infanticidal behavior.[75]

Management

Individual psychotherapy is recommended as a treatment option for all women with PPD. In cases of mild to moderate symptom severity, individual psychotherapy alone may be sufficient. However, for more severe and/or prolonged PPD, the first-line treatment approach involves the administration of a SSRI. In cases, where extreme anxiety or insomnia is a prominent feature, supplementation with a benzodiazepine may also be considered.

While some studies suggest that exogenous estrogen may help alleviate symptoms of PPD, it is not currently considered a first-line therapy unless there is proven estrogen deficiency or when other treatment options have been ineffective or insufficiently beneficial.[76,77]

BABY BLUES

The baby blues typically resolve on their own and usually do not require the use of psychotropic medications. However, in some cases where women are experiencing difficulty in sleeping even when the baby is asleep, a sleep aid may be considered. Zolpidem (5–10 mg) or a medium half-life benzodiazepine such as lorazepam (0.5–2 mg) can be prescribed for several nights to help break the cycle of independent insomnia from the infant's sleep cycle.

Providing emotional and physical support to the mother as she navigates the responsibilities of caring for a newborn while managing her previous obligations is crucial. It is important to recognize that the baby blues can potentially be a precursor to PPD. Therefore, all patients should be advised to contact their obstetrician if their symptoms worsen or cause significant distress or cause further distress.[78]

TREATMENT OF ANXIETY DISORDERS IN PREGNANCY AND POSTPARTUM

The prevalence of perinatal anxiety disorders ranges widely from study to study (8.7–30%) In general, anxiety disorders and depression are highly co-morbid conditions, and this co-morbidity may be common in the perinatal period as well.[79–84]

Symptoms of Anxiety Disorders

Panic Disorder[85,86]

Panic disorder is characterized by the occurrence of unexpected panic attacks in women, which are marked by intense fear and the sudden onset of physical symptoms like shortness of breath, palpitations, and dizziness. The diagnostic criteria for panic disorder also include several additional elements. These include (a) anticipatory worry about the possibility of experiencing further panic attacks, (b) concern regarding the consequences of such attacks (*e.g.* fears of dying or going crazy), and (c) behavioral changes resulting from the attacks (*e.g.* avoidance behaviors).

If there is significant avoidance of situations where panic attacks are feared, agoraphobia may also be diagnosed alongside panic disorder. Examples of such situations may include being home alone or being in crowded places. In the context of panic disorder, it is common for women to misinterpret these normal physiological sensations in catastrophic ways, believing that they are encountering a serious medical event such as a heart attack.

Obsessive Compulsive Disorder[87–89]

Obsessive compulsive disorder (OCD) is characterized by two main components. First, individuals experience unwanted intrusive thoughts, ideas, images, doubts, or impulses that generate anxiety, known as obsessions. Second, they feel compelled to engage in certain behavioral or mental acts to neutralize or alleviate the distress caused by these obsessions, known as compulsive rituals.

During pregnancy and the postpartum period, obsessions in OCD commonly revolve around concerns related to the well-being of the baby. Examples include persistent thoughts about the baby's death or sudden infant death syndrome (SIDS), as well as unwanted impulses to harm the child.

Differentiating between postpartum OCD and postpartum psychosis is crucial, particularly since both conditions may involve thoughts about harming the newborn. Despite some surface-level similarities, there are notable distinctions between the two. Postpartum psychosis often involves hallucinations (*e.g.* seeing smoke and fire emanating from the baby's nose and ears) and delusions (*e.g.* belief that the devil is targeting the baby), which are typically absent in cases of postpartum OCD.

Post-traumatic Stress Disorder (PTSD)[90,91]

People who undergo significant distress after being exposed to or witnessing a life-threatening event, and subsequently exhibit certain symptoms such as re-experiencing the event (*e.g.* nightmares, flashbacks), avoiding stimuli associated with the event, and experiencing heightened arousal (*e.g.* irritability, sleep disturbances), are diagnosed with post-traumatic stress disorder (PTSD).

Prevalence estimates of PTSD in pregnant women vary widely, ranging from 1.7% to 8.1%.

Generalised Anxiety Disorder (GAD)

It is diagnosed when an individual consistently experiences excessive and uncontrollable worry for more than half of the days over a period of at least 6 months. These worries extend to various aspects of life, including work, relationships, health, and finances. Alongside the persistent worry, individuals with GAD often encounter a range of physical symptoms such as restlessness, irritability, and muscle tension.

During the perinatal period, the experience of GAD may be further complicated by additional physical symptoms like sleep disturbances and muscle aches. Additionally, psychosocial stressors specific to this period, such as changes in roles, concerns about child health, and financial issues, can contribute to the complexity of the condition.

Social Phobia

Individuals who suffer from social phobia undergo significant distress in social or performance settings due to their fear of being embarrassed or negatively evaluated by others. When faced with such situations, these individuals tend to either completely avoid them or endure them while experiencing intense distress. The avoidance and distress associated with social anxiety significantly hinder their ability to function normally in their work or social lives.

In the context of miscarriage, pregnancy loss has been identified as a potential risk factor for heightened symptoms of anxiety or the onset of an anxiety disorder.[92–94]

Treatment of Anxiety Disorders

The preferred psychological approach for addressing clinical anxiety disorders, is cognitive behavior therapy (CBT), which can also be extended to perinatal anxiety problems. CBT operates on the fundamental principle that emotional responses are not solely caused by situations themselves, but rather by an individual's beliefs and interpretations of those situations. Specific emotions are associated with particular types of beliefs and interpretations. CBT is a time-limited treatment, typically consisting of 12–16 weekly sessions for anxiety disorders.

Experts in the fields of psychiatry and clinical psychology recommend CBT as the primary therapeutic option for pregnant and postpartum women dealing with anxiety disorders. Studies consistently support the effectiveness of CBT in treating OCD. The key elements of this intervention involve exposure to stimuli that evoke obsessions while avoiding engaging in compulsive rituals or other neutralizing strategies (safety behaviors) used to alleviate anxiety. Exposure-based therapy for OCD has been found to be more effective than relaxation techniques, anxiety management, and the use of the antidepressant clomipramine.

Treatments incorporating cognitive re-structuring and exposure have shown positive outcomes for social anxiety disorder, surpassing the results of no treatment or nonspecific therapies. Women diagnosed with PTSD often benefit from interventions that include stress inoculation training and traditional CBT. Stress inoculation training incorporates cognitive techniques, such as thought-stopping, challenging negative self-cognitions, relaxation techniques, modeling, and role-playing.

The effectiveness of CBT components for GAD is not as well-defined as for other anxiety disorders.

In terms of pharmacotherapy, SSRIs which are a class of antidepressant medications, are preferred during the perinatal period. SSRIs are easy to administer and carry a low risk of toxicity in case of overdose. Therefore, they are recommended as the first-line pharmacological treatment for PPD, postpartum panic disorder, and OCD.[95–106]

BIPOLAR ILLNESS DURING PREGNANCY AND POSTPARTUM

Bipolar disorder is characterized by drastic shifts in mood, encompassing episodes of mania, depression, and periods of stability. These episodes commonly endure for several weeks or even months.

During the manic phase, individuals may experience intense feelings of happiness, elation, or overwhelming joy. They tend to speak rapidly, exhibit heightened energy levels, and feel a sense of self-importance. They may generate numerous innovative ideas and develop grandiose plans. Manic individuals often find it challenging to maintain focus, easily becoming irritated or agitated. They may also experience delusions, hallucinations, and exhibit disordered or illogical thinking. Sleep disturbances, loss of appetite, and engaging in impulsive, reckless behaviors with severe consequences (such as excessive spending) are also common.

Decision-making and communication may become uncharacteristically risky or harmful according to others' observations.

Episodes of depression manifest as described earlier, involving prolonged periods of low mood, feelings of sadness, hopelessness, and loss of interest or pleasure in activities.

If mood-stabilizing medication is discontinued during pregnancy, there is a high risk of relapse. Research has indicated that bipolar women who were in a stable mood state at conception and chose to discontinue mood stabilizers were twice as likely to experience a relapse compared to those who continued their medication. The relapse duration was five times longer for the group who discontinued their mood stabilizers.[107]

However, others have found illness severity more than medication changes in pregnancy to be a predictor of relapse.[108]

Treatment[109]

For women who have enjoyed an extended period without experiencing a relapse, it may be worth considering the option of transitioning to a safer antipsychotic medication or even discontinuing treatment before conception and continuing to abstain during the initial trimester of pregnancy. Abruptly ceasing medication poses a significant risk of relapse both before and after childbirth.

When it comes to mood stabilizers, no particular option can be deemed unequivocally safe. The National Institute for Health and Care Excellence (NICE) recommends the use of mood-stabilizing antipsychotics as a preferable alternative to continuing with a mood stabilizer. Women who suffer from severe mental illness or are prone to rapid relapses following the discontinuation of a mood stabilizer should be advised to maintain their medication regimen after a thorough discussion of the associated risks.

If lithium is considered essential for a woman planning to conceive, she must be informed about the potential risk of fetal heart malformations during the first trimester, as well as the risk of toxicity in the baby if lithium usage continues during breastfeeding. Throughout pregnancy and the postnatal period, lithium plasma levels should be monitored more frequently, and the medication should be ceased during active labor. Close collaboration with fetal medicine services is crucial to appropriately monitor the fetus for Ebstein's anomaly in women prescribed lithium.

NICE strongly advises against the use of valproate during pregnancy, emphasizing the need for discontinuation before conception. Women taking valproate, who plan to become pregnant, should be counseled to gradually discontinue the drug due to the high risk of fetal malformations and adverse neurodevelopmental outcomes associated with any exposure during pregnancy. In cases where valproate is the only effective treatment option for a specific woman and is deemed necessary during pregnancy, a comprehensive explanation of the risks should be provided, and she should sign a consent form indicating her understanding of the potential for malformations and developmental delays.

If a woman is planning a pregnancy or becomes pregnant while taking carbamazepine, it is advisable to discuss the possibility of discontinuing the medication. In instances, where carbamazepine is used, prophylactic administration of vitamin K to both the mother and the newborn should take place following delivery.

For women using lamotrigine, frequent monitoring of lamotrigine levels is recommended during pregnancy and the postnatal period due to significant variations during these stages.

In cases of acute mania during pregnancy, antipsychotics should be employed, and if ineffective, electroconvulsive therapy (ECT) may be considered. For bipolar depression during pregnancy, CBT is recommended for moderate depression, while selective SSRIs are considered for more severe depression. Lamotrigine can also be an option in such cases.

Breastfeeding[110]

The well-established advantages of breastfeeding on the physical well-being and cognitive growth of children, are widely recognized. It is commonly recommended that women engage in breastfeeding for a minimum of 6 months. An important consideration that can impact a mother's choice to breastfeed is the safety of the medication used during this period.

The presence of psychotropic substances in breast milk is evident, although the extent of excretion varies. Obtaining precise data on infant exposure, such as direct measurements of infant plasma levels, is infrequent. However, using maternal plasma levels of antipsychotic medications can serve as a helpful approximation of the level of exposure experienced by the infant.

Prescribing psychotropic medication while breastfeeding involves adhering to certain guidelines:

1. When considering prescribing psychotropics, it is crucial to assess the safety of individual drugs for breastfeeding women who are contemplating pregnancy.

2. Discussions about drug safety during breastfeeding should ideally take place early on, preferably before conception or in the early stages of pregnancy.

3. Decisions regarding drug use during pregnancy should also include discussions about breastfeeding. It is not advisable to switch medications near the end of pregnancy or immediately after giving birth due to the high risk of relapse.

4. If a mother has been taking a specific psychotropic medication during pregnancy and until delivery, it is generally appropriate to continue with the drug while breastfeeding. This approach can help minimize

withdrawal symptoms in the infant, with a few exceptions to be noted. However, the benefits of breastfeeding for both the mother and the infant should always be weighed against the potential risk of drug exposure to the infant.

5. Unless the currently prescribed drug is contraindicated for breastfeeding, it is typically inappropriate to discontinue breastfeeding. In cases, where the prescribed drug is not suitable for breastfeeding, the priority is still the treatment of maternal mental illness. In such situations, the mother should be advised to bottle feed with formula milk while continuing treatment.

6. When initiating drug treatment after childbirth, several factors should be considered: The mother's previous response to treatment, avoidance of psychotropics with high reported levels in infants' blood plasma, and the half-lives of the drugs. Drugs with long half-lives can accumulate in breast milk and the infant's serum.

7. Neonates and infants have limited capacity to clear drugs from their systems compared to adults. Premature infants and those with renal, hepatic, cardiac, or neurological impairments face a higher risk from drug exposure.

8. It is essential to monitor infants for specific adverse effects of the drugs, as well as abnormalities in feeding patterns, growth, and development. If adverse effects or suspected toxicity arise, monitoring infant plasma levels becomes necessary.

9. Women taking sedating medication should be strongly advised not to breastfeed in bed, as falling asleep and rolling onto the baby could pose a risk of hypoxia. Sedation may also affect a woman's ability to interact with her children, necessitating close monitoring.

In summary, the following practices should be followed whenever possible:

- Administer the lowest effective dose.
- Avoid using multiple medications simultaneously (polypharmacy).
- Continue the medication regimen prescribed during pregnancy.

Antidepressants

When initiating an antidepressant, postpartum sertraline and mirtazapine may be chosen. Escitalopram and fluvoxamine can be used.

Antipsychotics

Women on clozapine should be explained risks of breastfeeding and clozapine should be continued. When initiating an antipsychotic postpartum olanzapine or quetiapine may be considered. Other drugs such as risperidone, paliperidone, amisulpiride and ziprasidone can be given.

Mood Stabilisers

Women taking lithium should be advised against breastfeeding and lithium should be continued. When starting a mood stabiliser postpartum a mood-stabilising antipsychotic, such as olanzapine or quetiapine may be considered. Valproate maybe used with caution postpartum and during breastfeeding. Other drugs such as carbamazepine, topiramate and lamotrigine can be used.

Sedatives

Avoid sedatives. If necessary, use drug with shortest half-life. Lorazepam may be given. Zolpidem and zopiclone maybe used in lowest doses.

References

1. Neurobiological changes during the peripartum period: implications for health and behavior Emilia F Cárdenas, Autumn Kujawa, Kathryn L Humphreys Social Cognitive and Affective Neuroscience, Volume 15, Issue 10, October 2020, Pages 1097–1110, https://doi.org/10.1093/scan/nsz091

2. Altshuler LL, Hendrick V, and Cohen L. Course of mood and anxiety disorders during pregnancy and the postpartum period. J. Clin. Psychiatry 1998;59:29–33.

3. Creasy RK and Resnik R. Maternal-Fetal Medicine: Principles and Practice, 3rd ed. Philadelphia, WB Saunders, 1994; 96–97.

4. Hernandez-Diaz S, Werler MM, Walker AM, et al. Folic acid antagonists during pregnancy and the risk of birth defects. N. Engl. J. Med. 2000;343, 1608–1614.

5. Munk-Olsen T, et al. New parents and mental disorders: a population-based register study. JAMA 2006; 296:2582–2589.

6. Mahon PB, et al. Genome-wide linkage and follow-up association study of postpartum mood symptoms. Am J Psychiatry 2009; 166:1229–1237.

7. Stein A, et al. Effects of perinatal mental disorders on the fetus and child. Lancet 2014; 384:1800–1819.

8. Yonkers KA, et al. The management of depression during pregnancy: a report from the American Psychiatric Association and the American College of Obstetricians and Gynecologists. Gen Hosp Psychiatry 2009; 31:403–413. 55.

9. Engelstad HJ, et al. Perinatal outcomes of pregnancies complicated by maternal depression with or without selective serotonin reuptake inhibitor therapy. Neonatology 2014; 105:149–154.

10. Beck AT. An inventory for measuring depression. Arch. Gen. Psychiatry 1961;4:53–61.

11. Beck AT, Rush HA, Shaw BF, and Emery G. Cognitive Therapy of Depression. New York: Guilford Press. 1979. 15. Holcomb, W. L., Stone, L. S., Lustman, P. J., et al. (1996) Screening for depression in pregnancy: characteristics of the Beck Depression Inventory. Obstet. Gynecol. 88, 1021–1025.

12. Salamero M, Marcos T, Gutierrez F, et al. Factorial study of the BDI in pregnant women. Psychol. Med. 1994;24, 1031–1035.

13. Cox JL, Holden JM, and Sagovsky R. Detection of postnatal depression: development of the Edinburgh Postnatal Depression Scale. Br. J. Psychiatry 1987;150:782–786.

14. Murray D and Cox JL. Screening for depression during pregnancy with the Edinburgh depression scale (EPDS). J. Reprod. Infant Psychol. 1990;8, 99–107.

15. Spitzer RL, Williams JB, Kroenke K, et al. Validity and utility of the PRIME-MD patient health questionnaire in assessment of 3000 obstetric-gynecology study. Am. J. Obstet Gynecol. 2000;183:759–769.

16. Spinelli MG. Interpersonal psychotherapy for depressed antepartum women: a pilot study. Am. J. Psychiatry 1997;154:1028–1030.

17. Spinelli MG and Endicott J. Controlled trial of interpersonal psychotherapy versus parenting education program for depressed women. Am. J. Psychiatry 2003;160:555–562.

18. Kelly RH., Zatzick DF, and Anders TF. The detection and treatment of psychiatric disorders and substance use among pregnant women cared for in obstetrics. Am. J. Psychiatry 2001; 158:213–219.

19. Paarlberg KM, Vingerhoets JJ, Passchier J, et al. Psychosocial factors and pregnancy outcome: a review with emphasis on methodological issues. J. Psychosom. Res. 1995;39:563–595.

20. National High Blood Pressure Education Working Group. National High Blood Pressure Education Working Group report on high blood pressure in pregnancy. Am. J. Obstet. Gynecol. 1990;163:1689–1712

21. Kurki T, Hilesmaa V, Raitasalo R, et al. Depression and anxiety in early pregnancy and risk for pre-eclampsia. Obstet. Gynecol. 2000;95, 487–490.

22. Kelly RH, Danielsen B, Golding J, et al. Adequacy of prenatal care among women with psychiatric diagnoses giving birth in California in 1994 and 1995. Psychiatr. Serv. 1999;50:1584–1590.

23. Pajulo M, Savonlahti E, Sourander A, et al. Antenatal depression, substance dependency and social support. J. Affect. Disord. 2001;65, 9–17.

24. Ban L, et al. Maternal depression, antidepressant prescriptions, and congenital anomaly risk in offspring: a population-based cohort study. BJOG 2014;121:1471–1481.

25. Lundy B, Jones NA, Field T, et al. Prenatal depression effects on neonates. Infant Behav. Dev. 1999;22:119–129.

26. Davis RL, et al. Risks of congenital malformations and perinatal events among infants exposed to antidepressant medications during pregnancy. Pharmacoepidemiol Drug Saf 2007;16:1086–1094.

27. Cohen LS, Heller VL, Bailey JW, et al. Birth outcomes following prenatal exposure to fluoxetine. Biol. Psychiatry 2000;48:996–1000.

28. Simon GE, Cunnignham ML, and Davis RL. Outcomes of prenatal antidepressant exposure. Am. J. Psychiatry 2002;159:2055–2061.

29. Gentile S. Selective serotonin reuptake inhibitor exposure during early pregnancy and the

risk of birth defects. Acta Psychiatr Scand 2011; 123:266–275. Robert, E. (1996) Treating depression in pregnancy [editorial]. N. Engl. J. Med. 335, 1056–1058.

30. Hallberg P, et al. The use of selective serotonin reuptake inhibitors during pregnancy and breast-feeding: a review and clinical aspects. J Clin Psychopharmacol 2005;25:59–73.

31. Gentile S. The safety of newer antidepressants in pregnancy and breastfeeding. Drug Saf 2005; 28:137–152.

32. Kallen BA, et al. Maternal use of selective serotonin re-uptake inhibitors in early pregnancy and infant congenital malformations. Birth Defects Res A Clin Mol Teratol 2007; 79:301–30.

33. Einarson TR, et al. Newer antidepressants in pregnancy and rates of major malformations: a meta-analysis of prospective comparative studies. Pharmacoepidemiol Drug Saf 2005; 14:823–827.

34. Thormahlen GM. Paroxetine use during pregnancy: is it safe? Ann Pharmacother 2006; 40:1834–1837.

35. Myles N, et al. Systematic meta-analysis of individual selective serotonin reuptake inhibitor medications and congenital malformations. Aust NZJ Psychiatry 2013; 47:1002–1012.

36. Berard A, et al. The risk of major cardiac malformations associated with paroxetine use during the first trimester of pregnancy: a systematic review and meta-analysis. Br J Clin Pharmacol 2016; 81:589–604.

37. Berard A, et al. First trimester exposure to paroxetine and risk of cardiac malformations in infants: the importance of dosage. Birth Defects Res B Dev Reprod Toxicol 2007; 80:18–27.

38. Davis RL, et al. Risks of congenital malformations and perinatal events among infants exposed to antidepressant medications during pregnancy. Pharmacoepidemiol Drug Saf 2007; 16:1086–1094.

39. Loughhead AM, et al. Placental passage of tricyclic antidepressants. Biol Psychiatry 2006; 59:287–290.

40. Loughhead AM, et al. Antidepressants in amniotic fluid: another route of fetal exposure. Am J Psychiatry 2006; 163:145–147.

41. Maschi S, et al. Neonatal outcome following pregnancy exposure to antidepressants: a prospective controlled cohort study. BJOG 2008; 115:283–289.

42. Hendrick V, et al. Management of major depression during pregnancy. Am J Psychiatry 2002; 159:1667–1673.

43. Figueroa R. Use of antidepressants during pregnancy and risk of attention-deficit/hyperactivity disorder in the offspring. J Dev Behav Pediatr 2010; 31:641–648.

44. Forsberg L, et al. School performance at age 16 in children exposed to antiepileptic drugs in utero – a population-based study. Epilepsia 2010; 52:364–369.

45. Hviid A, et al. Use of selective serotonin reuptake inhibitors during pregnancy and risk of autism. N Engl J Med 2013; 369: 2406–2415.

46. Rai D, et al. Parental depression, maternal antidepressant use during pregnancy, and risk of autism spectrum disorders: population based case-control study. BMJ 2013; 346:f2059.

47. Brown HK, et al. Association between serotonergic antidepressant use during pregnancy and autism spectrum disorder in children. JAMA 2017; 317:1544–1552.

48. Sujan AC, et al. Associations of maternal antidepressant use during the first trimester of pregnancy with preterm birth, small for gestational age, autism spectrum disorder, and attention-deficit/hyperactivity disorder in offspring. JAMA 2017; 317:1553–1562.

49. Castro VM, et al. Absence of evidence for increase in risk for autism or attention-deficit hyperactivity disorder following antidepressant exposure during pregnancy: a replication study. Trans Psychiatry 2016; 6:e708.

50. Mezzacappa A, et al. Risk for autism spectrum disorders according to period of prenatal antidepressant exposure: a systematic review and meta-analysis. JAMA Pediatrics 2017; 171:555–563.

51. Kieviet N, et al. Risk factors for poor neonatal adaptation after exposure to antidepressants in utero. Acta Paediatr 2015; 104:384–391.

52. Brandlistuen RE, et al. Behavioural effects of fetal antidepressant exposure in a Norwegian cohort of discordant siblings. Int J Epidemiol 2015; 44:1397–1407.

53. Pregnancy and breastfeeding, CHAPTER 7. De Vera MA, et al. Antidepressant use during pregnancy and the risk of pregnancy-induced hypertension. Br J Clin Pharmacol 2012; 74:362–369.

54. Zakiyah N, et al. Antidepressant use during pregnancy and the risk of developing gestational hypertension: a retrospective cohort study. BMC Pregnancy Childbirth 2018; 18:187.

55. Palmsten K, et al. Antidepressant use and risk for preeclampsia. Epidemiology 2013; 24:682–691.

56. Bruning AH, et al. Antidepressants during pregnancy and postpartum hemorrhage: a systematic review. Eur J Obstet Gynecol Reprod Biol 2015; 189:38–47.

57. Hanley GE, et al. Postpartum hemorrhage and use of serotonin reuptake inhibitor antidepressants in pregnancy. Obstet Gynecol 2016; 127:53–61.

58. Grzeskowiak LE, et al. Antidepressant use in late gestation and risk of postpartum haemorrhage: a retrospective cohort study. BJOG 2016; 123:1929–1936.

59. Palmsten K, et al. Use of antidepressants near delivery and risk of postpartum hemorrhage: cohort study of low income women in the United States. BMJ 2013; 347:f4877.

60. Lupattelli A, et al. Risk of vaginal bleeding and postpartum hemorrhage after use of antidepressants in pregnancy: a study from the Norwegian Mother and Child Cohort Study. J Clin Psychopharmacol 2014; 34:143–148.

61. Uguz F. Is there any association between use of antidepressants and preeclampsia or gestational hypertension? A systematic review of current studies. J Clin Psychopharmacol 2017; 37:72–77.

62. Miller LJ. Use of electroconvulsive therapy during pregnancy. Hosp Community Psychiatry 1994; 45:444–450

63. Jennings KD, Ross S, Popper S, et al. Thoughts of harming infants in depressed and nondepressed mothers. J. Affect. Disord. 1999 ;54(1–2), 21–28.

64. O'Hara MW, Schlechte JA, Lewis DA, et al. Prospective study of postpartum blues. Biologic and psychosocial factors. Arch. Gen. Psychiatry 1991;48:801–806.

65. Sugawara M, Toda MA, Shima S, et al. Premenstrual mood changes and maternal mental health in pregnancy and the postpartum period. J. Clin. Psychol. 1997;53:225–232.

66. Campbell JC, Poland ML, Waller JB, et al. Correlates of battering during pregnancy. Res. Nurs. Health 1992 ;15:219–226.

67. Cox JL. Medical management, culture, and mental illness. Br. J Hosp Med 1982 ;27:533–537.

68. O'Hara M.WSocial support, life events, and depression during pregnancy and the puerperium. Arch. Gen. Psychiatry 1986;43: 569–573.

69. O'Hara MW, Rehm, L. P., and Campbell SB Postpartum depression. A role for social network and life stress variables. J. Nerv. Ment. Dis. 1983;171:336–341.

70. Paykel ES, Emms EM, Fletcher J, et al. Life events and social support in puerperal depression. Br. J. Psychiatry 1980;136:339–346.

71. Kendell RE. Emotional and physical factors in the genesis of puerperal mental disorders. J. Psychosom. Res. 1985;29:3–11.

72. Turton P, Hughes P, Evans CDH, et al. Incidence, correlates and predictors of post-traumatic stress disorder in the pregnancy after stillbirth. Br. J. Psychiatry 2001;178:556–560.

73. O'Hara MW, Rehm LP, and Campbell SB. Predicting depressive symptomatology: cognitive-behavioral models and postpartum depression. J. Abnorm. Psychol. 1982;91:457–461.

74. Playfair HR and Gowers JI. Depression following childbirth—a search for predictive signs. J. Roy. Coll. Gen. Pract. 1981;31:201–208.

75. Chandra PS, Venkatasubramanian G, and Thomas T. Infanticidal ideas and infanticidal behavior in Indian women with severe postpartum psychiatric disorders. J. Nerv. Ment. Dis. 2002;190:457–461.

76. Epperson CN, Wisner KL, and Yamamoto B. Gonadal steroids in the treatment of mood disorders. Psychosom. Med. 1999;61:676–697.

77. Gregoire AJ, Kumar R, Everitt B, et al. Transdermal oestrogen fo treatment of severe postnatal depression. Lancet 1996;347:930–933.

78. C Neill Epperson and Jennifer Ballew, Psychiatric disorders in pregnancy and the postpartum: principles and treatment/edited by Victoria Hendrick. 67–68.

79. Birndorf CA, Madden A, Portera L, et al. Psychiatric symptoms, functional impairment, and receptivity toward mental health treatment among obstetrical patients. Int. J. Psychiatry Med. 2001;31:355–365.

80. Kelly RH, Zatzick DF, and Anders TF. The detection and treatment of psychiatric disorders and substance use among pregnant women cared for in obstetrics. Am. J. Psychiatry 2001;158:213–219.

81. Stuart S, Couser G, Schilder K, et al. Postpartum anxiety and depression: Onset and comorbidity in a community sample. J. Nerv. Ment. Dis. 1998;186:420–424.

82. Wenzel A, Haugen EN, Jackson LC, and Brendle, JR. Anxiety symptoms and disorders at eight weeks postpartum. J. Anxiety Disord. 2005;19, 295–311.

83. Rapkin AJ, Mikacich JA, Moatakef-Imani B, and Rasgon N. The clinical nature and formal diagnosis of premenstrual, postpartum, and perimenopausal affective disorders. Curr. Psychiatry Rep. 2002;4:419–428.

84. Matthey S, Barnett B, Howie P, and Kavanagh DJDiagnosing postpartum depression in

mothers and fathers: Whatever happened to anxiety? J Affect Disord. 2003;74:139–147.

85. Cowley DS and Roy-Byrne PP. Panic disorder during pregnancy. J. Psychosom. Obstet. Gynaecol. 1989 ;10:193–210.

86. Wisner KL, Peindl KS, and Hanusa BH. Effects of childbearing on the natural history of panic disorder with comorbid mood disorder. J. Affect. Disord. 1996;41:173–180.

87. Abramowitz JS, Schwartz SA, and Moore KM. Obsessional thoughts in postpartum females and their partners: content, severity and relationship with depression. J. Clin. Psychol. Med. Settings 2003;10:157–164.

88. Sichel DA, Cohen LS, Dimmock JA, et al. Postpartum obsessive compulsive disorder: a case series. J. Clin. Psychiatry 1993;54:156–159.

89. Suri R and Burt V. The assessment and treatment of postpartum psychiatric disorders. J. Pract. Psychiatry Behav. Health 1997;3:67–77

90. Smith MV, Rosehheck, R. A., Cavaleri, M. A, et al. Screening for and detection of depression, panic disorder, and PTSD in public-sector obstetrics clinics. Psychiatr. Serv. 2004;55:407–414.

91. Ayers S and Pickering AD. Do women get posttraumatic stress disorder as a result of childbirth? A prospective study of incidence. Birth 2001;28:111–118.

92. Geller PA, Klier CM, and Neugebauer R Anxiety disorders following miscarriage. J. Clin. Psychiatry 2001;62:432–438.

93. Frost M, and Condon JT. The psychological sequelae of miscarriage: a critical review of the literature. Aust. NZ J. Psychiatry 1996 ;30, 54–62.

94. Geller PA, Kerns D, and Klier CM. Anxiety following miscarriage and the subsequent pregnancy: a review of the literature and future directions. J. Psychosom. Res. 2004;56:35–45.

95. Shear K and Mammen O. Anxiety disorders in pregnant and postpartum women. Psychopharmacol. Bull. 1995;31:693–703.

96. Brown CS. Depression and anxiety disorders. Obstet. Gynecol. Clin. North Am. 2001;28: 241–268.

97. Weisberg RB and Paquette JA. Screening and treatment of anxiety disorders in pregnant and lactating women. Women's Health Issues 2002;12, 32–36.

98. McGrath C, Buist A, and Norman TR. Treatment of anxiety during pregnancy: effects of psychotropic drug treatment on the developing fetus. Drug Safety 1999;20:171–186.

99. Burt VK and Hendrick VC. Clinical Manual of Women's Mental Health. Washington, DC: American Psychiatric Publishing Inc. 2005.

100. Abramowitz JS. Variants of exposure and response prevention in the treatment of obsessive compulsive disorder: a meta-analysis. Behav. Ther. 1996;27:583–600.

101. Fals-Stewart W, Marks AP, and Schafer JA. Comparison of behavioral group therapy and individual behavior therapy in treating obsessive-compulsive disorder. J. Nerv. Ment. Dis. 1993;181:189–193.

102. Lindsay M, Crino R, and Andrews G. Controlled trial of exposure and response prevention in obsessive-compulsive disorder. Br. J. Psychiatry 1997;171:135–139.

103. Foa EB, Liebowitz MR, Kozak MJ, et al. Treatfent of obsessive compulsive disorder by exposure and ritual prevention, clomipramine, and their combination: a randomized, placebo controlled trial. Am. J. Psychiatry. 2005;162: 151–161.

104. Barlow DH, Raffa SD, and Cohen EM. Psychosocial treatments for panic disorders, phobias, and generalized anxiety disorder. In: Nathan PE and Gorman JM, eds. A Guide to Treatments That Work, 2nd ed., New York: Oxford University Press, 2002;pp. 301–335.

105. Wisner KL, Parry BL, and Pointek CM Postpartum depression. N. Engl. J. Med. 2002; 347:194–199.

106. Boerner R and Moeller H. The importance of new antidepressants in the treatment of anxiety and depressive disorders. Pharmacopsychiatry 1999;32:119–126.

107. Viguera AC, et al. Risk of recurrence in women with bipolar disorder during pregnancy: prospective study of mood stabilizer discontinuation. Am J Psychiatry 2007; 164:1817–1824.

108. Taylor CL, et al. Predictors of severe relapse in pregnant women with psychotic or bipolar disorders. J Psychiatr Res 2018; 104:100–107.

109. National Institute for Health Care and Excellence. Antenatal and postnatal mental health: clinical management and service guidance. Clinical guideline [CG192] 2014 (Last updated February 2020); https://www.nice.org.uk/guidance/cg192

110. Breastfeeding, The Maudsley® Prescribing Guidelines in Psychiatry 14th Edition David M. Taylor, Thomas R. E. Barnes, and Allan H. Young 702–706.

Medical Management of Ectopic Pregnancy

• Siddesh Iyer • Parikshit Tank

Introduction

Ectopic pregnancy has a worldwide incidence of about 1 to 2%.[1]

Management options include observation, medical care, and surgery. It is vital to understand the medical treatment options. Whether to treat a particular patient with medical management or surgical treatment is an important aspect of management.

Although mortality has decreased to a significant extent, ectopic pregnancy remains a major cause of maternal morbidity. Methotrexate forms the backbone of this treatment.

Pharmacology of methotrexate: Methotrexate, a folate antagonist inactivates the enzyme dihydrofolate reductase and blocks synthesis of DNA. It acts mainly in the S-phase of the cell cycle. It acts on trophoblasts, at the transplantation site.[2]

Methotrexate (indications and contra-indications): Absolute contraindications are long-standing liver disease, lung disease, pre-existing blood dyscrasias, peptic ulcer, and immunodeficiency.

Hypersensitivity to the drug, pregnant and lactating mothers are not candidates for methotrexate therapy.

According to the National Institute for Health and Care Excellence (NICE) guideline NG126, systemic methotrexate should be offered to women who are not pregnant [confirmed by ultrasonography (USG) and are compliant for follow-up.

MEDICAL TREATMENT PROTOCOLS

Literature shows ectopic pregnancy successfully treated with methotrexate and leucovorin in alternating doses.[3–7]

The dose being 1 mg/kg intramuscular methotrexate with leucovorin factor rescue. Leucovorin or folinic acid, the active form of folate, it protects cells from the effects of methotrexate and reduces its side effects. This alternate day regimen continues until human chorionic gonadotropin (hCG) levels fall by 15% in 2 days. Patients can receive up to 4 doses, but they do not have to receive all 4 doses.

The success rate of such multiple-dose treatment in the study by Stovall, et al., was 96%.[7,8]

The 1991 single-dose protocol stated that on day 0, patient received 50 mg/m^2 methotrexate. It consisted of testing a series of hCG values 4 to 7 days after. A successful treatment is 15% reduction in hCG levels between 4th and 7th days **(Table 19.1)**.

In case, if a 15% reduction is not observed and patient is clinically stable, a repeat dose could be given on day 7.

Table 19.1: Different methotrexate regimens used to treat ectopic pregnancy (modified from Barnhart, et al.)[8]

Protocol	Dose MTX	Regimen	hCG measurement days	Treatment success	When to administer additional dose
Multidose	1 mg/kg and 0.1 mg/kg LEU	Alternate doses of each	0, 1, 3, 5, 7	hCG declines 15% from previous value	2nd, 3rd or 4th dose given if hCG does not decline by 15% from previous value. Maximum 4 doses
Single-dose	50 mg/m^2	Day 0	0, 4, 7	hCG declines 15% between day 4 and 7	Repeat dose on day 7, if hCG does not decline 15%
Two-dose	50 mg/m^2	Day 0, Day 4	0, 4, 7	hCG declines 15% between day 4 and 7	Repeat course on day 7, if hCG does not decline 15%

MTX: Methotrexate; LEU: Leucovorin

29 out of 30 patients (96.7%) who were enrolled in this study, were successfully treated.[9]

The convenience of this method made it popular. In 1993, an extended study of 120 patients with single dose of methotrexate treatment was reported of whom 113 (94.2%) were successfully treated. Of these, 4 patients required a second dose of methotrexate on day 7.[10]

The overall success rate for single-dose protocols was 88.1% as per one meta analysis with 95% CIs of 86 to 90%.[8] Single-dose protocols require fewer visits and fewer injections.

A new protocol was introduced in 2007 to increase effectiveness and maintain convenience.[11] The goal of this treatment was to administer methotrexate on day 0 and day 4, while continuing to monitor hCG levels the same days. Therefore, no additional visits were required.

A reduction in hCG from day 4 to day 7 by 15% was considered successful treatment in this protocol. The second cycle was performed on day 7, if adequate hCG lowering was not observed. If 15% decline was not found between days 11 and 14, the patient needed referral for surgical treatment. Out of a total 101 patients 88% were medically treated.[12] Of those undergoing surgical management, only 3% had a ruptured ectopic pregnancy. There has not been a well-powered comparative study between the two-dose protocol and the single-dose protocol, or the multidose protocol.

Choice for Medical Management

hCG values above 5,000, moderate-large free fluid on ultrasound, fetal heart activity, serum hCG rising over a 48 hour period are poor candidates for medical management **(Table 19.2)**.[13] Mol, et al.[14] recommend single-dose methotrexate for initial hCG values <1,500 and multidose methotrexate for initial values <3,000.

What treatment to choose, medical or surgical, depends on the discussion between the doctor and the patient. There is no true cut-off below which methotrexate therapy will be more successful. As the hCG value increases, the success rate decreases. One must modify consent to use methotrexate in women with high hCG as per the hCG value, and patients need to understand that these are candidates more likely to fail.

Methotrexate use requires multiple doctor's visits and several weeks of hCG monitoring. Women do not prefer multiple visits due to competing demands for time.

Table 19.2: Choice for medical treatment

Contraindicated	Good candidate	Poor candidate
• Hemodynamically not stable • Suspected ruptured ectopic • Sensitivity to the drug • Intrauterine pregnancy • Breastfeeding • Active lung disease • Kidney disease • Chronic liver disease • Pre-existing blood dyscrasia • Immunodeficiency • Peptic ulcer • Unable to comply with visits and follow-up	• Hemodynamically stable • Low-beta-hCG (<5000 mIU/ml) • Size of mass <3.5 cm • Unruptured mass • Certainty that there is no IUP • No embryonic cardiac activity • Willingness for follow-up • No known sensitivity to MTX	• High-beta-hCG (>5000 mIU/ml) • Size of mass >3.5 cm • Presence of embryonic cardiac activity • Significant abdominal pain • IUP has not been ruled out • Not sure if she will come for all outpatient visits

As per a study evaluating compliance with methotrexate therapy, only 45.5% of patients completed follow-up[15] Only one-fifth of them completed 'adequate' follow-up, defined as days 4, 7, and weekly until beta-hCG levels were not detectable. 24% of patients in this group required surgery. It is not right to offer single-dose therapy to women who may have compliance issues because it is a 'single dose'. A drawback of the single dose is that a woman may be falsely reassured that treatment for an ectopic pregnancy is complete after the injection and so may not comply with the required follow-up care.

As per another study, patients of lower socioeconomic status were more likely to fail methotrexate treatment by about five times.[16] Whether the cause of this increased failure rate was a delayed disease course, poor compliance, or whether it is due to a true biological disorder, it is not clear.

Risks of Methotrexate Treatment

One must know the risks and side effects when administering methotrexate therapy. Risk of rupture ranges from 7 to 14%. How fast the hCG rises is a predictor of rupture.[17] Most ruptures occurred when increase of hCG was at least by two-thirds or 66% after 48 hours or continued to rise in spite of treatment.

The commonest side effects are mild and include nausea, vomiting, mouth sores, diarrhea, and hepatic derangement. Rare but serious side effects include nephrotoxicity, interstitial pneumonitis, and alopecia dermatitis. Side effects are dose and treatment limited.

Risks of Treating Intrauterine Pregnancy

An intrauterine pregnancy is an absolute contraindication to use methotrexate. Despite this, treatment of pregnancies of unknown locations with methotrexate is quite common.[18]

About 50% with high hCG and no evidence of intrauterine pregnancy on ultrasound may have an intrauterine pregnancy rather than an ectopic pregnancy.[19–21]

There are reports documenting intrauterine pregnancies after women have been treated with methotrexate. In many cases, treatment of intrauterine pregnancies leads to miscarriage. However, in some women treated for undiagnosed ectopic pregnancies, there have been offsprings with birth defects. There are reports documenting teratogenicity of methotrexate. There have been instances in patients with psoriasis who have taken oral methotrexate for short-term, in low doses during early pregnancy where fetuses have had craniofacial, skeletal, cardiovascular, and gastrointestinal abnormalities.[22–24]

Inappropriate treatment with methotrexate, hence is a cause of medical liability.

SUMMARY

Methotrexate as a drug is safe and effective in well-selected cases. Methotrexate allows patients to avoid surgery, but it also has some drawbacks. Treatment requires extensive patient follow-up and can be difficult for some women. Patients must be followed clinically until serum hCG becomes undetectable. However, one must remember that this requires number of visits that consumes valuable time for both patients and physicians. A few studies suggest that ovarian function may worsen with methotrexate in the short term, while others do not agree on this.[25,26]

In conclusion, case selection is paramount for the treatment of ectopic pregnancy with methotrexate.

Confirming the diagnosis is essential to avoid unnecessary administration of the drug, as it does have significant effects on the mother and the fetus.[27]

Serum hCG or ultrasound at follow-up can avoid unnecessary administration of methotrexate. In addition, patients should be counseled well, and must be willing to follow-up, and have no absolute contraindications to methotrexate.

References

1. Creanga AA, Shapiro-Mendoza CK, Bish CL, Zane S, Berg CJ, Callaghan WM. Mortality trends from ectopic pregnancy in the United States: 1980-2007. Obstetrician and gynecologist. 2011; 117:837–43. [PubMed][Google Scholar]

2. Barnhart K, Coutifaris C, Esposito M. The pharmacology of methotrexate. expert opinion 2001;2:409–17. [PubMed] [Google Scholar]

3. ACOG Practice Bulletin No. 94: Medical Management of Tubal Pregnancy. Obstetrician and gynecologist. 2008;111:1479–85. [PubMed] [Google Scholar]

4. Tanaka T, Hayashi H, Kutsuzawa T, Fujimoto S, Ichinoe K. Treatment of interstitial ectopic pregnancy with methotrexate: a successful case report. 1982;37:851–2. [PubMed] [Google Scholar]

5. Rodi IA, Sauer MV, Gorrill MJ, et al. Medical management of non-ruptured ectopic pregnancy with methotrexate and citrobolam rescue: preliminary experience. fertile sterile 1986;46:811–3. [PubMed] [Google Scholar]

6. Stovall TG, Ling FW, Buster JE. Exogenous chemotherapy for unruptured ectopic pregnancy. Fertile sterile. 1989;51:435–8. [PubMed] [Google Scholar]

7. Stovall TG, Ling FW, Gray LA, Carson SA, Buster JE. Methotrexate treatment of uninterrupted ectopic pregnancy: 100 reports. Obstetrician and gynecologist. 1991;77:749–53. [PubMed] [Google Scholar]

8. Barnhart KT, Gosman G, Ashby R, Sammel M. Medical management of ectopic pregnancy: a meta-analysis comparing 'single dose' and 'multiple dose' therapy. Obstetrician and gynecologist 2003; 101:778–84. [PubMed] [Google Scholar]

9. Stovall TG, Ling FW, Gray LA. A single dose of methotrexate to treat ectopic pregnancy. Obstetrician and gynecologist. 1991;77:754–7. [PubMed] [Google Scholar]

10. Stovall TG, Ling FW. Single-Dose Methotrexate: An Extended Clinical Trial. American Journal of Obstetrics and Gynecology. 1993; 168: 1759–62. Discussion 62–5. [PubMed] [Google Scholar]

11. K Barnhart, AC Hummel, MD Sammel, S. Menon, J. Jain, N. Chakhtoura. Fertile sterile. 2007;87:250–6. [PubMed] [Google Scholar]

12. Lipscomb GH, McCord ML, Stovall TG, Huff G, Portera SG, Ling FW. Predictors of methotrexate treatment success in women with ectopic pregnancy. N Engl J Med 1999;341:1974–8. [PubMed] [Google Scholar]

13. Menon S, Collins J, Bernhardt KT. Establishing human chorionic gonadotropin limits for guidance in the treatment of ectopic pregnancy with methotrexate: a systematic review. Fertile sterile. 2007;87:481–4. [PubMed] [Google Scholar]

14. Mol F, Mol BW, Ankum WM, van der Veen F, Hajenius PJ. Current evidence on surgery, systemic methotrexate, and follow-up in the treatment of ectopic pregnancy: a systematic review and meta-analysis. Renewal of human reproduction. 2008, 14:309–19. [PubMed] [Google Scholar]

15. Jaspan D, Giraldo-Isaza M, Dandolu V, Cohen AW. Adherence to methotrexate therapy for suspected ectopic pregnancy in an urban population. Fertile sterile. 2010;94:1122–4. [PubMed][Google Scholar]

16. Butts SF, Gibson E, Sammel MD, Shaunik A, Rudick B, Barnhart K. Race, socioeconomic status, response to methotrexate treatment of ectopic pregnancies in an urban population. Fertile sterile. 2010;94:2789–92. [PMC free article] [PubMed] [Google Scholar]

17. Dudley PS, Heard MJ, Sangi-Haghpeykar H, Carson SA, Buster JE. Characterization of an ectopic pregnancy that ruptures despite treatment with methotrexate Fertile sterile. 2004;82:1374–8. [PubMed] [Google Scholar]

18. Barnhart KT, Fay CA, Suescum M, et al. Clinical factors affecting the accuracy of ultrasonography during early symptomatic pregnancy. Obstetrician and gynecologist. 2011; 117:299–306. [PubMed] [Google Scholar]

19. Barnhart KT, Katz I, Hummel A, Gracia CR. Suspected diagnosis of ectopic pregnancy. Obstetrician and gynecologist. 2002; 100:505–10. [PubMed][Google Scholar]

20. Chung K, Chandavarkar U, Opper N, Barnhart K. Reassessing the role of dilatation and cruttage in the diagnostic of unknown location of a pregnancy diagnosis. Fertile sterile. 2011;96:659–62. [PubMed] [Google Scholar]

21. Shaunik A, Kulp J, Appleby DH, Collection MD, Barnhart KT. Usefulness of dilation and curettage in diagnosing unplaced pregnancies. American Journal of Obstetrics and Gynecology. 2011;204:130, e1-6. [PubMed] [Google Scholar]

22. Nguyen C, Duhl AJ, Escallon CS, Blakemore KJ. Multiple abnormalities in fetuses exposed to low-dose methotrexate in early pregnancy. Obstetrician and gynecologist. 2002;99:599–602. [PubMed] [Google Scholar]

23. Addar MH. Methotrexate embryopathy in a surviving intrauterine fetus after diagnosis of suspected ectopic pregnancy: A case report. J Obstet Gynaecol Can. 2004;26:1001–3. [PubMed] [Google Scholar]

24. Usta IM, Nassar AH, Unis KA, Abu-Musa AA. Methotrexate embryopathy after treatment of a misdiagnosed ectopic pregnancy. International Journal of Gynecology and Obstetrics: Official body of the International Union of Gynecology and Obstetrics. 2007;99:253–5. [PubMed] [Google Scholar]

25. McLaren JF, Burney RO, Milki AA, Westphal LM, Dahan MH, Lathi RB. Effects of methotrexate exposure on subsequent fertility in women undergoing controlled ovarian stimulation. Fertile sterile. 2009;92:515–9. [PubMed] [Google Scholar]

26. Oriol B, Barrio A, Pacheco A, Serna J, Zuzuarregui JL, Garcia-Velasco JA. Systemic methotrexate used to treat ectopic pregnancy affects ovarian reserve. not give Fertile sterile. 2008;90:1579–82. [PubMed] [Google Scholar]

27. ASRM Practice Bulletin.Treatment of ectopic pregnancy. Fertile sterile. 2006;86:S96–102. [PubMed] [Google Scholar]

Micronutrient Supplementation in Obstetrics and Gynecology

• Komal Chavan • Anusha Devalla

Introduction

The intake of micronutrients has a role to play in all the stages of a woman's reproductive period. This is especially true during the periods of pregnancy and lactation and the formative years of a child development as 'the first thousand days' of life contribute to the phenotypic development. During this period, they are particularly susceptible to the various environmental factors which can adversely affect the genome. The levels of fat-soluble vitamins can vary as the fat storage content increases towards mid-gestation. Here, can be significant shifts in the serum levels of the important trace elements and minerals. Adequate micronutrient supplementation is also essential in women planning conception and those in their menopause. A paradigm shift in the diet to poor habits have dramatically increased the obesity rates, especially in the developing countries. Bariatric surgery further compromises the absorption of these micronutrients. Expectedly, it is also noticed in the pregnant women from underdeveloped countries, who face nutritional insufficiency including micronutrient deficiency leading to poor perinatal outcomes and long-term adverse effects in the foetus (Barker hypothesis). World Health Organization (WHO) in collaboration with the United States, has introduced the Every Newborn action plan to mitigate the adverse birth outcomes. Table 20.1 shows the various outcomes related to micronutrient deficiency.

Table 20.1: Antenatal nutritional interventions and outcomes of interest[1]

Maternal outcome	Fetal/Neonatal outcomes
Infections	Neonatal infections
Anemia	Small for gestational age
Pre-eclampsia/eclampsia	Low birthweight
Gestational diabetes mellitus	Preterm birth
Increased maternal mortality	Increased fetal/neonatal mortality
Improper lactation	Nutritional deficiencies in the neonate
Impaired fertility (poor oocyte quality)	Non-communicable diseases in adulthood
Delayed wound healing	

MINERALS

1. Iron

Deficiency: Maternal nutritional anaemia amounts to 40% prevalence of anaemia globally, highest in the South-east Asian population. Anaemia has been associated with increased pregnancy-related complications, especially pre-eclampsia, intrauterine growth restriction, labour dystocia and postpartum hemorrhage. Iron requirements can increase to more than twice the pre-pregnancy requirements mainly owing to rapid expansion of fetoplacental and maternal red cell mass. Supplementation with iron to about 30–60 mg/day will meet the steadily increasing requirements from 0.8 mg in the first trimester to >6 mg/day in the last 3 months, as also supported by WHO.[2] Prophylactic supplementation with iron has shown to reduce maternal mortality by 70% but the results cannot be equally extrapolated to the non-anaemic women.[3]

Excess: Excessive iron intake can lead to type-2 diabetes, hypertension, metabolic syndrome causing adverse cardiovascular risk profile secondary to inflammation. In pregnancy, such changes have been linked to pregnancy-induced hypertensive disorders. It has been shown to increase platelet aggregation and thrombosis as well as linked to inflammatory signalling and colorectal tumourogenesis. Targetted iron supplementation therapies around periconceptional period can effectively reduce the possible risks.[4]

Multiple micronutrient supplementation (MMS), including iron and folic acid, commonly prescribed in various programmes is not currently recommended by WHO.[5]

Menorrhagia is undoubtedly the most important cause of anaemia. Therefore, women experiencing heavy blood loss should consume iron-rich foods, such as cooked green leafy vegetables, dried fruits, beans, cooked chicken, liver and kidneys and Brewer's yeast. Yogurt, citrus fruits and sour foods can aid in the absorption of iron.

2. Folic Acid

The US Preventive Services Task Force recommends daily supplementation of 400–800 micrograms folic acid in order to prevent neural tube defects.[6]

Deficiency: Increased requirements of folic acid to be started pre-conceptional at doses around 5 mg are required for those women who are on anticonvulsants, previous baby affected with neural tube defect and known maternal diabetes and hemoglobinopathies.[7]

A reduction in the incidence of autism spectrum disorders around 33% has been observed in a recent meta-analysis,[8] in addition to decrease in the incidence of small-for-gestational age babies.[9]

Simultaneous supplementation of vitamin B_{12} and folic acid is essential as the latter might precipitate B_{12} deficiency.

Excess: Despite the known benefits, excess consumption has been linked to certain reactive airway diseases, insulin resistance, and variable fetal development and carcinogenesis.[10] Currently, there is no change in the consensus on folic acid recommendation.

Reproductive performance and consequent reduced fertility are believed to be a result of poor intake of micronutrients and healthy lifestyle patterns with adequate omega 3 and folic acid is found to be beneficial to achieve better fertility outcomes and live birth rates.[11]

3. Calcium

Calcium is an essential micronutrient required for fetal skeletal development; especially in the third trimester. Studies on various micronutrients have provided insights on the role of prevention of pre-eclampsia with calcium supplementation with recommended daily dose being 1000 mg. WHO recommends daily intake in the range of 1.5–2 g.[4] However, there is variable sub-optimal intake of calcium as per regional differences.[12] A pooled analysis conducted on 28,000 women concluded that there is a reduction of about 46%, 53% and 50% in the incidence of pre-eclampsia, respectively. This favourable observation is not clinically evident in healthy nulliparous women with adequate calcium intake and is found controversial with respect to preterm birth and low-birth weight.[10]

Calcium is considered to play an important role in follicular development and maturation. It also has been hypothesized that vitamin D receptor (VDR) has been associated with calcium. Most polycystic ovarian syndrome (PCOS) patients have been found associated with calcium deficiency. Calcium levels have been found to be reduced in obese women with PCOS compared with healthy individuals. Recently, the role of vitamin D supplementation in combination with calcium 1500 mg for 6 months has been highlighted to improve the body mass index in PCOS women.[13]

4. Iodine

Deficiency has been known to be associated with fetal and neonatal hypothyroidism as well as adverse effects on neonatal cognitive development. WHO recommends daily consumption of 250 µg of iodine in the diet. The significance of this was emphasized and promotion of iodized salt in the last decade.

Excess consumption of iodine can lead to fetal goitre, as reported in Japanese women whose diet is high in seaweeds, but studies suggesting a safe upper limit in pregnancy are sparse.

5. Selenium

Selenium is essential to convert the inactive to active form of thyroid hormones as well as is incorporated in enzymes for protein synthesis, antioxidative and immunomodulatory mechanisms.[4]

Deficiency: Various observational studies quoted daily recommended intake up to 60 mg and women with lower levels have higher probability of early pregnancy loss, intrahepatic cholestasis of pregnancy and pre-eclampsia. These can be due to various suggested mechanisms such as markedly reduced antioxidative protective mechanisms that lead to implantation disorders, but results need further validation.

Selenium supplementation in the antenatal and postnatal period can reduce the incidence of thyroiditis and thus hypothyroidism, probably by complex interactions among the various enzymes in the thyroid hormone synthesis pathway and this negates the counterbalance seen in the postpartum immunological rebound.[4]

Excess: On the contrary, various epidemiological studies report high serum-selenium levels and its association to hyperglycaemia, type-II diabetes mellitus and dyslipidaemia, possibly because of interplay between selenoproteins and insulin-directed signalling pathways. This mechanism is also implicated in the pathogenesis of PCOS.

PCOS: Selenium, being an antioxidant mineral, helps in curbing the free radicals that is considered important for the normal functioning of reproductive tissues. Hence, its lower levels has been linked to increased levels of luteinizing hormones, androgens such as testosterone.

Its excess has also been implicated in nervous system abnormalities, gastrointestinal symptoms, rash and hair damage; noted at levels >850 µg/day.

6. Magnesium

Magnesium is known to play a vital function in cardiac, muscular and nervous excitability, DNA and protein synthesis and body temperature regulation.

Deficiency: Normally, its deficiency is extremely rare but may occur in high demand and dilutional states, such as pregnancy. Higher first trimester intake may lead to higher birthweight, while it is known to mitigate the risk of intrauterine growth restriction and pre-eclampsia.

In vitro fertilization (IVF): An observational study has shown that higher levels of magnesium have proven to have better reproductive outcomes and its supplementation is beneficial prior to IVF procedures.[15]

7. Zinc

Zinc is a crucial element participating in antioxidant protective mechanisms, protein and carbohydrate metabolism, synthesis of nucleic acids and various steps of embryogenesis.

Deficiency: Disturbance in zinc homeostasis may have deleterious effects on pregnancy outcome, including pre-eclampsia, fetal growth restriction, intrauterine death and prolonged labour. Randomized double blind controlled trials say 25 mg daily supplementation is recommended in pregnancy.

Recent studies from Turkey and India emphasize the need for zinc intake in pregnancy, as the deficiency has been postulated to pre-eclampsia possibly to abnormal lipid metabolism and peroxidation, increased zinc binding-protein and estrogen levels. Its deficiency in the pathogenesis of pre-eclampsia is still not clear.[4]

PCOS: Lower levels of zinc have been reported in women with PCOS and treating this is suggested to improve insulin sensitivity.

8. Manganese

Manganese acts as a cofactor in the enzymes involved in the metabolic and detoxification processes in the placenta. The main source is through diet and circulating serum manganese concentrations have been observed to be lower in women with fetal growth restriction as mentioned by Zota, et al., indicating the manganese in maintaining fetal growth amongst all the micronutrients. It has been demonstrated by Than, et al., that manganese deficiency can lead to premature uterine contractions. Further studies on the role of manganese are required to highlight its importance as a supplement in pregnancy.[4]

9. Chromium

Chromium has been postulated to play an important role in lipid and carbohydrate

Table 20.2: Recommended dietary allowances (RDA) supplementation of micronutrients in pregnancy[14]

S. No.	Micronutrient	Recommended intake
1.	Vitamin A (µg)	800
2.	Vitamin D (IU)	200
3.	Vitamin E (mg)	10
4.	Niacin (mg)	18
5.	Folic acid (µg)	400
6.	Vitamin B_1 (mg)	1.4
7.	Vitamin B_2 (mg)	1.4
8.	Vitamin B_6 (mg)	1.9
9.	Vitamin B_{12} (µg)	2.6
10.	Vitamin C (mg)	70
11.	Zinc (mg)	15
12.	Iron (mg)	30
13.	Selenium (µg)	65
14.	Copper (mg)	2
15.	Iodine (µg)	150

metabolism. It might not improve the reproductive function but has shown to benefit patients with hirsutism.

Table 20.2 shows Recommended dietary allowences (RDA) supplementation of micronutrients in pregnancy.

VITAMINS

1. Vitamin A

Excess: In humans, isotretinoin, a synthetic retinoid but not β-carotene (precursor of Vitamin A), poses a 25 times increased risk of congenital malformations, mainly affecting the development of neural crest cells. Vitamin A may become toxic, if the dose in pregnancy exceeds 10,000 IU daily or 25,000 IU weekly. Therefore, due to uncertainty in the vitamin A content fortified in some foods, they should be best avoided in pregnancy (eggs, liver). The symptoms of acute vitamin A toxicity dizziness, nausea, vomiting, headaches, skin exfoliation, blurred vision, vertigo, reduced muscle coordination, weight loss and fatigue.[12]

Adult women suffering from menorrhagia may have reduced serum levels of vitamin A. One study in which vitamin A at a dose of 60,000 U for 35 days was used to treat women with menorrhagia showed a considerable reduction in blood loss compared to the placebo group.

Vitamin A has shown to have an inverse correlation with the risk of uterine fibroids, mainly associated with preformed vitamin A derived from animal sources. Modern studies reveal no significant correlation between intake of vitamins C and E and the incidence of leiomyoma. Vitamin D is significantly associated, unlike other vitamins, specific to white women and uterine leiomyoma and can serve as a potent pharmacological agent in future.[16]

With regards to micronutrient consumption, extensive literature is available suggesting that risk of cervical dysplasia is significantly reduced with higher intake of vitamin A, E and E apart from folate, lycopene and beta-carotene. Biologically, they may have a role as an antioxidant and HPV persistence and defective DNA synthesis.[16]

2. Vitamin C, E

Vitamin C (ascorbic acid and dehyroascorbic acid), is an essential water-soluble vitamin found widely in fruit and vegetables; it has important roles in collagen synthesis, antioxidant, wound healing and prevention of anaemia. Vitamin E (α-tocopherol) is a lipid-soluble vitamin acting with the lipid membrane and with synergistic interactions with vitamin C. Vitamin C is commonly included in low doses (<200 mg/day) within multivitamin preparations for pregnancy, but has also been given in higher doses (up to 1000 mg/day) as a supplement, alone or in combination with vitamin E.

A considerable interest exists regarding prevention of maternal and perinatal morbidity with vitamins C and E. However, the most recent meta-analysis of ten trials (6533 women) published in 2008 of antioxidant supplementation (including vitamin C and E but also other supplements, such as lycopene) showed no difference in the relative risk (RR) of pre-eclampsia (RR 0.73, 95% CI 0.51 to 1.06), pre-term birth (before 37 weeks) (RR 1.10, 95% CI 0.99 to 1.22), SGA infants (RR 0.83, 95% CI 0.62 to 1.11), or any baby death (RR 1.12, 95% CI 0.81 to 1.53). In the absence of further evidence, routine supplementation with higher dose vitamin C and E is not recommended as they can be potentially dangerous in high concentrations.

3. Vitamin D

Vitamin D is a fat-soluble hormone that plays a pivotal role in calcium, magnesium, and phosphate homeostasis and as an anti-proliferative and immunomodulatory mediator.

It is primarily obtained via skin production from sunlight exposure and only one-fifth via nutritional intake, consuming fortified milk or juice, fish oils, and dietary supplements. It also is produced endogenously in the skin with exposure to sunlight. Physiologically, active form of vitamin D is 1,25-dihydroxyvitamin D. This active form is essential to promote absorption of calcium from the gut and enables normal bone mineralization and growth.

The risk factors for vitamin D deficiency in pregnancy include Asian/black ethnicity, maternal low sun exposure, maternal obesity and choices of clothing. Vitamin D deficiency can lead to multiple obstetric complications, such as pre-eclampsia, disorders of bone formation in fetus, gestational diabetes, preterm labour and birth and higher risk of caesarean section.

International bodies like British National formulary have recommended daily Vitamin D supplementation of 400 IU. On the other hand, the WHO does not support universal supplementation. High-quality randomised trials are still required to assess the effect of vitamin D supplementation on pregnancy and newborn outcomes.

Optimum serum levels in pregnancy are still a matter of debate and some studies have come to a consensus of at least 20 ng/ml (50 nmol/L) to maintain bone health. There is inconsistent evidence to recommend universal screening for vitamin D levels in pregnant women. For those who are at an increased risk for vitamin D deficiency as mentioned before, maternal serum levels can be measured and individualized treatment offered. When identified, it must be treated with a dose of 1000–2000 IU per day in pregnancy. Lesser studies are available to supplement it routinely to prevent pre-eclampsia.

It is typically a part of the prenatal vitamins containing 400 IU of vitamin D per tablet. Most prenatal vitamins, typically contain 400 international units of vitamin D per tablet. Deriving the conclusions from recent studies, the authors in a recent clinical report from the Committee on Nutrition of American Academy of Pediatrics have suggested a daily intake to maintain the serum vitamin D levels in pregnancy.[17]

Conflicting results have been seen regarding the beneficial effects of vitamin D supplementation in PCOS women. It is thought to reduce the serum total testosterone, free androgen index, hirsutism and C-reactive protein levels apart from a significant increase in sex hormone binding globulin when compared to placebo, with improved menstrual regularity, but no significant difference in BMI or waist and hip circumference has been observed. Further research is needed to validate the use of Vitamin D supplementation in subfertile patients and PCOS patients due to limited benefit.[15,16]

Observational studies and meta-analysis have identified a potential association of breast cancer with vitamin-D deficiency. Some recent observations, however, refute any such association and therefore warrant further investigation.[16]

Vitamin D has shown to decrease the pro-inflammatory cytokines, *in vitro* and thus has been suggested to stop the cascade causing primary dysmenorrhea.

4. Vitamin K

Menorrhagia: A few studies have investigated vitamin K (phylloquinone) injection to treat primary dysmenorrhea. Treatment with phylloquinone is thought to reduce the blood loss, hence may be helpful to treat primary dysmenorrhea, due to its action on prothrombin.[15]

Changes in micronutrient absorption after bariatric surgery: Appropriate gap after undergoing a bariatric surgery is important, as this has been linked to cause small-for-gestational age babies due to micronutrient deficiencies.[4] The Paleo diet promoted post-surgery, focusses on fat-excess and low carbohydrate diet which can improve

Table 20.3: Recommended dietary allowances of micronutrients in postmenopausal women.[19]

S. No.	Nutrient	Reference intake
1.	Vitamin A (μg)	700
2.	Vitamin E (mg)	15
3.	Vitamin D (μg)	15
4.	Vitamin K (μg)	90
5.	Thiamine (mg)	1.1
6.	Riboflavin (mg)	1.1
7.	Niacin (mg)	14
8.	B_6 (mg)	1.5
9.	B_5 (mg)	5
10.	B_{12} (μg)	2.4
11.	Vitamin C (mg)	75
12.	Biotin (μg)	30
13.	Iron (mg)	8
14.	Folate (μg)	400
15.	Zinc (mg)	8
16.	Magnesium (mg)	320
17.	Selenium (μg)	55
18.	Calcium (mg)	1200
19.	Phosphorus (mg)	700
20.	Potassium (mg)	4700

glucose tolerance and anaemia; but published studies also show that it can lead to low-birth weight.[4] Less gastric acid, bile and pancreatic enzymes are available for the absorption of nutrients.[18]

Postmenopausal women, often under-estimated, require supplementation of micronutrients for their good health. **Table 20.3** shows the RDA of micronutrients in postmenopausal women and **Table 20.4** shows vitamin requirement of a non-pregnant woman.

Table 20.4: Recommended dietary allowances of micronutrients in non-pregnant woman[14]

S. No.	Micronutrient	Reference intake
1.	Vitamin A (ug)	700
2.	Vitamin D (ug)	15
3.	Vitamin E (mg)	15
4.	Vitamin B_1 (mg)	1.1
5.	Vitamin B_2 (mg)	1.1
6.	Vitamin B_3 (mg)	14
7.	Vitamin B_6 (mg)	1.3

References

1. Beulen YH, Super S, de Vries JHM, Koelen MA, Feskens EJM, Wagemakers A. Dietary Interventions for Healthy Pregnant Women: A Systematic Review of Tools to Promote a Healthy Antenatal Dietary Intake. Nutrients. 2020 Jul 3;12(7):E1981.

2. Bothwell TH. Iron requirements in pregnancy and strategies to meet them. Am J Clin Nutr. 2000 Jul;72(1 Suppl):257S-264S.

3. Cantor AG, Bougatsos C, Dana T, Blazina I, McDonagh M. Routine iron supplementation and screening for iron deficiency anemia in pregnancy: a systematic review for the US. Preventive Services Task Force. Ann Intern Med. 2015 Apr 21;162(8):566–76.

4. Mistry HD, Williams PJ. The Importance of Antioxidant Micronutrients in Pregnancy. Oxid Med Cell Longev. 2011 Sep 13;2011:e841749.

5. Caniglia EC, Zash R, Swanson SA, Smith E, Sudfeld C, Finkelstein JL, et al. Iron, folic acid, and multiple micronutrient supplementation strategies during pregnancy and adverse birth outcomes in Botswana. Lancet Glob Health. 2022 Jun 1;10(6):e850–61.

6. Jun S, Gahche JJ, Potischman N, Dwyer JT, Guenther PM, Sauder KA, et al. Dietary Supplement Use and Its Micronutrient Contribution During Pregnancy and Lactation in the United States. Obstet Gynecol. 2020 Mar;135(3):623–33.

7. Folic Acid Supplementation for the Prevention of Neural Tube Defects: An Updated Evidence Report and Systematic Review for the US Preventive Services Task Force | Guidelines | JAMA | JAMA Network [Internet]. [cited 2022 Aug 28]. Available from: https://jamanetwork.com/journals/jama/fullarticle/2596299

8. Wang M, Li K, Zhao D, Li L. The association between maternal use of folic acid supplements during pregnancy and risk of autism spectrum disorders in children: a meta-analysis. Mol Autism. 2017;8:51.

9. Hodgetts VA, Morris RK, Francis A, Gardosi J, Ismail KM. Effectiveness of folic acid supplementation in pregnancy on reducing the risk of small-for-gestational age neonates: a population study, systematic review and meta-analysis. BJOG Int J Obstet Gynaecol. 2015 Mar;122(4):478–90.

10. Parisi F, di Bartolo I, Savasi VM, Cetin I. Micronutrient supplementation in pregnancy: Who, what and how much? Obstet Med. 2019 Mar;12(1):5–13.

11. Gaskins AJ, Chavarro JE. Diet and fertility: a review. Am J Obstet Gynecol. 2018 Apr; 218(4):379–89.

12. Heppe DHM, Medina-Gomez C, Hofman A, Franco OH, Rivadeneira F, Jaddoe VWV. Maternal first-trimester diet and childhood bone mass: the Generation R Study. Am J Clin Nutr. 2013 Jul;98(1):224–32.

13. Kadoura S, Alhalabi M, Nattouf AH. Effect of Calcium and Vitamin D Supplements as an Adjuvant Therapy to Metformin on Menstrual Cycle Abnormalities, Hormonal Profile, and IGF-1 System in Polycystic Ovary Syndrome Patients: A Randomized, Placebo-Controlled Clinical Trial. Adv Pharmacol Sci. 2019 Jul 1;2019:e9680390.

14. Oh C, Keats EC, Bhutta ZA. Vitamin and Mineral Supplementation During Pregnancy on Maternal, Birth, Child Health and Development Outcomes in Low- and Middle-Income Countries: A Systematic Review and Meta-Analysis. Nutrients. 2020 Feb 14;12(2):491.

15. Ciebiera M, Esfandyari S, Siblini H, Prince L, Elkafas H, Wojtyła C, et al. Nutrition in Gynecological Diseases: Current Perspectives. Nutrients. 2021 Apr 2;13(4):1178.

16. Afrin S, AlAshqar A, El Sabeh M, Miyashita-Ishiwata M, Reschke L, Brennan JT, et al. Diet and Nutrition in Gynecological Disorders: A Focus on Clinical Studies. Nutrients. 2021 May 21;13(6):1747.

17. Vitamin D: Screening and Supplementation During Pregnancy [Internet]. [cited 2022 Jul 16]. Available from: https://www.acog.org/en/clinical/clinical-guidance/committee-opinion/articles/2011/07/vitamin-d-screening-and-supplementation-during-pregnancy

18. Devlieger R, Guelinckx I, Jans G, Voets W, Vanholsbeke C, Vansant G. Micronutrient Levels and Supplement Intake in Pregnancy after Bariatric Surgery: A Prospective Cohort Study. PLOS ONE. 2014 Dec 3;9(12):e114192.

19. Mansour A, Ahadi Z, Qorbani M, Hosseini S. Association between dietary intake and seasonal variations in postmenopausal women. J Diabetes Metab Disord. 2014 Apr 25;13:52.

Prevention and Treatment of Postpartum Haemorrhage including Carbetocin

• Pradnya Changede • Rahul Mayekar

Introduction

Postpartum haemorrhage (PPH) is an important cause of maternal morbidity and mortality in low-income countries. At a global level 25% of maternal deaths occur due to PPH. PPH is responsible for 38% of maternal deaths in India. PPH is reported in 2–4% of vaginal deliveries and in 6% caesarean deliveries. 295,000 women died during antepartum period or during childbirth in 2017. PPH is responsible for 99% of maternal deaths occurring in low- and middle-income countries.[1]

Definition of PPH[2]

Table 21.1 shows different definitions of PPH.

TYPES OF PPH

1. *Primary PPH:* Postpartum haemorrhage occurring in first 24 hours after delivery
2. *Secondary PPH:* Postpartum haemorrhage occurring from 24 hours post-delivery to 12 weeks after delivery.[2]

Incidence of PPH: The incidence of PPH is 5% of deliveries (when blood loss is not

Table 21.1: Definitions of PPH

1. World Health Organisation 2. French College of Gynaecologists and Obstetricians	Blood loss >500 ml irrespective of route of delivery.
3. International Federation of Gynecology and Obstetrics 4. Chinese ministry of health and Queensland health authority 5. German society of Gynecology and Obstetrics	Blood loss of 500 ml or more during vaginal birth or Blood loss of 1000 ml or more during caesarean birth
6. The American College of Obstetrics and Gynecologists	Cumulative blood loss of at least 1000 ml of blood or any amount of blood loss accompanied by signs and symptoms of hypovolemia within 24 hours of birth
7. Royal College of Obstetricians and Gynecologists	Blood loss >500 ml irrespective of route of delivery. (mild PPH blood loss of 500–1000 ml, major PPH blood loss of >1000 ml) Major PPH is subdivided as moderate PPH in which there is blood loss of 1001–2000 ml and severe PPH as blood loss of >2000 ml)

PPH: Postpartum haemorrhage

correctly assessed) and 10% when blood loss is correctly assessed.[3]

Methods to Quantify Blood Loss[3]

1. Visual estimation (not so accurate)
2. Volumetric
3. Gravimetric
4. Colorimetry
5. Visual aids (charts are available)

The ratio of heart rate to systolic blood pressure is called shock index (SI).

Increased mortality is noted, when SI $\geq$0.9. More blood transfusion is required when SI >1.

International Federation of Gynecology and Obstetrics (FIGO) recommends shock index for the diagnosis and management of PPH. SI is used as a marker for predicting severity of PPH.

Rule of 30

Approximate blood loss of 30% is normal, which is 70 ml/kg in adults or 100 ml/kg throughout pregnancy, causes

- 30% fall in haematocrit
- 30% fall in haemoglobin (approximately 3 g/dl)
- Decrease in systolic blood pressure by 30 mm Hg
- Rise in pulse rate (30 beats per minute)

Causes

4 Ts (Tone, Tissue, Trauma and Thrombin)[4]
1. Tone—atonic uterus (80%).
2. Tissue—retained placental bits (tissue).
3. Trauma—genital tract trauma.
4. Thrombin—abnormalities of coagulation.

40% of PPH occurs in low-risk women. PPH prophylaxis is recommended for use in all women (both high-risk and low-risk cases). One should remember that each and every woman giving birth is at risk of PPH. As entire blood loss may not be visualised externally, estimation of blood loss remains a challenge. Amniotic fluid gets mixed with blood which hampers estimation of blood loss.

RISK FACTORS FOR PPH[5]

- Multiparity (>4 births)
- Anaemia
- Patients with prolonged labor
- Patients with previous history of PPH (in subsequent pregnancy, there is 18% chance of recurrence of PPH. The risk of recurrence increases to 27% after two consecutive pregnancies)
- Placenta accreta spectrum
- Large for gestational age
- Operative vaginal delivery
- Hypertensive disorders in pregnancy
- Multiple gestations

Various scores are available to predict PPH.

PPH PREVENTION

Active management of third stage of labour for all patients (AMTSL) is recommended by WHO. In AMTSL, 10 U IM or IV oxytocin (uterotonic agent) is administered prophylactically during third stage of labor. It also includes delayed clamping of umbilical cord (1–3 minutes after birth) and placenta removal by controlled traction of the umbilical cord in the presence of skilled birth attendants. Use of uterotonics is the most crucial step in active management of third stage of labour. It is not recommended to give continuous uterine massage for prevention of PPH.

WHO Recommendations for Prevention of PPH[6,7]

1. Uterotonic agents should be used for PPH prevention during the third stage of labour. It is recommended for use during all births. For PPH prevention, various drugs, such as oxytocin, carbetocin, ergometrine, methylergometrine, misoprostol, or fixed-dose combination of oxytocin and ergometrine can be used.
2. 10 IU oxytocin, IM/IV has been recommended for the prevention of PPH for all deliveries (high risk as well as low risk) (vaginal delivery and caesarean

both). Since ages, oxytocin has been the uterotonic of choice for PPH prevention. 100 µg carbetocin, administered IM/IV is also recommended for use in prevention of PPH, when its cost is comparable to other effective uterotonics. Where availability of skilled health personnel is a concern, misoprostol (600 µg, PO) is recommended for PPH prevention. Skilled health personnel are required to administer injectable uterotonics. Ergometrine/methylergometrine (200 µg, IM/IV) can be used for the prevention of PPH, when diagnosis of hypertensive disorders in pregnancy has been excluded. Combination of oxytocin and ergometrine (5 IU/500 µg, IM) has been used for the prevention of PPH in the absence of hypertension. Prostaglandins like carboprost and sulprostone are not recommended for PPH prevention.

3. When all uterotonics are freely available, oxytocin (10 IU, IM/IV) is the uterotonic agent of choice for the prevention of PPH for all births. When intravenous access is available, 10 IU oxytocin slow, IV is preferred to IM route. When oxytocin is not available or quality of oxytocin cannot be guaranteed, *e.g.* cold chain has not been maintained other uterotonics, such as carbetocin, ergometrine/methylergometrine, or oxytocin and ergometrine fixed-dose combination or oral misoprostol can be used for the prevention of PPH. When availability of skilled health personnel to administer injectable uterotonics is an issue, misoprostol (600 µg, PO) can be administered by community health workers and lay health workers for the prevention of PPH. Antenatal distribution of misoprostol to pregnant women for self-administration is recommended when women deliver outside health facility. Monitoring and evaluation for prevention of PPH should be carried out in these women.

4. During caesarean section, blood loss can be decreased by using oxytocin which is the recommended uterotonic drug of choice for PPH prevention. During caesarean section, controlled cord traction is preferred over manual removal of placenta.

PPH TREATMENT

Uterotonics play an important role in PPH treatment. Intravenous administration of oxytocin is the first choice of uterotonic. Other uterotonics, such as ergometrine, fixed dose of oxytocin and ergometrine or sublingual misoprostol 800 µg are recommended when oxytocin is not available or if bleeding continues despite use of oxytocin. Fluid resuscitation with crystalloids and massage of atonic uterus is recommended for treatment of PPH. Tranexamic acid is recommended in refractory atonic and trauma-related bleeding. Uterine balloon tamponade is recommended in absence of uterotonics or if bleeding persists. Temporary measures of bimanual uterine compression, external aortic compression and anti-shock garments are recommended. Where facilities are available uterine artery embolization (UAE) should be considered. Surgical intervention should be carried out without delay if bleeding continues. If controlled cord traction (CCT) and oxytocin fail to deliver placenta, manual removal placenta manual removal of placenta (MRP) should be done. Prophylactic antibiotics, such as ampicillin or first-generation cephalosporin are used to prevent infection. Prostaglandin-$F_{2\alpha}$ and ergometrine are not recommended in retained placenta. Uterine packing has no role in treatment of atonic PPH after vaginal delivery. Only in research settings, oxytocin injection in umbilical vein is tried in cases of retained placenta.

DRUGS USED FOR PPH

1. Oxytocin

Oxytocin is the gold standard drug for PPH prevention and treatment. It is administered routinely for active management of third stage of labour. WHO recommends use of

10 international units (IU) of oxytocin IV or IM for PPH prevention. Use of oxytocin is recommended for all births (vaginal as well as cesarean deliveries). IV oxytocin is recommended for the treatment of PPH. In 1977, WHO model list of essential medicines (EML) included oxytocin as an essential medicine.

History: Uterotonic effect of extract from posterior pituitary of humans was found by Sir Henry Dale in 1906. In 1950, Vincent du Vigneaud an American biochemist discovered that oxytocin is made-up of 9 amino acids. The molecular structure of oxytocin was determined in 1952. It was the first polypeptide hormone to be sequenced. Oxytocin was first synthesized in 1953 and Du Vigneaud received Nobel prize for it in 1955.

Synthesis: It is synthesized in cell bodies of magnocellular neurons located in the para ventricular nucleus of the hypothalamus. Nerve axons transport it to the posterior pituitary where it is stored and released into the circulation.

Pharmacokinetics: It is a synthetic cyclic peptide. Chymotrypsin renders it ineffective, if drug is administered by oral route. If drug is given by IM route, onset of action is within 3–7 min, but effect lasts long for >1 hour. If drug is administered by intravenous route, onset of action is within 1 min and effect lasts up to 3–5 min. Shorter half-life requires continuous infusion for uterotonic activity.

Oxytocin receptors are present in low concentration from 13 to 17 weeks and rises up to 12-fold by 37 to 41 weeks. Receptor concentration is maximal at onset of labour. It causes physiological contraction–fundal contraction and cervical relaxation. Oxytocinase present in placenta, uterus and plasma of pregnant female degrades oxytocin. Oxytocin is removed by liver and kidneys from circulation.[8]

Mechanism of action: Synthetic oxytocin has action similar to endogenous oxytocin.

It increases the permeability of uterine muscles to sodium-stimulating contraction of uterine muscle. When oxytocin receptors are activated myometrial contractions are increased. Intracellular calcium increases and decidua produces prostaglandin thereby increasing myometrial contraction. The action of oxytocin is proportionate to estrogen level and period of gestation. The response increases from 20 to 30 weeks and then plateaus from 34 weeks till term when sensitivity increases. More number of receptors are present in fundus than lower uterine segment. Large doses result in drop in blood pressure with reflex tachycardia.

Dosage in PPH[9]

For prevention: 10 IU, intramuscular route

For treatment parenteral route (intravenous route-preferred or intramuscular) or intravenous (infusion)

Drug is administered by:
- Initial dose: 20 U in 500 ml NS over 1 hour (can be increased to—40 units)
- Maintenance dose: 2.5 units per hour (20 U in 1 litre NS over 8 hours solution—125 ml per hour)

Preparations
1. Injection 10 IU per ml
2. *Combination drug:* Syntometrine (syntocinon 5 U and ergometrine 0.5 mg)
3. Intranasal solution—40 units/ml
4. Buccal 50 IU

Storage: It must be stored under cold conditions (2 to 8°C) and needs protection from light to prevent drug degradation and maintain quality.

Side effects of oxytocin include flushing, nausea, vomiting, hypotension, tachycardia, hyponatremia due to antidiuretic effect.

Uses
1. Induce and augment labor (not a part of this chapter)
2. PPH (prevention and treatment)
3. Lactation—milk let down

Contraindications

Hypersensitivity to drug.

2. Carbetocin

It is a newer heat-stable analogue of oxytocin. It is a long-acting analogue of oxytocin. It is a synthetic octapeptide. It has agonistic action at oxytocin receptor. Though oxytocin is the preferred drug for preventing PPH. It must be stored and transported at 2–8°C (cold chain has to be maintained), making access to this lifesaving drug difficult. Heat exposure makes the drug less effective. Refrigeration is not required for carbetocin as it is heat-stable.[10]

Indication

It is used in prevention of PPH (atonic uterus).

WHO recommends use of carbetocin in PPH prevention when

- Its cost is comparable to other uterotonics.
- Unavailability of oxytocin.
- No guarantee of quality of oxytocin.

Preparation—1 vial contains 100 µg of carbetocin in 1 ml solution for injection. In India, it is available as room temperature stable formulation with shelf life of 2 years when it is stored at 30°C and relative humidity of 75%.

Refrigeration is not required for room temperature-stable formulation. It can be kept at high temp without losing potency for 2 years. It has same ingredients as original preparation but differs in excipients. It remains stable at 30°C for 3 years, 40°C for 6 months, 50°C for 3 months and 60°C for 1 month.

Pharmacokinetics: Single IV injection of carbetocin causes uterine activity within 2 minutes and action lasts for 1 hour. The median terminal elimination half-life of Carbetocin is 33 minutes and 55 minutes after IV and IM administration, respectively. After IM administration peak concentration is reached after 30 min and <1% of dose is excreted unchanged. After drug administration within 2 minutes sustained uterine contractions lasting for 6 minutes

are produced. After intravenous injection, rhythmic contractions for 60 minutes are noted. When intramuscular injection is given sustained uterine contractions last for 11 minutes and rhythmic contractions last for 120 minutes. It was created by making several modifications to the oxytocin structure which prolongs half-life and reduces enzymatic degradation.

Dose: 100 µg, IV or IM, can be given slowly over 1 minute. A single dose is recommended. No further doses are required.

Mechanism of action: It binds to oxytocin receptors and increases rate and force of uterine contractions.

1. Phospholipase C is activated, which yields diacylglycerol. Membrane calcium channels are thus activated allowing its entry into intracellular space.
2. Calcium is released by activation of inositol triphosphate. Inositol triphosphate acts on sarcoplasmic reticulum-releasing calcium.

Advantages

1. Greater effect (biological) has been seen.
2. Long half-life (as compared to oxytocin).
3. More heat-stable than oxytocin, which is of prime importance in resource-poor settings (no cold storage required).
4. Designed for more sustained contractility.
5. Avoids need for continuous infusion.
6. Reduced need for additional uterotonics.
7. Good tolerability.
8. Longer half-life (40 minutes) resulting in longer duration of action.
9. Similar efficacy.
10. Similar onset of action.

Carbetocin HAeMorrhage PreventION (CHAMPION) trial[10]

For blood loss of at least 500 ml, when heat-stable carbetocin was compared to oxytocin for prevention of PPH or for the use of additional uterotonic agents carbetocin was found to be noninferior to oxytocin. For the outcome of blood loss of 1000 ml noninferiority was not demonstrated.

Table 21.2: Comparison of oxytocin and carbetocin

Parameter	Carbetocin IV	Carbetocin IM	Oxytocin IV	Oxytocin IM
Onset of action	1–2 min	2–3 min	Immediate effect	2–5 min
Duration of action	60 min	119	3–5 min	30 min
Half-life	40 min	40 min	3–5 min	3–5 min

Contraindication

- Use for induction of labour—not recommended
- Pregnancy and labor before baby delivery
- Epilepsy
- Hypersensitivity
- Renal, hepatic and cardiovascular disease.

Efficacy

Equally effective as oxytocin in reducing risk of PPH or severe PPH (similar safety profile comparable to ergot and misoprostol with better tolerability.

Future[11]

The 2019 international consensus statement (on use of uterotonic agents) recommends that at present both oxytocin and carbetocin are recommended for routine administration during caesarean section. In future, carbetocin may become the preferred first-line uterotonic drug.

Due to prolonged duration of action of carbetocin, use of infusion is not required.

Carbetocin 100 µg, intravenously, has been recommended over oxytocin infusion for prevention of PPH during elective caesarean section by the 2018 Society of Obstetricians and Gynecologists of Canada guideline.

During vaginal delivery, use of carbetocin 100 µg, intramuscularly is recommended as this decreases need for uterine massage and PPH prevention in patients having one risk factor for PPH.

In the 2017 Royal College of Obstetricians and Gynecologists (RCOG) guideline (guideline includes result of a 2012 Cochrane review), it has been noted that there is significant reduction in the use of other uterotonics at caesarean section when carbetocin is used.

Oxytocin is recommended as the first-line uterotonic for the treatment of PPH. Carbetocin is considered a second-line uterotonic.

Oxytocin is recommended to prevent PPH (after caesarean section) based on professional consensus according to the 2016 French guideline.

A comparison of oxytocin and carbetocin is shown in **Table 21.2**.

3. Prostaglandins (PGs)

Von Euler first described it in 1935. They act as local hormones. Subscript numeral indicates degree of unsaturation.

A. Carboprost (15 methyl $PGF_{2\alpha}$)

It is a prostaglandin used for treatment of PPH.

Mechanism of action: $PGF_{2\alpha}$ acts on myometrium and causes change in myometrial cell permeability. It alters membrane-bound calcium. It increases amplitude and frequency of uterine contractions. It increases GI motility. It promotes myometrial contraction. The mechanism of action of prostaglandins is via cyclic adenosine monophasphate (cAMP)-mediated calcium release. Addition of a methyl group results in longer duration of action.

Pharmacokinetics: It is rapidly absorbed and metabolised in lungs and liver. Plasma levels peaked 20 minutes after IM injection and declined slowly. It crosses placenta. It undergoes omega oxidation and is excreted in urine (83% as metabolites). It is a Category C drug.

Dose: 0.25 mg can be given IM, every 15 minute (interval of 15–90 minute) recommended up to 8 doses. Maximum 2 g can be given intra-myometrial, especially during C section. Storage—refrigerator 2–8°C.

Use: Treatment of PPH.

Contraindication: Asthma, cardiac, respiratory, hepatic and renal disease.

Side effects (noted in 20% patients): Diarrhoea, hypertension, vomiting, fever, flushing, headache, tachycardia and broncho-constriction. It is not recommended for use in asthmatic and in those with suspected amniotic fluid embolism.

B. Misoprostol

It is a prostaglandin E_1 analogue. It was initially used for treatment of peptic ulcer disease. FIGO, RCOG, American College of Obstetricians and Gynecologists (ACOG) and International Confederation of Midwives (ICM) endorse use of misoprostol. WHO recommends use of misoprostol for preventing and treating PPH in the absence of qualified health providers to administer oxytocin. Misoprostol has been distributed during antenatal care visit when delivery may occur outside hospitals. Community health workers and birth attendants may distribute this drug during home visits for PPH prevention. It is incorporated in WHO list of essential medicines.

Route of administration:[12] Sublingual miso-prostol is the only tested route in randomised controlled trials (RCTs). Evidence of rectal administration is limited.

Pharmacokinetics: Sublingual (SL) route has rapid action, is easy to administer, has faster absorption and greater bioavailability resulting in high serum concentration. Bioavailability of vaginal misoprostol was 3 times more than oral. Absorption of vaginal route is inconsistent and addition of water can improve absorption. It is soluble in water. Sublingual route achieves maximum serum concentration. Time to peak was shorter in sublingual and oral route than vaginal route.

Oral route resulted in higher serum levels as compared to vaginal route. Sublingual has better action due to the absence of first pass metabolism after sublingual route. Good supply under tongue and neutral pH is another contributing factor. Levels lasted longer after vaginal administration.[12]

Mechanism of action: Uterotonic effects are caused by binding of prostaglandin to smooth muscle cells in the uterine lining. Its uterotonic properties are useful in PPH.

Advantages: Oxytocin requires refrigeration, sterile equipment and skilled personnel. Misoprostol is available as a tablet and remains stable at room temperature. It is available and affordable and does not require skilled personnel for administration of drug. FIGO guidelines suggest misoprostol the best alternative to oxytocin when refrigeration and sterile equipment are not available in low resource settings. Misoprostol is cost-effective and has a long shelf life. It may be more effective for the prevention of PPH (500 ml) when compared with oxytocin, however higher risk of adverse effects is observed when other uterotonic drugs are combined with misoprostol.

Disadvantage: Misoprostol can absorb moisture from areas of high humidity and degrade. Side effects include high fever and shivering. Nausea, vomiting, and diarrhoea are also noted with use of this drug.

Dose: 800 µg sublingual dose is used for treatment of PPH. Useful in settings, where there is no access to oxytocin and skilled personnel is not available for administration of uterotonics.

If PPH occurs in women who have already received prophylactic misoprostol orally (600 µg), there is no role of using additional dose of misoprostol for treatment of PPH.

Side effects: Include fever, shivering, nausea and vomiting.

Contraindication: Allergic reaction.

4. Tranexamic Acid (TXA)

Invented by Utako Okamoto and her husband Shouske from Japan in 1962. WHO recommends 1 g of IV injection of tranexamic acid as soon as possible after giving birth for management of PPH. If bleeding persists after 30 minutes or restarts within 24 hours, a second dose is recommended. TXA reduces hemorrhage deaths by one-third. Survival benefits fall by 10% for every 15-minute delay. It is incorporated in WHO list of essential medicines.

Pharmacokinetics: It is heat-stable, cost effective, has long shelf life, is excreted unchanged and half-life is 2 hours. 30–50% drug is bioavailable after oral administration. IM route can be used as alternative to IV route.

Median time to reach therapeutic concentration is 3.5 minutes for IM and 66 minutes for oral route.

Most elimination takes place in 8 hours. It is primarily excreted by urine, 95% in unchanged form. 90% of IV drug and 39% orally administered is excreted in 24 hours.

Mechanism of action: The breakdown of fibrin blood clots is inhibited by tranexamic acid thus reducing bleeding. Fibrin breakdown occurs when plasminogen produced by liver is activated to plasmin by tissue plasminogen activator (tPA). Plasmin splits the fibrin blood clot into fibrin degradation product (FDP). It competitively and reversibly inhibits activation of plasminogen. The conversion of plasminogen to plasmin is decreased which prevents fibrin degradation. The framework of fibrin matrix is thus stabilised.

In 2009, World Maternal Antifibrinolytic (WOMAN) trial was launched. It was a multicentre, randomised, double-blind, placebo-controlled trial to study effect of tranexamic acid.[13,14]

It was noted that deaths due to PPH reduced significantly with use of tranexamic acid. The rate of thromboembolic events or complications was not increased. Decreased mortality due to bleeding was noted when tranexamic acid was administered within 3 hours of childbirth. Such reduction in deaths due to bleeding was not noted when tranexamic acid was given after 3 hours.

Dose: 1 g of tranexamic acid in 10 ml (100 mg/ml) is given intravenously at a rate of 1 ml per minute. A second dose is recommended after 30 minutes if bleeding continues or recurs, within 24 hours of the first dose.

Contraindication

- Allergy
- History of seizures
- Thromboembolism (venous or arterial)
- Active thromboembolic disease
- Kidney impairment

5. Methergin

Ergonovine maleate and methylergonovine are ergot alkaloid derivatives which have strong uterotonic activity.

Mechanism of action: Calcium channel mechanism and actin–myosin interaction cause myometrial contractions.

Dose: 0.2 mg, IM doses. Additional dose can be given every 15-minute up to maximum 3 doses. If given IV may cause life-threatening hypertension.

Fixed dose—5U oxytocin with 0.5 U ergometrine.

Dose—1 ml, IM.

Pharmacokinetics: Onset of action is within 2–5 min.

Duration of action—3 hours (30–120 minutes)

Advantage: Sustained myometrial contraction and rapid onset of action.

Side effects: Nausea, vomiting and rise in BP.

Contraindication: Hypertension, pre-eclampsia and heart disease.

In case of failure of uterotonic agents, other measures to control bleeding can be used.

1. *Bimanual compression:* Bimanual compression of uterus is done. One hand is kept in vagina and other hand on anterior abdominal wall.

Table 21.3: Comparison of various uterotonic drugs

	Oxytocin	Carbetocin	Misoprostol	Ergometrine	Carboprost
Dose	Prevention of PPH—10 IU, IM or IV treatment 40 units, IV	Only for prevention—100 µg, IM or IV (single dose)	Prevention—600 µg, PO treatment 800 µg	0.2 mg, IM Fixed dose 5U oxytocin with 0.5 U ergometrine	250 µg, every 15 min (max. 8 doses 2 mg)
Onset of action	IV within 1 min IM route within 3–7 min	IV within 2 min IM within 11 min	Within 10–15 min Oral, sublingual rapid onset	Within 2–5 min	IM 15–60 min Can be given intramyometrial
Duration of action	IV up to 3–5 min Peak after 30 min, IM, effect lasts longer for >1 hour	IV within 60 min IM within 120 min (4 to 10 times longer than oxytocin)	Rectal route Prolonged duration Oral peak 30 min Vaginal 70–80 min	3 hours	Peak after 20 min in IM Declined slowly
Half-life	1–6 min	40 min	20–40 min	30–120 min	3 hours
Side effects	Uterine hyper-stimulation, flushing , antidiuretic, hypotension	Flushing Hypotension Caution in epilepsy, asthma and hypertension	Shivering, fever	Nausea, vomiting, rise in BP contraindicated hypertension and pre-eclampsia and heart disease	GI side effects, bronchospasm, contraindicated asthma, active cardiac, renal and hepatic disease, acute PID

2. *Uterine artery embolization (UAE):*[14] FIGO recommends UAE for bleeding not controlled by medical and nonsurgical treatment (refractory hemorrhage). Disadvantages include cost, trained personnel and equipments for using this technology. UAE can be considered when it is important to preserve the patient's fertility.

3. *Uterine balloon devices*[14]: Uterine balloon tamponade is recommended by FIGO in cases of refractory PPH. It is an effective nonsurgical technique which can help treat PPH. *Types:* Shivkar's pack, Bakri balloon and Ellavi balloon.

4. *Nonpneumatic antishock garment (NASG):* The WHO recommends NASG as a temporary measure to stop bleeding until appropriate care is available. It is a lower body compression device comprising of six (articulated neoprene and hook-and-loop) fastener segments. Counterpressure is provided by lower body which improves cardiac output and blood pressure. Recommended for transfer of patient to tertiary centre.[14]

A comparison of various uterotonic drugs is given in **Table 21.3**.

Surgical interventions: Compression sutures and systematic pelvic devascularization

The technique of B-Lynch suture was first described by Christopher B-Lynch in 1997. It apposes anterior and posterior walls using vertical brace sutures put around uterus. Success rate of B lynch is 86%, as it works by applying pressure on placental bed. It is a life and fertility sparing surgery.[15–17]

Internal hypogastric artery ligation was first described by Sagarra M, et al. in early 1960, bilateral uterine artery ligation was described by O' Leary in 1966 and stepwise devascularisation was described by Abd Rabbo.

Systematic pelvic devascularization consists of uterine artery ligation (unilateral followed by bilateral), followed by ovarian artery ligation (unilateral followed by bilateral), followed by internal iliac artery ligation (unilateral followed by bilateral).

Uterine artery ligation. Uterus receives 90% of its blood supply from the uterine arteries, hence ligation of these arteries helps reduce ongoing blood loss. Success rate is 80%.

Ovarian artery ligation procedure involve ligation of utero-ovarian vessel anastomosis to reduce uterine blood supply. Ligate the utero-ovarian artery just below where ovarian suspensory ligament joins uterus.

Internal Iliac Artery Ligation

Internal iliac artery is the main vessel supplying pelvic organs. Bilateral ligation of internal iliac artery results in 85% reduction in pulse pressure. 50% reduction in blood flow is observed in the arteries distal to the ligation. Efficacy is 84%.

Hemostatic Resuscitation[18–20]

Due to the resemblance with whole blood, packed red blood cells (PRBCs), fresh frozen plasma (FFP), and platelets are transfused in a 1:1:1 ratio. Better patient survival outcomes are noted with this method. The complication rate is also decreased with the use of this ratio for transfusion. When PRBC is not available, whole blood can be used in case of massive hemorrhage.

In hemorrhages, fibrinogen concentration decreases. Component replacement should be started when values of <200 mg/dl are reached. FFP, cryoprecipitate, and fibrinogen concentrates are used for replacing fibrinogen. As variable concentration of fibrinogen is found in FFP, fibrinogen replacement with cryoprecipitate is recommended. 2 g fibrinogen for each 100 ml is contained in one unit of cryoprecipitate. One unit of cryoprecipitate will increase serum fibrinogen level by 10 mg/dl. Cryoprecipitate are usually transfused as a dose of 10 units. Serum fibrinogen level increases by 100 mg/dl when 10 units of cryoprecipitate are administered **(Table 21.4)**. Massive blood transfusion (MBT) **(Table 21.5)** is defined as:

1. Transfusion requirement of >4 PRBC units (some articles consider ≥10 PRBC within 24 hours)
2. Replacement of total volume of blood within 24 hours or replacement of 50% of blood volume within 3 hours.

Typical one round of transfusion in massive transfusion consists of 6 units PRBC, 6 units FFP, 6 units platelet counts or 1 plateletpheresis and 10 units of cryoprecipitate.

Factor 7 (NoVo Seven):[21,22] Recommended for approval for treatment of severe PPH by European Medicines agency. Considered as a rescue therapy in life-threatening bleeding unresponsive to standard therapy. Initial dose 200 µg/kg followed by 100 µg/kg at 1 hour and 3 hours.

Calcium[23]

Hypocalcaemia is a result of use of citrate as blood anticoagulant in transfusion. 97% of patients getting MBT have hypocalcaemia.

It is recommended to add 1–2 grams of IV calcium chloride or 3–6 grams of IV calcium gluconate when administering one round of massive transfusion is required.

SUMMARY

Mnemonic 'HAEMOSTASIS' has been suggested for management of PPH **(Flowchart 21.1)**.[24,25]

H—ask for help

A—assess vitals

E—establish aetiology and ensure availability of blood and uterotonics

M—massage uterus

O—oxytocin and prostaglandins

S—shift to theatre

T—tamponade test

A—apply compression sutures

S—systematic pelvic devascularization

Flowchart 21.1: Management of PPH[25]

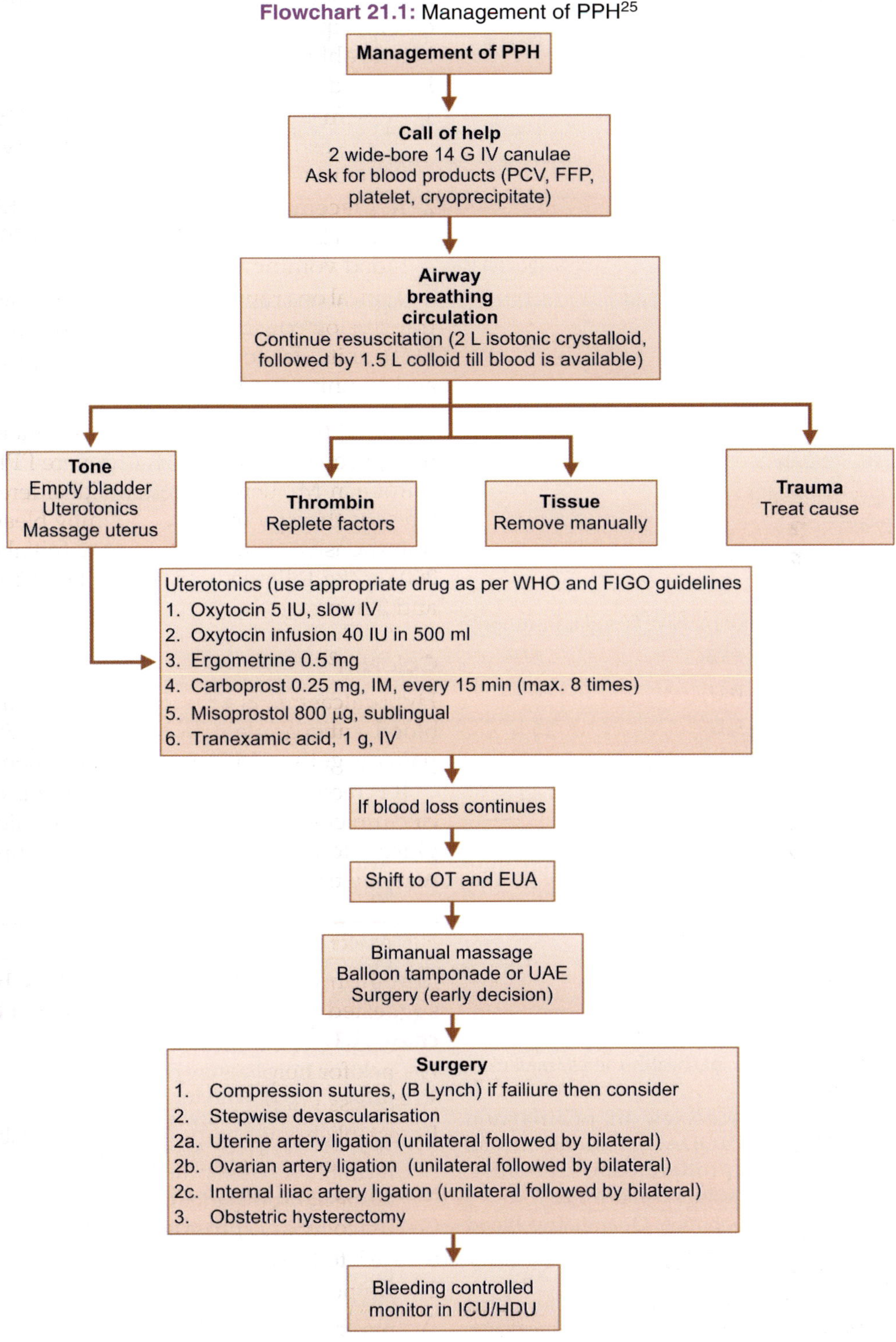

Table 21.4: Blood component therapy[20]

Component	Volume of blood for preparation	Volume of product	Storage	Shelf life	Preparation time	Increase in blood parameter	Matching
1 unit RBC	450–500 ml	200 ml +100 ml (preservative)	1–6°C	35–42 days	None	Hgb 1 to 1.5 g/dl	ABO and Rh
1 unit platelets	450–500 ml	50 ml	Room temp. (20–24°C)	5 days	None	20,000–40,000 platelets/µl	Unmatched
1 unit plasma	450–500 ml	250 ml	–18°C	1 year	Thaw at 37°C	Factors 2,7,9 and 10 are given which normalise PT, INR	ABO and Rh
1 unit cryo precipitate	450–500 ml	15 ml	–18°C	1 year	Thaw at 37°C	5–10 mg/dl of fibrinogen	Suggested ABO

RBC: Red blood cell; PT: Prothrombin time; INR: International normalised ratio; Hgb: Hemoglobin

Table 21.5: Protocol for massive blood transfusion[14]

	PRBCs	FFP	Platelets	Cryoprecipitate
Round 1	6 U	6 U	6 U	10 U
Round 2	6 U	6 U	6 U	10 U
Round 3	Tranexamic	Acid	1 g IV	Over 10 min
Round 4	6 U	6 U	6 U	

I—interventional radiology/internal iliac artery zigation
S—subtotal/total hysterectomy)

References

1. World Health organization. Maternal health WHO incidence of deaths. Available from: https://www.who.int/health-topics/maternal-health#tab=tab_1
2. Belfort M A. Overview of postpartum haemorrhage. UPTODATE. Available from: https://www.uptodate.com/contents/overview-of-postpartum-hemorrhage
3. ACOG committee opinion. Quantitative Blood Loss in Obstetric Hemorrhage. Committee Opinion CO, Number 794, December 2019.
4. Janice M. Anderson, Duncan Etches, Prevention and Management of Postpartum Hemorrhage. Am Fam Physician. 2007;75(6) p.875–882. Available from. https://www.aafp.org/pubs/afp/issues/2007/0315/p875.html
5. Oberg A S, Diaz S H. Pattern of recurrence. American Journal of Obstetrics and Gynaecology. VOLUME 210, ISSUE 3, MARCH 01, 2014 P229.E1-229.E8.
6. World Health Organization. WHO recommendations Uterotonics for the prevention of postpartum haemorrhage. Available from https://apps.who.int/iris/bitstream/handle/10665/277276/9789241550420-eng.pdf
7. World Health Organization. WHO recommendations for the prevention and treatment of postpartum haemorrhage. Available from.https://apps.who.int/iris/bitstream/handle/10665/75411/9789241548502_eng.pdf
8. Fuchs RA, Fuchs F, Husslein P, Soloff MS, Oxytocin receptors in the human uterus during pregnancy and parturition. American Journal of Obstetrics and Gynaecology, VOLUME

150, ISSUE 6, NOVEMBER 15, 1984 P734-741. Available from. Oxytocin receptors in the human uterus during pregnancy and parturition - American Journal of Obstetrics and Gynecology (ajog.org)

9. UpToDate, Steps in management of postpartum hemorrhage. Available from. https://www.uptodate.com/contents/image?imageKey=OBGYN%2F57307

10. Widmer M, Piaggio G, Thi MH Nguyen et al. Heat-Stable Carbetocin versus Oxytocin to Prevent Hemorrhage after Vaginal Birth. Available from https://www.nejm.org/doi/full/10.1056/nejmoa1805489 DOI: 10.1056/NEJMoa1805489

11. Chao YS, McCormack S. Carbetocin for the Prevention of Post-Partum Hemorrhage: A Review of Clinical Effectiveness, Cost-Effectiveness, and Guidelines [Internet]. Ottawa (ON): Canadian Agency for Drugs and Technologies in Health; 2019 Jul 29. Available from: https://www.ncbi.nlm.nih.gov/books/NBK546425/

12. Tang S O, Schweer H, Seyberth H W, et al. Pharmacokinetics of different routes of administration of misoprostol .Human Reproduction, Volume 17, Issue 2, February 2002, P. 332–336, https://doi.org/10.1093/humrep/17.2.332

13. Picetti, R., Miller, L., Shakur-Still, H. et al. The WOMAN trial: clinical and contextual factors surrounding the deaths of 483 women following post-partum haemorrhage in developing countries. BMC Pregnancy Childbirth 20, 409 (2020). https://doi.org/10.1186/s12884-020-03091-8

14. Escobar M F , Nassar A, Theron G. et al FIGO recommendations on the management of postpartum hemorrhage 2022. Int J Gynaecol Obstet. 2022 Mar;157 Suppl 1:P. 3-50. https://obgyn.onlinelibrary.wiley.com/doi/10.1002/ijgo.14116

15. Zheng, J and Xiong, X and Ma, Q and Zhang, X and Li, M. A new uterine compression suture for postpartum haemorrhage with atony. BJOG: an international journal of obstetrics and gynaecology 2011 Feb;118(3):P.370-4.

16. Mehdi M, Chandraharan E, Glob. libr. women's med., Diagnosis and Management of Shock in Postpartum Hemorrhage. ISSN: 1756-2228; Available from. https://www.glowm.com/article/heading/vol-13--obstetric-emergencies--diagnosis-and-management-of-shock-in-postpartum-hemorrhage/id/409603#.YwEHYXZBxPY. DOI 10.3843/GLOWM.409603

17. Talaulikar V S, Arul Kumaran S. Uterus sparing surgical or radiological treatment of major postpartum hemorrhage: efficacy and implications for future fertility. The Global Library of Women's Medicine's Welfare of Women Global Health Programme.

18. Muñoz M, Stensballe J, Ducloy-Bouthors AS, et al. Patient blood management in obstetrics: prevention and treatment of postpartum haemorrhage. A NATA consensus statement. Blood Transfus. 2019 Mar;17(2): p.112-136. Available from https://www.ncbi.nlm.nih.gov/pmc/articles/PMC6476742/. doi: 10.2450/2019.0245-18.

19. Patil V, Shetmahajan M. Massive transfusion and massive transfusion protocol. Indian J Anaesth. 2014 Sep;58(5):p.590-5. Available from https://www.ncbi.nlm.nih.gov/pmc/articles/PMC4260305/. doi: 10.4103/0019-5049.144662.

20. Kogutt BK, Vaught AJ. Postpartum hemorrhage: Blood product management and massive transfusion. Semin Perinatol. 2019 Feb;43(1): p. 44-50. Available from https://pubmed.ncbi.nlm.nih.gov/30527516/. doi: 10.1053/j.semperi.2018.11.008.

21. Magon N, Babu KM, Kapur K, Chopra S, Joneja GS. Recombinant activated factor VII in post-partum haemorrhage. Niger Med J. 2013 Sep;54(5):p. 289-94. Available from https://www.ncbi.nlm.nih.gov/pmc/articles/PMC3883225/. doi: 10.4103/0300-1652.122328.

22. S. Sobieszczyk and G. H. Breborowicz. The Use of Recombinant Factor VIIa* Available from. https://www.glowm.com/pdf/PPH_2nd_edn_Chap-50.pdf

23. Chakraborty A, Can AS. Calcium Gluconate. [Updated 2022 Jun 4]. In: StatPearls [Internet]. Treasure Island (FL): StatPearls Publishing; 2022 Jan-. Available from: https://www.ncbi.nlm.nih.gov/books/NBK557463/

24. Sebghati M, Chandraharan E. An update on the risk factors for and management of obstetric haemorrhage. Womens Health (Lond). 2017 Aug;13(2):34-40. doi: 10.1177/1745505717716860. Epub 2017 Jul 6. PMID: 28681676; PMCID: PMC5557181 Available from https://www.ncbi.nlm.nih.gov/pmc/articles/PMC5557181/

25. Mavrides E, Allard S, Chandraharan E, Collins P, Green L, Hunt BJ, Riris S, Thomson AJ on behalf of the Royal College of Obstetricians and Gynaecologists. Prevention and management of postpartum haemorrhage. BJOG 2016;124:e106–e149.

Thyroid Disorders in Pregnancy

• Shreya Prabhoo • Neha Mathews • Prabhat Kumar Agrawal

Introduction

Endocrine disorders frequently affect women during their reproductive age group. Out of these, thyroid disorders are the second most common only preceded by diabetes among pregnant women. Timely diagnosis and management are imperative not only for optimization of the woman's health but also for the wellbeing of the growing fetus.

THYROID PHYSIOLOGY IN PREGNANCY

Learning the thyroid physiology in pregnancy is important for the understanding of site of action of various drugs used in disorders of the gland. Following are the important physiological adaptations that occur during pregnancy **(Fig. 22.1)**:

1. Raised thyroid-binding globulin (TBG) level owing to the hyper estrogenic state

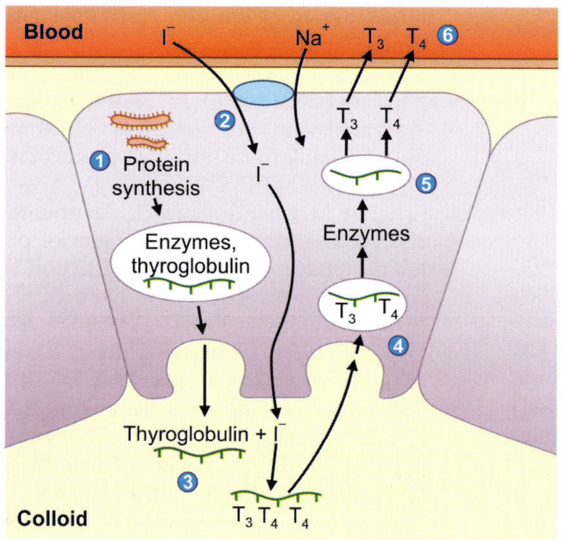

Fig. 22.1: Thyroid hormone synthesis[1]

Table 22.1: Classification of thyroid disorders in pregnancy

Hypothyroidism	*Hyperthyroidism*
Primary	Autoimmune causes, *e.g.* Graves' disease
Iodine deficiency	
Autoimmune disease, *e.g.* Hashimoto's and atrophic thyroiditis	Subacute thyroiditis
Transient causes, *e.g.* postpartum thyroiditis and de Quervain's thyroiditis	Iodine therapy
Iatrogenic causes, *e.g.* radioactive iodine therapy, contrast agent exposure, antithyroid drugs, thyroidectomy	Toxic nodular goitre
Secondary, *e.g.* tumor of the pituitary or pituitary failure	Toxic adenoma
Tertiary, *e.g.* hypothalamic failure	Iatrogenic, *e.g.* drugs like amiodarone, lithium

which leads to increase in the total triiodo-thyronine (T_3) and thyroxin (T_4).

2. Increased demand for dietary iodine
3. Raised glomerular filtration rate (GFR) in pregnancy is responsible for increased iodine clearance.
4. Raised beta human chorionic gonadotropin (β-hCG) levels causing cross reactivity with thyroid-stimulating hormone (TSH) receptors causing hyperthyroidism in the first trimester.
5. Placental deiodinase inactivates T_4 to its inactive form reverse T_3.

Various thyroid disorders in pregnancy are listed in **Table 22.1**.

HYPOTHYROIDISM IN PREGNANCY

Symptoms

- Muscle weakness and fatigue
- Weight gain
- Increased sensitivity to cold
- Constipation
- Puffy face
- Dry skin
- Hoarseness of voice.

Effects of hypothyroidism during pregnancy:
Maternal: Anemia, pre-eclampsia, placental abruption, pre-term labor, low-birth weight infant.
Fetal/neonatal: Cognitive impairment, respiratory distress, hyperbilirubinemia.

Treatment

Levothyroxine

Oral levothyroxine is primarily used for treatment, but parenteral dosage is at times required in severe hypothyroidism.

The tablet should be consumed 30–60 minutes prior to breakfast on an empty stomach with advise to avoid simultaneous consumption of iron, calcium, antacids or proton pump inhibitors within 4 hours.

In pregnant women, an initial dose of 1.8 µg/kg is started and dose is adjusted as per 4 weekly TSH report. In women with pre-gestational hypothyroidism, a dose increment of 25 µg is made at the confirmation of pregnancy to meet the initial T_4 demand,[2] postpartum the dose is decreased to 1.6 µg/kg.[3]

Levothyroxine has the US Food and Drugs Administration (FDA) approval for pituitary thyrotropin suppression in thyrotropin-dependent well-differentiated thyroid cancer in adjunct to surgery.[4] Injectable levothyroxine has been approved to treat myxedema coma or severe hypothyroidism.[5] Myxedema coma—start 200 to 400 µg, IV loading dose, followed by a daily dose of 1.2 µg/kg/day (use lower doses in patients with a history of cardiac disease, arrhythmia, or older patients). Once symptoms resolve switch to oral therapy (8 µg/kg/day).[6]

Adverse effects of the drug include:
- Angina pectoris
- Tachycardia
- Palpitations
- Arrhythmia
- Weight loss
- Diarrhoea
- Alopecia
- Decreased bone mineral density.

Contraindications to Use
- Acute myocardial infarction
- Active arrythmias
- Uncorrected adrenal insufficiency.

HYPERTHYROIDISM

Symptoms of hyperthyroidism:
- Palpitations
- Weight loss
- Tachycardia and arrythmia
- Increased appetite
- Tremors
- Nervousness, anxiety and irritability.

Effects of Hyperthyroidism during Pregnancy

Maternal: Pre-eclampsia, preterm labor, anesthesia-related complications, tachycardia, congestive cardiac failure, thyroid storm.

Fetal/neonatal: Tachycardia, intrauterine growth restriction (IUGR) and goitre.

Drugs used in Hyperthyroidism and Graves' Disease

1. Thioamides like propylthiouracil and methimazole (metabolite of carbimazole) are the drugs used for treatment of hyperthyroidism.
2. Propylthiouracil (PTU)
   Initial dose: 300–450 mg/day (orally in three divided dosevs)
   Maintenance dose: 100–150 mg/day (orally in three-divided doses)
3. Methimazole
   Initial dose: 15–40 mg/day to be administered orally in divided doses in mild and moderate cases, 60 mg/day in severe cases.
   Maintenance dose: 5–30 mg/day to be administered orally in three-divided doses.
4. For Graves' disease
   - PTU—
     Initial dose: 50–150 mg, orally, three times a day.
   - *Maintenance dose:* 50 mg to be administered orally twice or three times a day.[1]
   - Methimazole
     Initial dose: 10–20 mg/day to be administered orally once a day.
     Maintenance dose: To be changed as per the reduction in thyroid function tests
5. Advantages of propylthiouracil over carbimazole are:
   - More plasma protein bound
   - Lower placental transfer
   - Smaller amount of secretion in breast milk
6. Carbimazole has better patient compliance due to longer half-life.
7. Initial aggressive therapy with high-dose carbimazole (10–20 mg, BD) or PTU (150 mg, TID) is started and gradually reduced to 5 mg and 50 mg, respectively.[7] It takes 3–8 weeks for normalization of thyroid function tests due to previously stored T_3 and T_4.
8. FT_4 should be measured 4 weekly and dose adjusted to maintain it in upper one-third of normal.
9. Beta-blockers are used when symptoms of tachycardia and palpitations are present and aim is to maintain resting pulse between 70–90 beats per min.[8]
10. Radioactive iodine therapy is contra-indicated in pregnancy, however up to 10 weeks gestation it does not compromise thyroid function and hence termination

Thioamides
Thyroid gland
Peroxidase
Thyroglobulin
I⁻
I⁻
I°
MIT-DIT—T_3, T_4
Iodides
Transport
Proteolysis
Iodides,
thioamides
Peripheral
tissues
T_4, T_3
T_4, T_3
Blood
Iodinated contrast media,
β-blockers, amiodarone
thioamides
T_3

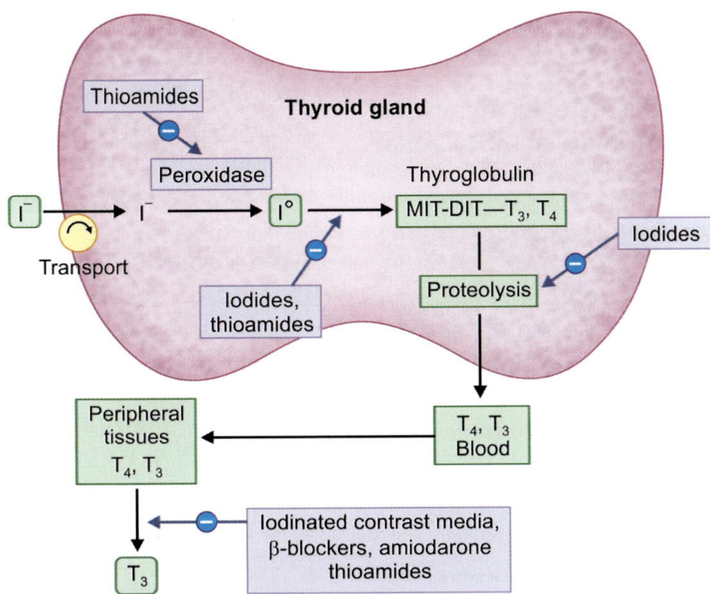

Fig. 22.2: Drug action on thyroid physiology (Katzung BG, editor: Basic and Clinical Pharmacology, 11th ed. McGraw-Hill, 2009: Fig. 38.1). MIT: Monoiodotyroisine; DIT: di-iodotyrosine

Flowchart 22.1: Algorithm for thyroid storm in pregnancy[10,11]

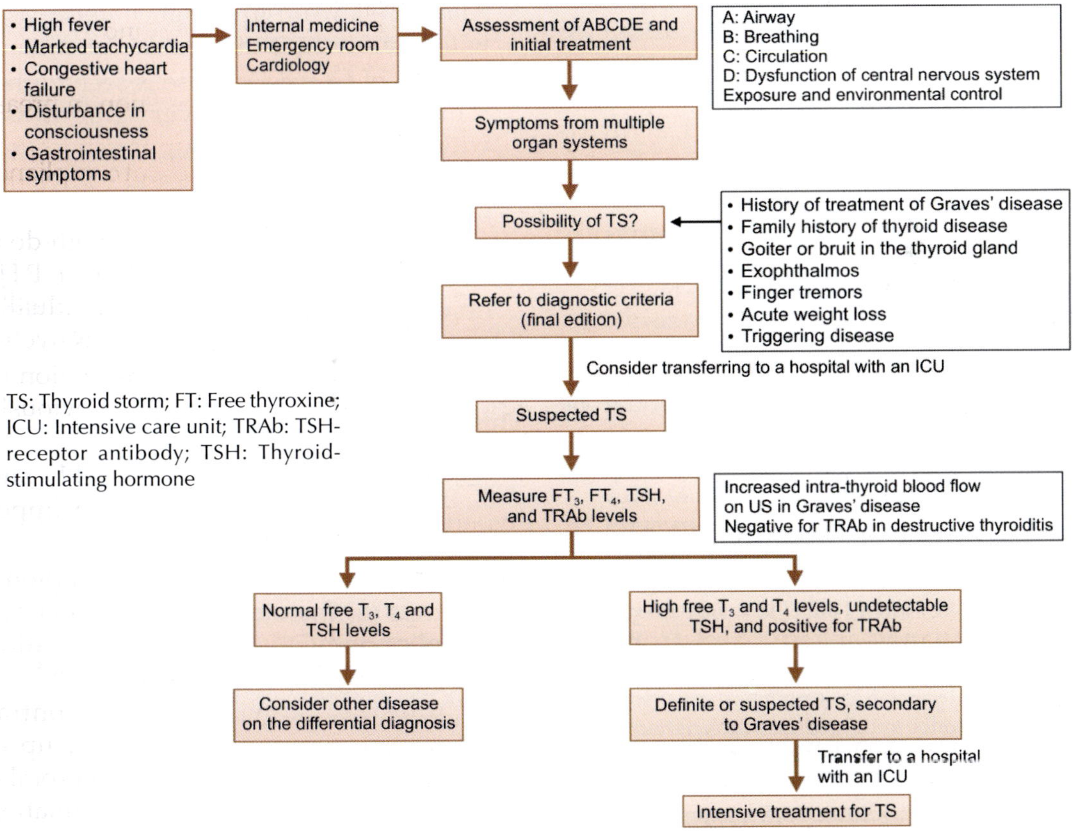

• High fever
• Marked tachycardia
• Congestive heart failure
• Disturbance in consciousness
• Gastrointestinal symptoms
Internal medicine
Emergency room
Cardiology
Assessment of ABCDE and initial treatment
A: Airway
B: Breathing
C: Circulation
D: Dysfunction of central nervous system
Exposure and environmental control
Symptoms from multiple organ systems
Possibility of TS?
• History of treatment of Graves' disease
• Family history of thyroid disease
• Goiter or bruit in the thyroid gland
• Exophthalmos
• Finger tremors
• Acute weight loss
• Triggering disease
Refer to diagnostic criteria (final edition)
Consider transferring to a hospital with an ICU
Suspected TS
Measure FT_3, FT_4, TSH, and TRAb levels
Increased intra-thyroid blood flow on US in Graves' disease
Negative for TRAb in destructive thyroiditis
Normal free T_3, T_4 and TSH levels
High free T_3 and T_4 levels, undetectable TSH, and positive for TRAb
Consider other disease on the differential diagnosis
Definite or suspected TS, secondary to Graves' disease
Transfer to a hospital with an ICU
Intensive treatment for TS

TS: Thyroid storm; FT: Free thyroxine; ICU: Intensive care unit; TRAb: TSH-receptor antibody; TSH: Thyroid-stimulating hormone

is not advised in case of inadvertent administration.

Adverse reactions: Rash, fever, hepatitis, systemic lupus erythromatosus (SLE) like syndrome, agranulocytosis.

National and international guidelines guiding therapy [National Guidelines for Screening of Hypothyroidism during Pregnancy, India (MOHFW) 2014]: Screening should be done for women who are at high risk for hypothyroidism.

- Residing in an area of known iodine insufficiency (moderate-to-severe)
- Obesity [body mass index (BMI)]—30 kg/m^2
- Prior thyroid dysfunction or surgery
- Symptoms or the presence of neck swelling (goitre)
- Family history of thyroid disease (parents/siblings/children)
- Mental retardation in family/previous births
- Known case of autoimmune diseases like type-I diabetes/systemic lupus erythematosus/rheumatoid arthritis (RA)/Addison's disease/coeliac disease, etc.
- History of adverse obstetric outcomes like recurrent miscarriages, pre-term delivery, intrauterine demise, pre-eclampsia/eclampsia, abruptio placentae
- History of subfertility
- Exposure to medications like amiodarone or lithium, iodinated radiologic contrast.

Diagnostic Criteria for Guiding Therapy in Pregnancy

TSH levels during pregnancy are lower as compared to TSH levels in a non-pregnant state. Pregnancy-specific and trimester specific reference levels for TSH are as follows:

- First trimester—0.1–2.5 mIU/L
- Second trimester—0.2–3 mIU/L
- Third trimester—0.3–3 mIU/L

Sub-clinical hypothyroidism (SCH) is defined as a serum TSH between 2.5 and 10 mIU/L with normal FT$_4$ concentration.

In cases with TSH between 4–10 mIU/L treatment with levothyroxine is indicated if thyroid peroxidase antibody (TPOAb) is positive.

Also consider treatment for women with TPOAb negative with TSH between 4–10 mIU/L and those with TPOAb positive with TSH 2.5–4 mIU/L as this is associated with improved reproductive outcomes.

Overt hypothyroidism (OH) is defined as serum TSH >2.5–3 mIU/L with low FT$_4$ levels or TSH >10 mIU/L irrespective of FT$_4$.

- The patient should be switched to the prepregnant dosage and TSH levels rechecked after 6 weeks.
- In women with dose requirement within 50 µg, therapy can be safely discontinued and Sr-TSH rechecked after 6 weeks.
- Annual follow-up is recommended in cases with autoimmune thyroid dysfunction.
- Relapse of Graves' disease is seen within 3 months of their delivery due to the withdrawal of immunosuppressive effect of pregnancy, hence TSH and FT$_4$ values need to be monitored at 6 weeks and 12-week interval.
- PTU and methimazole both are generally excreted in breast milk.

POSTPARTUM THYROIDITIS

This autoimmune phenomenon manifests in about 20% women postpartum in the first year with variable manifestations of hypo/hyperthyroidism, most often presenting with a swollen gland.

Guidelines for Thyroid Nodules and Malignancy

For nodules larger than 1 cm detected in pregnancy, free needle aspiration cytology (FNAC) is recommended.

If nodules are malignant, surgery should be offered in the second trimester. Most well-differentiated thyroid cancers are slow growing and postpartum surgical treatment is unlikely to adversely affect prognosis.

[131]Iodine should not be given to lactating women. Contraception should be offered for 6 months to 1 year in them.[7]

CONCLUSION

It can thus be concluded that screening, early diagnosis and appropriate therapy with monitoring play a pivotal role in optimizing reproductive outcomes in pregnant women. Routine monitoring and postpartum follow-up have an equally important role in preventing long-term sequelae of the disease.

References

1. The Pharmaceutical journal, PJ, June 2021, Vol 306, No 7950;306(7950):DOI: 10.1211/PJ.2021.1.88261

2. Thangaratinam S, Tan A, Knox E, Kilby MD, Franklyn J, Coomarasamy A. Association between thyroid antibodies and miscarriage and preterm birth :meta-analysis of evidence BMJ 2011;342:d2616

3. Alexander EK, Marqusee E, Lawrence J, Jarolim P, Fischer GA, Larsen PR. Timing and magnitude of increases in levothyroxine requirements during pregnancy in women with hypothyroidism. N Engl J Med. 2004 Jul 15;351(3):241–9. [PubMed]

4. Haugen BR, Alexander EK, Bible KC, Doherty GM, Mandel SJ, Nikiforov YE, Pacini F, Randolph GW, Sawka AM, Schlumberger M, Schuff KG, Sherman SI, Sosa JA, Steward DL, Tuttle RM, Wartofsky L. 2015 American Thyroid Association Management Guidelines for Adult Patients with Thyroid Nodules and Differentiated Thyroid Cancer: The American Thyroid Association Guidelines Task Force on Thyroid Nodules and Differentiated Thyroid Cancer. Thyroid. 2016 Jan;26(1):1–133. [PMC free article] [PubMed]

5. Ono Y, Ono S, Yasunaga H, Matsui H, Fushimi K, Tanaka Y. Clinical characteristics and outcomes of myxedema coma: Analysis of a national inpatient database in Japan. J Epidemiol. 2017 Mar;27(3):117–122. [PMC free article] [PubMed]

6. Jonklaas J, Bianco AC, Bauer AJ, Burman KD, Cappola AR, Celi FS, Cooper DS, Kim BW, Peeters RP, Rosenthal MS, Sawka AM, American Thyroid Association Task Force on Thyroid Hormone Replacement. Guidelines for the treatment of hypothyroidism: prepared by the american thyroid association task force on thyroid hormone replacement. Thyroid. 2014 Dec;24(12):1670–751. [PMC free article] [PubMed]

7. Nelson-Piercy C. Thyroid and parathyroid disease. In: Handbook of Obstetric Medicine. Oxford: ISIS Medical Media 1997;80–94.

8. Pruyn SC, Phelan JP, Buchanan GC. Long-term propanolol therapy in pregnancy: Maternal and fetal outcome. Am J Obstet Gynecol 1979;135:485–489.

Tocolysis

• Sana Ismail • Ruchika Garg

Introduction

Tocolysis is an obstetrical procedure to prolong gestation in patients who are experiencing preterm labor. This is achieved by inhibiting contractions of uterine smooth muscle using medications such as calcium channel blockers, beta-adrenergic agonist receptors, cyclo-oxygenase inhibitors, and magnesium sulfate, etc.

Tocolysis is given when the gestational age is <34 weeks to allow the steroid cover to have its action when there is no maternal and fetal compromise.

In the meta-analysis, tocolysis has not been able to improve perinatal outcome, but it prolongs pregnancy by at least 48 hours which allows the betamethasone to be administered and to do its action and the patient can be shifted to a center equipped with better neonatal facilities.

Use of Progestogens in the Management of Preterm Birth

17 Alpha-Hydroxy-Progesterone Caproate (17-OHP)

It was first introduced in 1950, synthetic progesterone with a longer half-life of 7 days, administered intramuscularly with a dose of 250 mg/week. It is the only United States Food and Drug Administration (US-FDA) approved progestin for prevention of preterm birth.

Mechanism of Actions of Progestogens

It decreases the gap junction, antagonizes oxytocin, causes relaxation of smooth muscle, has anti-inflammatory effects, and maintains cervical integrity.

Cyclo-oxygenase (COX-2) Inhibitors

Indomethacin acts by inhibiting prostaglandins to reduce uterine contractions, and binds reversibly to COX (5–6 hours).

Maternal side effects: Platelet dysfunction, bleeding disorder, renal, GI dysfunction, asthma.

Fetal and neonatal side effects: In utero constriction of the ductus arteriosus, oligohydramnios, neonatal pulmonary hypertension, reduced fetal renal blood flow and increased chances of necrotising enterocolitis and intraventricular hemorrhage.

ATOSIBAN

It is an oxytocin antagonist. It prevents oxytocin-stimulated increases in inositol triphosphate production. This prevents release of stored calcium from the sarcoplasmic reticulum and subsequent opening of voltage-gated calcium channels.

This cytosolic calcium increase prevents contractions of the uterine muscle, reducing the frequency of contractions and inducing uterine quiescence. It acts as an antagonist of Gq-coupling, explaining the inhibition of the inositol triphosphate pathway thought to be responsible for the effect on uterine contraction, but acts as an agonist of Gi-coupling. This agonism produces a pro-inflammatory effect in the human amnion, activating pro-inflammatory signal tranducer NF-κB.

Atosiban crosses the placenta and, at a dose of 300 µg/min, was found to have a 0.12 maternal/fetal concentration ratio. Atosiban has initial half-life (tα) of 0.21 hours and a terminal half-life (tβ) of 1.7 hours.

Dose: Initial bolus of 6.75 mg over 1 min followed by infusion of 18 mg/hr for 3 hours then 6 mg/hr for up to 45 hours (to a max. of 330 mg).

There is concern with its safety.

Minor side effects: Nausea, hyperglycaemia, headache, dizziness and palpitations. Since data do not strongly recommend one tocolytic over another on the basis of delivery delay or outcome, maternal tolerance is important. Atosiban has a lower rate of adverse effects than other tocolytics and is therefore better tolerated by patients. There is no relationship between atosiban and fetal distress and it may be useful in the management of acute fetal hypoxia suggested by a cardiotocograph.

The risk or severity of adverse effects can be increased when droxidopa, arbutamine epinephrine, etafedrine, formoterol fenoterol, dobutamine, and celiprolol is combined with atosiban.

When to Give Atosiban?

Atosiban is indicated in women with regular uterine contractions of at least 30 seconds duration at a rate of 4 per 30 minutes or cervical dilatation of 0–3 cm and effacement of 50% between 24 and 33 completed weeks of gestation and with normal fetal heart. The patient should be >18 years of age.

NIFEDIPINE (CALCIUM CHANNEL BLOCKER)

Calcium channel blockers should be considered as first-line tocolytic agents in the developing countries. The benefits of calcium channel blocker in reducing neonatal respiratory distress syndrome and neonatal jaundice are even more important in developing countries because of the limited capacities of neonatal intensive care facilities.

It is given orally, initial oral dose of 20 mg followed by 3 to 4 times daily up to 48 hours. There is increased chances of adverse reaction if dose >60 mg per day is used. Side effects include maternal hypotension, headache, nausea and flushing. It should not be combined with betamimetics (*e.g.* ritodrine) or magnesium sulphate. Nifedipine enhances neuromuscular blocking effects of magnesium which can interfere with pulmonary and cardiac functions.

BETAMIMETICS FOR TOCOLYSIS

Ritodrine Hydrochloride

Ritodrine hydrochloride was approved by FDA (USA) for preterm labour. It is a phenylethylamine derivative with plasma half-life of 2.5 hours and is preferentially active on beta-2-receptors.

Dose: Start with 0.05 mg/min (5 drops/min) till contractions cease usually at a dose of 0.15 mg/min (15 drops/min). But maximum of 0.30 mg/min (30 drops/min) and continued for 48 hours. Effective dose is 0.05 to 0.15 mg/min.

Complications of ritodrine: Maternal tachycardia, hypotension, palpitations or chest pain, pulmonary edema, fetal tachycardia, hypokalemia.

Terbutaline

Terbutaline has replaced ritodrine because of its easy administration, it is given as IV bolus of 250 µg followed by 10–50 µg/min until the labour stops. Then administer subcutaneously 0.25–0.5 mg, every 2–4 hours for 12 hours. A maintenance dose of 2.5–5 mg, orally, may be given 4–6 times a day. Side effects and contraindications are like ritodrine.

ROLE OF MAGNESIUM SULPHATE FOR TOCOLYSIS AND NEUROPROTECTION

$MgSO_4$ has modest neuroprotective effect, earlier the gestational age at delivery, better is the effect of $MgSO_4$ and neonatal outcome. The actual mechanism is not clearly understood, however, the different modes of protective functions are:

$MgSO_4$ crosses the placenta and it causes cerebral vasodilatation, reduces inflammatory cytokines, inhibits calcium influx into the cells, inhibits/delays ischemic cell death, reduces free radicals during hypoxic perfusion, it decreases cord blood cytokine production. It increases the levels of brain-derived neurotrophic factor (BDNF) (cord blood) (<34 weeks).

International guidelines on the use of $MgSO_4$ for neuroprotection [Royal College of Obstetricians and Gynecologists (RCOG), National Institute for Health and Care Excellence (NICE)] in pregnancy: <30 weeks— 4 g, IV bolus, 1 g/hr, IV for up to 24 hours or up to delivery whichever is earlier.

Most trials recommend to follow existing pre-eclampsia (PE) regimen, 4 g, IV bolus for 30 minutes, then 1 g/hr intravenous until birth or maximum up to 24 hours, whichever is shorter.

Maternal side effects: Flushing, perspiration, headache and muscle weakness.

Neonatal side effects: Lethargy, hypotonia and rarely respiratory depression.

Side Effects of Tocolytics

Maternal
- *General:* Tachycardia, tremor, hypotension

- *Metabolic:* Hyperglycemia, hypokalemia
- *Cardiovascular system (CVS):* Chest discomfort, palpitation
- *Pulmonary:* Pulmonary edema, dyspnea

Neonatal
- *Metabolic:* Hypoglycemia and hypocalcemia
- Ileus.

Contraindications

Absolute contraindications
- Thyrotoxicosis
- Cardiac disease
- Fetal compromise
- Chorioamnionitis
- Antepartum hemorrhage.

Relative contraindications
- Diabetes mellitus
- Hypertension
- Ruptured membranes
- Cervix >3 cm dilated.

Suggested Reading

1. American College of Obstetricians and Gynaecologists: Management of Preterm Labour. Practice bulletin No. 171, October 2016.
2. Anotayanonth S, Subhedar NV, Garner P, et al. Beta-mimetics for inhibiting preterm labour. Cochrane Database Syst Rev.2004;(4): CD004352.
3. Combs CA, Garite T, Maurel K, et al. Failure of 17-hydroxyprogesterone to reduce neonatal morbidity or prolong triplet pregnancy: A double-blind, randomized clinical trial. Am J Obstet Gynecol. 2011;204:166.
4. Dodd JM, Crowther CA, Dare MR, et al. Oral beta-mimetics for maintenance therapy after threatened preterm labour. Cochrane Database Syst Rev. 2006;(1):CD003927.
5. Doyle LW, Crowther CA, Middleton P, et al. Magnesium sulphate for women at risk of preterm birth for neuroprotection of the fetus. Cochrane Database Syst Rev. 2009;(1):CD004661.
6. Gyetvai K, Hannah ME, Hodnett ED, ET AL. Tocolytics for preterm labour: a systematic review. Obstet Gynecol. 1999;94(5 Pt 2):869–77.

Sildenafil in Obstetrics and Gynecology

• Rana Choudhary • Kairavi H Gokani • Kedar N Ganla

Introduction

Sildenafil (compound UK-92,480) was synthesized at Pfizer's research facility in England. It was initially studied for use in hypertension and angina pectoris. However, phase-I clinical trials under suggested the drug caused marked penile erections. It was therefore marketed for erectile dysfunction and patented in 1996, approved for use in erectile dysfunction by the Food and Drug Administration (FDA) in 1998. It became the first oral treatment approved to treat erectile dysfunction.

PHARMACOKINETICS

The bioavailability of sildenafil after oral intake is 41% (mean). It has a protein-binding of approximately 96%. After administration it is metabolized primarily in the liver CYP3A4 (major route), CYP2C9 (minor route). The metabolite formed is N-desmethylsildenafil which has a potency of approximately 50% potency for phosphodiesterase type-5 (PDE5). If taken with a high-fat meal, absorption is reduced; the time taken to reach the maximum plasma concentration increases by around one hour, and the maximum concentration itself is decreased by nearly one-third.

The onset of action after oral intake is after 20 minutes and the elimination half-life is 3–4 hours. It is excreted in Feces (~80%) and urine (~13%).

MECHANISM OF ACTION: SILDENAFIL CITRATE (Fig. 24.1 and Flowchart 24.1)

Sildenafil protects cyclic guanosine mono-phosphate (cGMP) from degradation by

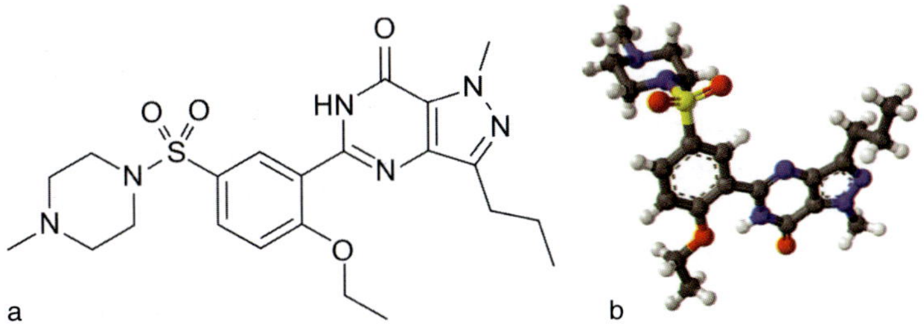

Formula: $C_{22}H_{30}N_6O_4S$
Molar mass: 474.58 g · mol^{-1}

Figs 24.1a and b: Molecule of sildenafil citrate

Flowchart 24.1: Mechanism of action—Sildenafil citrate

Sildenafil citrate
→ Selective inhibitor of cGMP-specific PDE type 5
→ ↑Nitric oxide
→ Smooth muscle relaxation
→ ↑Inflow of blood

- Corpus cavernosum → ↓Erectile dysfunction
- ↑Uterine blood flow → ↑Endometrial thickness
- ↑Uteroplacental flow → ↑IUGR

IUGR: Intrauterine growth restriction; PDE: Phosphodiesterase type-5

cGMP-specific PDE5. Nitric oxide (NO) binds to guanylate cyclase receptors, which results in increased levels of cGMP, leading to smooth muscle relaxation (vasodilation). This smooth muscle relaxation leads to vasodilation and increased inflow of blood. The molecular mechanism of smooth muscle relaxation involves the enzyme cGMP-dependent protein kinase, also known as PKG. This kinase is activated by cGMP and it phosphorylates multiple targets in the smooth muscle cells, namely myosin light chain phosphatase, RhoA, IP3-receptor, phospholipase C and others. Overall, this results in a decrease in intracellular calcium and desensitizing proteins to the effects of calcium, engendering smooth muscle relaxation. Sildenafil is a potent and selective inhibitor of cGMP-specific PDE5, which is responsible for degradation of cGMP. The molecular structure of sildenafil is similar to that of cGMP and acts as a competitive binding agent of PDE5, resulting in more cGMP.

Side Effects—Oral

Common side effects
- Nausea, headache, indigestion, nosebleed
- Temporary redness of face and neck, visible water retention.

Infrequent side effects
- Problems with eyesight
- Chronic trouble sleeping
- Diarrhea, dizzy, fever
- Flu-like symptoms, inflammation of the nose, joint pain
- Rash, redness of skin
- Sinus irritation and congestion, stuffy nose, trouble-breathing.

Precautions
- *Cardiac illness:* History of heart attack, angina, heart failure, stroke
- *Penial conditions:* Angulation, fibrosis/scarring, priapism
- Dizzy or cause vision problems
- Do not drive, use machinery, or any activity that requires alertness or clear vision until you are sure you can perform such activities safely.
- Limit alcoholic beverages.

USES OF SILDENAFIL CITRATE

I. Pulmonary Hypertension

Usual adult dose for pulmonary hypertension (oral)—initial dose: 5 or 20 mg, three times a day, 4 to 6 hourly. Maximum dose: 20 mg orally three times a day.

II. Male Infertility

- Erectile dysfunction
- Sperm motility.

How should sildenafil be used?

- Sildenafil should be taken orally about 1 hour before sexual activity.
- It takes about 1 hour to reach maximum concentration in the blood (30–120 minutes).
- Sildenafil has a half-life of 3–5 hours and is effective for up to 4 hours.
- Usual adult dose for erectile dysfunction— Initial dose: 50 mg orally once a day, as needed, 1 hour prior to sexual activity. Maintenance: 25 to 100 mg orally once a day, as needed, 1 hour prior to sexual activity.
- Usual geriatric dose for erectile dysfunction: Initial dose: 25 mg, orally, once a day, 1 hour prior to sexual activity.

A recent meta-analysis and systematic review (2017) showed that acute administration of PDE5 inhibitors had no effect on semen volume and sperm concentration (n = 1317).[1] However, the percentage of motile spermatozoa, the percentage of total progressive motility, and rapid progressive motility were increased after oral PDE5 inhibitors treatment. Interestingly, these significant changes were observed only in infertile men, but not in normal patients. The percentage of morphologically normal spermatozoa also increased in infertile men.

III. Female Sexual Dysfunction (FSD)

Pathophysiology

- Decrease in muscle relaxation
- Decrease in genital blood flow, uterine blood flow and increase oxidative stress
- Decrease in vaginal lubrication
- Increase in vaginal luminal pressure
- Dyspareunia, vaginimus
- Finally reduced libido and decreased satisfaction
- All these symptoms adversely affect their QoL.

Sildenafil–female sexual dysfunction

- Studies have shown that 50 mg of sildenafil citrate daily orally increased to max. 100 mg can be helpful if taken not >2 hours or <1 hour before sexual intercourse.[2]

Use of sildenafil in FSD helped with the below symptoms in 90% of women:[3,4]

- Effective duration
- Intensity of adequate arousal
- Lubrication
- Orgasmic function

Sildenafil can be used in menopausal women (naturally/surgically). It improves:[3-5]

- Genital arousal
- Satisfaction after intercourse.

IV. Thin Endometrium

- Sildenafil has benefited patients with thin endometrium undergoing *in vitro* fertilization (IVF).
- Patients were administered vaginal sildenafil citrate, 25 mg, QID, for 7 days
- These patients had previous failed cycles of IVF.
- They had a poor endometrial response and none achieved a lining >8 mm despite previous treatment with oestrogen
- Evaluated parameters were
  - Uterine artery pulsatility index (PI)
  - Endometrial thickness
- After using sildenafil citrate vaginally, the PI which was between 2.0 and 3.4, decreased to between 1.5 and 2.7 after 7 days of sildenafil, reflecting increased diastolic blood flow.
- The endometrial thickness developed to >10 mm in these patients after 7 days.

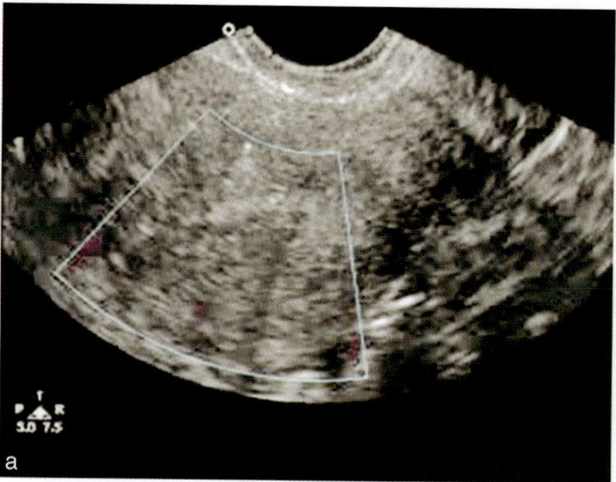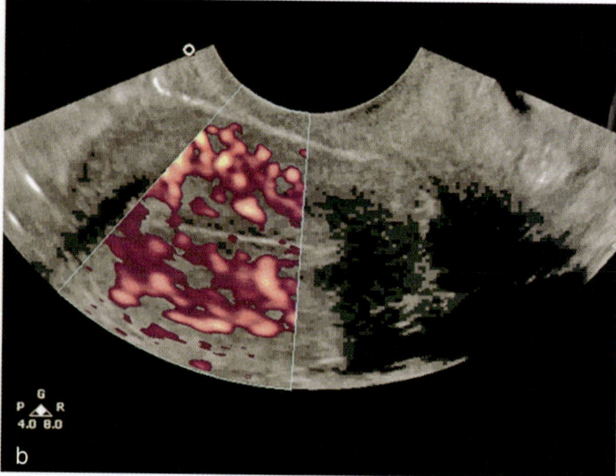

Figs 24.2a and b: Improvement in the endometrial flow after starting sildenafil citrate vaginally

- Use of sildenafil (25 or 100 mg) during the luteal phase of the menstrual cycle, demonstrated a significant increase in uterine volumetric blood flow.[6]

Various studies have shown that vaginal sildenafil citrate has improved outcome in previous failed IVF cycles due to thin endometrium **(Fig. 24.2)**.[7–9]

Conclusion

- Oral sildenafil citrate is a good way to improve the endometrial receptivity[9–11]
- Improvement of endometrial thickness and uterine blood flow with significant reduction of resistive index (RI) and PI were detected (68%), implantation were higher (26 *vs* 7%) and pregnancy rate were higher (40 *vs* 14%).
- Beneficial role of sildenafil citrate in thin endometrium and failed IVF embryo transfer (ET) cycles, assisted intrauterine inseminisation (IUI) cycles, or resistant endometrium, where it increased uterine receptivity.[11]
- Sildenafil when compared to estradiol valerate has better results as far as endometrial vascularity is concerned and marginally increased pregnancy outcome in patients undergoing IUI.[12]

V. Intrauterine Growth Restriction (IUGR) and Oligohydramnios

During the second and third trimesters, transport of nutrients from mother to fetus is predominantly dependent on utero-placental blood flow. Constriction of myometrial arteries reduces blood supply and transport of nutrients to fetus leading to IUGR and oligohydroamnios **(Flowchart 24.2)**.

Flowchart 24.2: Mechanism of IUGR and oligohydramnios

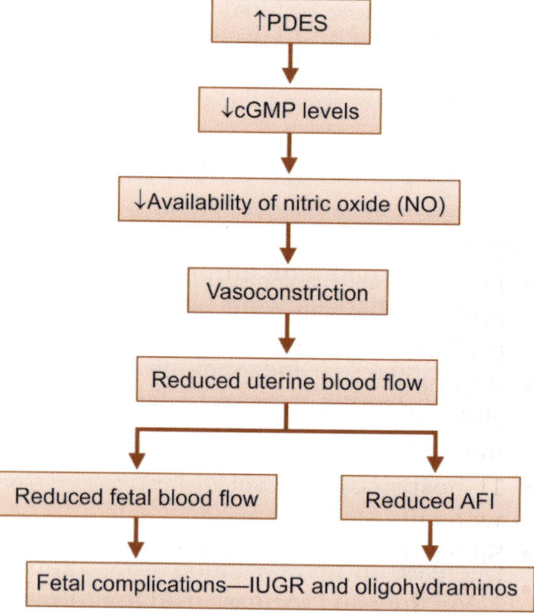

- Sildenafil citrate in these patients seems to:[13–15]
  - Decreased arterial pressure
  - Improved arterial perfusion in human placenta model
- *Literature review:* Sildenafil in IUGR[13–15]
  - Systematic meta-analysis to evaluate effects of sildenafil.
  - 22 animal studies and 2 human randomized controlled trials (RCTs).[13–15]
  - Sildenafil increases fetal growth during (FGR) and pre-eclampsia pregnancy compared with healthy pregnancy.
  - Effects were similar among different species and largest after oral and continuous administration.
  - Significant blood pressure-lowering effect of sildenafil is present during FGR/pre-eclampsia pregnancy only (P <0.01), with the effect size being highly dependent on baseline blood pressure and without effect in the absence of hypertension.
  - There was statistically significant difference in the mean birth weight at delivery with sildenafil citrate.[14,15]
  - Sildenafil was also associated with pregnancy prolongation (p = 0.0001), increased gestational age at delivery (p = 0.004), improved neonatal weight (p = 0.0001), and less admission to neonatal intensive care unit (p = 0.03). No adverse effects reported.[15]

STRIDER-DUTCH TRIAL[16]

- Dutch Sildenafil therapy in dismal prognosis early onset fetal growth restriction (STRIDER) RCT.
- Assess beneficial and harmful effects of sildenafil *vs* placebo on fetal and neonatal mortality with severe early-onset FGR.
- 11 hospitals, the Netherlands (*n* = 360 women)
- Sildenafil 25 mg or placebo, orally, TDS
- Primary outcome—death or major neonatal morbidity

- Secondary outcomes—neurodevelopmental impairment, etc.

The decision to halt this trial was made following a planned interim analysis conducted by an independent data and safety monitoring committee, which concluded the following:

1. There was a signal of potential harm relating to an increased incidence of persistent pulmonary hypertension of newborn and a non-significant trend towards an increase in neonatal death (but not stillbirth).
2. There was likely futility to show a significant beneficial effect in primary outcome: a composite of mortality and major neonatal morbidity at hospital discharge.

- Detailed review and validation of findings before any further exposure of women and fetuses to sildenafil.
- Findings in the Dutch trial do not seem to be consistent with those of completed STRIDER trials in UK and New Zealand/Australia.
- These previous trials, using almost identical methods, did not find any beneficial effect of sildenafil therapy in FGR, but also found no evidence of an association with postpartum hemorrhage (PPH) of newborn or neonatal death.

Pregnancy: Category B

- No adverse fetal outcomes were reported in pregnant women receiving sildenafil late in their pregnancy.
- No evidence of teratogenicity, embryotoxicity, or fetotoxicity was observed in pregnant rats or rabbits dosed with sildenafil during organogenesis.
- Human case reports have reported no deleterious effects on the mother or offspring.[17]

Sildenafil in Obstetrics

- Uteroplacental blood improves delivery of oxygen and other nutrients to fetus.[17–20]

- Augments feto-placental blood flow in setting of placental vascular insufficiency helps in increasing the amniotic fluid index (AFI), and this is one of the reasons why patients with oligohydramnios and FGR may benefit from sildenafil citrate.[18–20]
- Window of fetal maturity and hence reduces neonatal morbidity and mortality due to prematurity.[17–20]
- The amniotic fluid volume was higher in the sildenafil group at the final assessment (11.5 compared with 5.4 cm, P=.02).[18–20]
- The sildenafil group delivered later (38.3 compared with 36 weeks of gestation, P = 0.001), had a lower rate of cesarean delivery (28% compared with 73%), and their neonates were less.[17–20]
- Likely to be admitted to the neonatal intensive care unit (11% compared with 41%, P = 0.001).[17]

Dosage: Vaginal sildenafil citrate, 25 mg, TID, from the day of diagnosis of IUGR until delivery.[17–20]

OTHER RECENT USES

a. *Torsion:* Medical management in the form of vaginal sildenafil citrate may be useful in selected cases of early ovarian torsion by improving venous drainage, tissue perfusion, and decreasing tissue damage by preventing reperfusion injury.[21]

b. *Alzheimer disease:* Propensity score-stratified analyses confirmed that sildenafil is significantly associated with a decreased risk of Alzheimer disease (AD) across all four-drug cohorts tested (diltiazem, glimepiride, losartan and metformin) after adjusting for age, sex, race and disease comorbidities. We also found that sildenafil increases neurite growth and decreases phospho-tau expression in neuron models derived from induced pluripotent stem cells from patients with AD, supporting mechanistically its potential beneficial effect in AD.[22]

c. *Along with CC to improve pregnancy rate:* A randomized clinical trial of sildenafil plus clomiphene citrate showed that adding sildenafil citrate improved ovulation success rate and increased pregnancy rates in patients with unexplained infertility.[23–25]

d. *Along with granulocyte colony-stimulating factor (GCSF) for improving enometrial thickness:* Vaginal sildenafil improved endometrial thickness as compared GCSF alone or in combination with intrauterine infusion of granulocyte colony-stimulating factor (filgrastim, GCSF).[26]

e. *Recurrent first trimester abortion*: There are case reports on use of oral sildenafil citrate with nitric oxide patch for cases of spontaneous recurrent first trimester abortion.[27]

FUTURE USE OF SILDENAFIL

- Sildenafil citrate (60 mg/kg per day) or control gel diet (containing 0.3% salt) was administered from gestational-day 10 until birth.
- Echocardiographic parameters, glomerular filtration rate, and fractional electrolyte excretion were determined.
- Prenatal sildenafil treatment subtly improves cardiovascular but not renal function in the offspring of this FGR rat model.[28]

References

1. Tan P, Liu L, Wei S, Tang Z, Yang L, Wei Q. The Effect of Oral Phosphodiesterase-5 Inhibitors on Sperm Parameters: A Meta-analysis and Systematic Review. Urology. 2017 Jul;105:54–61. doi: 10.1016/j.urology.2017.02.032. Epub 2017 Mar 1. PMID: 28259808.

2. Gao L. Int J Gynaecol Obstet. 2016 May. Systematic review and meta-analysis of phosphodiesterase type 5 inhibitors for the treatment of female sexual dysfunction.

3. H. George Nurnberg et al. Sildenafil for Sexual Dysfunction in Women Taking Antidepressants. Am J Psychiatry 156:10, October 1999. https://doi.org/10.1176/ajp.156.10.1664

4. Dasgupta R, Wiseman OJ, Kanabar G et al. Efficacy of sildenafil in the treatment of female sexual dysfunction due to multiple sclerosis. J Urol. 2004 Mar;171(3):1189–93; discussion 1193. doi: 10.1097/01.ju.0000113145.43174.24. PMID: 14767298. Sildenafil significantly increases vaginal Vasocongestion (increased vascular blood flow) J Womens Health Gend Based Med. 2002

5. Hale SA, Jones CW, Osol G, Schonberg A, et al. Sildenafil increases uterine blood flow in nonpregnant nulliparous women. Reprod Sci. 2010 Apr;17(4):358–65. doi: 10.1177/1933719109354648. PMID: 20228381; PMCID: PMC2885136.Fertility And Sterility Vol. 78, No. 5, November 2002,1073–1076.

6. Kim, Kwang, Lee, Hee et el. (2010). Efficacy of luteal supplementation of vaginal sildenafil and oral estrogen on pregnancy rate following IVF-ET in women with a history of thin endometria: A pilot study. Journal of Women's Medicine. 3. 155.

7. Fetih AN, Habib DM, Abdelaal II, et al. Adding sildenafil vaginal gel to clomiphene citrate in infertile women with prior clomiphene citrate failure due to thin endometrium: a prospective self-controlled clinical trial. Facts Views Vis Obgyn. 2017 Mar;9(1):21–27. PMID: 28721181; PMCID: PMC5506766.

8. Dehghani Firouzabadi R, avi M. Effect of sildenafil citrate on endometrial preparation and outcome of frozen-thawed embryo transfer cycles: a randomized clinical trial. Iran J Reprod Med. 2013 Feb;11(2):151-8. PMID: 24639741; PMCID: PMC3941353.

9. Moini A, Zafarani F, Jahangiri N, Jahanian Sadatmahalleh SH, Sadeghi M, Chehrazi M, Ahmadi F. The Effect of Vaginal Sildenafil on The Outcome of Assisted Reproductive Technology Cycles in Patients with Repeated Implantation Failures: A Randomized Placebo-Controlled Trial. Int J Fertil Steril. 2020 Jan;13(4):289–295. doi: 10.22074/ijfs.2020.5681. Epub 2019 Nov 11. PMID: 31710189; PMCID: PMC6875854.

10. Li X, Luan T, Zhao C, Zhang M, Dong L, Su Y, Ling X. Effect of sildenafil citrate on treatment of infertility in women with a thin endometrium: a systematic review and meta-analysis. J Int Med Res. 2020 Nov;48(11):300060520969584. doi: 10.1177/0300060520969584. PMID: 33176524; PMCID: PMC7673063.

11. Benni JM, Patil PA. An overview on sildenafil and female infertility. Indian j health sci 2016;9:131–6.

12. Leah A. Garcia, Su M. Hlaing ET AL. Sildenafil Attenuates Inflammation and Oxidative Stress in Pelvic Ganglia Neurons after Bilateral Cavernosal Nerve Damage. International Journal of Molecular Sciences. June 2015.

13. Paauw ND. Sildenafil During Pregnancy: A Preclinical Meta-Analysis on Fetal Growth and Maternal Blood Pressure. Hypertension. 2017 Nov.

14. Maged M. Taiwan J Obstet Gynecol. 2018 Aug. Use of sildenafil citrate in cases of intrauterine growth restriction (IUGR); a prospective trial.

15. El-Sayed MA. J Matern Fetal Neonatal Med. 2018 Apr. Utero-placental perfusion Doppler indices in growth restricted fetuses: effect of sildenafil citrate.

16. Trials.2019 Jan. Detailed statistical analysis plan for the Dutch STRIDER randomised clinical trial on sildenafil versus placebo for pregnant women with severe early onset fetal growth restriction.

17. Villanueva-García D, Mota-Rojas D, Hernández-González R, Sánchez-Aparicio P, Alonso-Spilsbury M, Trujillo-Ortega ME, Necoechea RR, Nava-Ocampo AA. A systematic review of experimental and clinical studies of sildenafil citrate for intrauterine growth restriction and pre-term labour. J Obstet Gynaecol. 2007 Apr; 27(3):255–9. doi: 10.1080/01443610701194978. PMID: 17464805.

18. Choudhary R, Desai K, Parekh H, Ganla K. Sildenafil citrate for the management of fetal growth restriction and oligohydramnios. Int J Womens Health. 2016 Aug 9;8:367–72. doi: 10.2147/IJWH.S108370. PMID: 27563258; PMCID: PMC4984996.

19. Vora, Priyanka & Choudhary, Rana & Ganla, Kedar. (2020). Sildenafil citrate to improve colour doppler indices in patient with pre-eclampsia: a path less taken. International Journal of Reproduction, Contraception, Obstetrics and Gynecology. 9. 5124. 10.18203/2320-1770. ijrcog20205259.

20. Obstet Gynecol. 2017. Sildenafil Citrate Therapy for Oligohydramnios: A Randomized Controlled Trial.

21. Ganla KN, Choudhary RA, Vora PH, Athavale UV. Sildenafil Citrate: Novel Therapy in the Management of Ovarian Torsion. J Hum Reprod Sci. 2019 Oct-Dec;12(4):351-354. doi: 10.4103/jhrs.JHRS_52_19. Epub 2019 Dec 17. PMID: 32038089; PMCID: PMC6937764.

22. Fang J, Zhang P, Zhou Y, et al. Endophenotype-based in silico network medicine discovery combined with insurance record data mining

identifies sildenafil as a candidate drug for Alzheimer's disease. Nat Aging 1, 1175–1188 (2021) https://doi.org/10.1038/s43587-021-00138-z.

23. Mohamed TY. Oral Sildenafil for Treatment of Female Infertility among PCO Patients: Randomized Comparative Study. Austin J Obstet Gynecol. 2019; 6(3): 1143.

24. Ahmed A. Aboelroose, Zakia M. Ibrahim, et al. A randomized clinical trial of sildenafil plus clomiphene citrate to improve the success rate of ovulation induction in patients with unexplained infertility. International Journal of Gynecology and Obstetrics. 2020.https://doi.org/10.1002/ijgo.13159).

25. Li X, Su Y, Xie Q, Luan, et al. Gynecologic and Obstetric Investigation. The Effect of Sildenafil Citrate on Poor Endometrium in Patients Undergoing Frozen-Thawed Embryo Transfer following Resection of Intrauterine Adhesions: A Retrospective Study. T. 2021, Vol. 86, No. 3. July 2021.

26. Belapurkar P, Jaiswal A, Madaan S (June 29, 2022) Comparison of Efficacy Between Vaginal Sildenafil and Granulocyte-Colony Stimulating Factor (G-CSF) in Improving Endometrial Thickness (ET) in Infertile Women. Cureus 14(6): e26415. doi:10.7759/cureus.26415.

27. Gamea RMR, El-Bhoty SB, ElEbiary MT, El-Gharib MN. The Effects of Nitric Oxide Patch Versus Oral Sildenafil Citrate on First Trimester Pregnant Women with a History of Recurrent Miscarriage. Madridge J Case Rep Stud. 2018; 2(2): 67–70. doi: 10.18689/mjcrs-1000117).

28. Terstappen F. Hypertension. 2019 May Prenatal Sildenafil Therapy Improves Cardiovascular Function in Fetal Growth Restricted Offspring of Dahl Salt-Sensitive Rats.

Steroids in Obstetrics and Gynecology

• Geetha Balsarkar • Sunil Tambvekar

Introduction

Corticosteroids and Pharmaceutical Preparations

Steroids are hormones that are produced by the chemical process known as steroidogenesis. The steroid hormone's chemical structure is mostly derived from cholesterol, and they possess a structure known as 'the steroid ring.'

Corticosteroids are a class of steroid hormones that are produced primarily by the adrenal cortex, and other organs, like ovaries. Their equivalents that are produced in a lab are known as corticosteroids. The most common kinds of corticosteroids are known as glucocorticoids and mineralocorticoids, respectively. They are involved in a wide range of physiological process for life processes, some of the most important of which include the stress response, the immunological response, and the regulation of inflammation, as well as the metabolism of carbohydrates, blood electrolyte levels, protein catabolism, and behavior.[1] Dexamethasone and its derivatives are nearly pure glucocorticoids, but prednisone and its derivatives also contain some mineralocorticoid action in addition to the glucocorticoid effects.[2] Synthetic pharmaceutical medicines with corticosteroid-like actions are used to treat a wide range of illnesses.

Agonists of the glucocorticoid and/or mineralocorticoid receptors are corticosteroids. Some corticosteroids, in addition to their corticosteroid activity, may also have progestogenic activity, which may result in sexually-related adverse effects.[3]

A typical side effect of glucocorticoids is the induction of Cushing's syndrome by the use of medicine. Mineralocorticoids frequently cause side effects, such as atypically increased blood pressure, steroid-induced diabetes mellitus, psychosis, restless sleep, hypokalemia, hypernatremia without peripheral edema, metabolic alkalosis, and degradation of connective tissue.[4]

APPLICATIONS IN OBSTETRICS AND GYNECOLOGY AND CLINICAL GUIDELINES

Antenatal Corticosteroids for Fetal Lung Maturity

History

Graham Liggins, a researcher in the field of medicine, began his investigation into the effects of administering dexamethasone on the timing of labour in pregnant sheep in the year 1969. This experiment was carried out by Liggins in order to test his hypothesis, which states that the embryo, and not the mother, is responsible for the onset of labour.[6] In spite of the fact that dexamethasone led the expecting sheep to birth their fetuses early, Liggins found that the lamb fetus was delivered alive and breathing![5] This completely unrelated observation brought about fundamental shifts in the practice. The fields of obstetrics and neonatology were both irrevocably changed as a result of this chanced observation.

Liggins subsequently ran a similar experiment on 282 human mothers who were all projected to deliver their babies before their due date. This time, however, he enlisted the support of his colleague, paediatrician Ross Howie. This preliminary research found that giving corticosteroids, specifically betamethasone, resulted in immediate statistically significant improvements.[7] These improvements included a lower neonatal mortality rate, a lower incidence of respiratory distress syndrome, but only in fetuses who had undergone <32 weeks of gestation and were treated for a minimum of 24 hours prior to delivery, and a lower incidence of intraventricular cerebral haemorrhage.

In 1972, Sir Graham Liggins and Ross Howie were the first to demonstrate the efficacy of this corticosteroid medication on humans by conducting a randomised controlled experiment employing betamethasone. The trial was directed by Sir Graham Liggins.[7]

Nevertheless, these findings did not make their way into clinical practice in the United States until more than two decades after they were published.

Mechanism of Action

Antenatal corticosteroids have an effect on type-II pneumocytes, which are found in the alveoli of an infant's pulmonary tissue.[8]

Enhanced lung mechanics and gas exchange are the outcomes of accelerated pneumocyte morphologic development, which causes structural and biochemical alterations.

Glucocorticoids speed up the maturation process of cells and boost production of the mRNA that codes for the proteins necessary for the synthesis of surfactant.

These cellular and molecular modifications in the lung alveoli contribute to an even greater improvement in respiratory outcomes.

Adverse Effects

Early studies had shown that using corticosteroids before birth might have unfavorable long-term effects.[9] In animal studies, prenatal exposure to corticosteroids resulted in deleterious effects on the cardio-metabolic system, decreased brain growth, and increased issues with learning and memory. These effects were also exacerbated by the usage of the steroids.[10] It is not yet known whether human fetuses would experience the same effects; nonetheless, some study has found that human preterm fetuses treated with prenatal corticosteroids had a higher chance of having learning and memory impairments. This is the case even though it is not known whether human fetuses would suffer the same consequences. These medications are able to cross the placenta and enter the brain of the developing baby, which may have an effect on neurodevelopment.[9] According to research conducted on both humans and animals, receiving many doses of prenatal corticosteroids may raise the risk of developing long-term vision and hearing issues in the offspring.[11–13] However, there is no indication of such issues with the use of prenatal steroids for a single course, and it is recommended that multiple courses be avoided.

1. *Immediate effects on the fetus are:*
   - Transient FHR changes (non-reassuring) within 2–3 days administration
   - Transient improvement in end-diastolic flow (EDF) in the umbilical artery
2. *Infants:* No evidence of a rise in adverse infant outcomes
3. *Maternal:* Most women tolerate well.
   - Transient hyperglycemia does not increase the risk of death, chorioamnionitis, or puerperal sepsis.

Contraindications

Contraindications to antenatal corticosteroid administration include:[14]

- Systemic maternal infection
- Maternal chorioamnionitis

Concerns about 'risks in multiple course corticosteroid therapy':

- *Maternal Fetal Medicine Networks Unit trial:* A higher proportion of small-for-gestational age (SGA) fetuses in the repeated course group, a smaller placenta, and an increase in the incidence of cerebral palsy.[15]
- *Multiple courses of antenatal corticosteroid for preterm birth study:* Dose–response relationship between the number of corticosteroid courses and decrease in fetal growth.[16,17]

Guidelines for Clinical Practice

When the premature fetus is anticipated to be delivered within 24 to 48 hours, corticosteroids are administered. The optimal benefit period begins 24 hours after administration and lasts for 7 days.[7]

In obstetrics and neonatology, antenatal steroids, their effects, and optimal use have been the subject of active research over the past four decades. In the 1980s, one of the very first systematic evaluations and meta-analyses was conducted on the use of antenatal steroids for women at risk of preterm birth. The Cochrane logo is derived from this review and depicts how the forest plot analysis would have appeared in 1982, if the evidence had been analyzed collectively. In 1989, when the first comprehensive systemic review and meta-analysis were published, the conclusion was that steroids reduced the risk of death and serious illness in infants. However, there were still many uncertainties, and in the 30 years since then, more studies have been conducted and the review has been updated regularly.[33]

Consequently, numerous clinical organisations have established clinical guidelines for the administration of corticosteroids during pregnancy. In some regions of the globe, antenatal steroids are administered up to 36 weeks into the pregnancy.[18] The time between the administration of steroids and delivery may affect the effectiveness of the steroids.[19]

Government of India has issued operational guidelines for use of antenatal corticosteroids in preterm labour in 2014 **(Table 25.1)**.[27] Key points are as follows:

- A single injection regimen of dexamethasone will be administered to women with preterm labor (between 24 and 34 weeks of gestation) at all levels of public and private health facilities.
- Inject 6 mg of dexamethasone sodium phosphate intramuscularly four times, 12 hours apart.
- Indications: Conditions leading to imminent delivery, such as antepartum hemorrhage, preterm premature membrane rupture, and severe pre-eclampsia.
- It should be noted that the initial point of contact must make every effort to guarantee the administration of antenatal corticosteroids.
- Contraindications:
  - Frank chorioamnionitis
  - A repeat course of antenatal steroids is not recommended.

Choice of Drug

Although dexamethasone is typically suggested over betamethasone due to its enhanced efficacy and safety, wide availability, and low cost, betamethasone is more successful at avoiding the weakening of the brain in preterm fetuses. Dexamethasone is often recommended due to its increased efficacy and safety, wide availability, and low cost.[28] Both of these medications have extremely similar molecular structures and are able to pass through the placenta. In point of fact, the two steroids are exactly the same, with the exception of one additional methyl group found on betamethasone.[29] There is no evidence to show that betamethasone is

Table 25.1: Global perspective: Guidelines published on antenatal corticosteroids

Organisation (year published)	Gestational-age recommendations	Other inclusion criteria	Betamethasone or dexamethasone
World Health Organization (2015)[20]	24–34 weeks	Gestational age can be accurately assessed, preterm birth anticipated within 7 days, lack of maternal infection	Either betamethasone or dexamethasone
Government of India. Operational guidelines for use of antenatal corticosteroids in preterm labour (2014)[26]	24–34 weeks	Repeat course of antenatal steroids is not recommended.	Dexamethasone
Royal College of Obstetricians and Gynecologists (2015)[21]	24–33 weeks and 6 days	Anticipated preterm birth	Not specified
The American College of Obstetricians and Gynecologists (2020)[22]	24–33 weeks and 6 days	Preterm birth anticipated within 7 days	Betamethasone
Antenatal Corticosteroids Clinical Practice Guidelines Panel (2015)[23]	≤34 weeks and 6 days	Preterm birth anticipated in ≥7 days	Either betamethasone or dexamethasone
Australian and New Zealand Neonatal Network (2018)[24]	<34 weeks and 6 days	Preterm birth anticipated in 1–8 days	Not specified
Society of Obstetricians and Gynecologists of Canada (2018)[25]	24–34 weeks and 6 days	Preterm birth anticipated in ≥7 days	Either betamethasone or dexamethasone
Cochrane sytematic review (August 2022)[29]	-	-	No difference

preferable to dexamethasone, despite the fact that betamethasone has a longer half-life.

Cochrane systematic review was published in August 2022 regarding the selection of various corticosteroids and regimens. The authors concluded: "Overall, it remains uncertain whether there are significant differences between dexamethasone and betamethasone, or between regimens. For the majority of infant and early childhood outcomes, there may be no difference between these medications. However, for several important outcomes for the mother, infant, and child, the evidence was equivocal and did not exclude the possibility of significant benefits or risks. The evidence regarding various antenatal corticosteroid regimens is limited and does not support the use of one regimen over another."[29]

According to the research, there are no statistically significant differences between dexamethasone and betamethasone in terms of respiratory distress syndrome (RDS) or neonatal mortality. Both are efficacious, and their efficacy is comparable.

Choice of Steroids: Indian Context

In India, 'dexamethasone sodium phosphate' is the preferred medication.

The salt betamethasone acetate + phosphate, which only requires two doses every 12 hours, is unavailable in India. Betamethasone phosphate (commonly used, by the trade name: Inj. betnesol) is the salt available in India. It is short-acting and requires more frequent administration than the former salt. As a result, the dosage schedule for betamethasone phosphate is comparable to that of dexamethasone, and it offers no additional benefits over dexamethasone.

Additionally, betamethasone is more expensive and less stable than dexamethasone at high temperatures. In certain instances, however, inj., if dexamethasone is unavailable, the provider may substitute inj. betamethasone phosphate, provides newborns with the benefits of corticosteroids.

Evidence on usage of antenatal steroids after 34 weeks (late preterm) and prior term elective caesarian sections.

Systematic reviews and meta-analyses on the use of steroids in late preterm infants have suggested that moderate-quality evidence suggests that exposure reduces the need for respiratory support and increases the risk of hypoglycemia in late preterm neonates. To assess the benefits and hazards in this population, large, definitive trials with adequate neurodevelopmental follow-ups are required.[30] On the effectiveness of antenatal steroids before term elective caesarean sections, a Cochrane review was published in December 2021. With the exception of the outcome of admission to neonatal special care (all levels) for respiratory morbidity, the overall certainty of the evidence for the primary outcomes was determined to be low or very low.

Prior to caesarean section, additional research should investigate the efficacy of antenatal steroids at various gestational ages.[31] Recent studies have highlighted the lack of definitive evidence for such use.[32]

There are nine ongoing studies with prospective eligibility that could be included in future updates of Cochrane reviews.

AUTO-IMMUNE DISORDERS

Corticosteroids are typically prescribed in non-endocrine autoimmune diseases.

The non-endocrine autoimmune disorders due to auto-antibodies, encountered by obstetricians are systemic lupus erytematosus (SLE), antiphospholipid syndrome (APS), thrombocytopenia and less often, rheumatoid arthritis, myasthenia gravis and Addison's disease.

Systemic lupus erythematosus is a multi-system disease that predominantly affects reproductive-aged women. With a greater comprehension of the disease and its treatment with corticosteroids, antimalarials, and immunosuppressive drugs, pregnancy outcomes have vastly improved over time.[34]

Corticosteroids have been widely used to treat SLE in pregnant women. Although corticosteroid use during pregnancy does not increase the risk of severe malformations, the risk of oral clefts is nearly tripled.[35]

Prednisolone, prednisone, and methyl-prednisolone are the medications of choice in pregnancy due to their minimal placental transfer. With higher concentrations, there is a significant risk of developing hypertension and glucose intolerance during pregnancy, and calcium must be supplemented to compensate for bone mineral loss caused by chronic steroid use. High-dose steroid use during pregnancy (>20 mg/day) has been linked to an increased risk of preterm labour, premature membrane rupture, and fetal growth restriction.[34]

Immune thrombocytopenia during pregnancy, typically manifesting as idiopathic thrombocytopenic purpura (ITP), is one of the most difficult cases for obstetricians. In pregnancy, corticosteroids or intravenous immunoglobulin (IVIg) are the initial line of treatment. 21 days of standard initial treatment are recommended.[36,37]

The recommended initial dose of prednisolone ranges from 0.2 to 0.5 mg/kg per day to 1 mg/kg per day. Initial response occurs between 2 and 14 days, while maximal response occurs between 4 and 28 days.[34]

APPLICATIONS IN REPRODUCTIVE ENDOCRINOLOGY AND EARLY PREGNANCY

Prednisone

Prednisone is also an immunomodulatory agent with numerous beneficial effects in the treatment of autoimmune disorders and the initiation of early pregnancy.[38,39] Studies have shown that prednisone can inhibit the cytotoxicity of uterine natural killer (NK) cells and the release of cytokines in pre-implantation endometrium. Additionally, prednisone can enhance the secretion of human chorionic gonadotropin (hCG) and promote the proliferation and invasion of trophoblast.[38,40] This hints that prednisone may have a major impact on the likelihood of embryo implantation as well as the results of IVF. It is considered that the harmful effects caused by prednisone are low,[41] as only approximately 10% of the active substance makes it to the fetus.[42–44]

During assisted-reproductive technology (ART) procedures, prednisolone, is typically prescribed for **high-risk groups, repeated implantation failure, recurrent pregnancy loss, and anti-nuclear antibodies (ANA)/ double-stranded DNA (ds DNA) positivite status**. Tab. prednisolone, 5 mg, TID, should be initiated during the endometrial preparation cycle and continued until the beta-hCG levels are detected; it can then be tapered to BD for 5 days and OD for five days.

This is particularly advantageous for IVF attempts in women with coexisting autoimmune disorders, and it can be continued throughout pregnancy. Prednisolone has been shown to increase the success and live birth rates of IVF pregnancies in patients with auto-antibodies, such as those with **auto-immune hypothyroidism**.[45]

ADDITIONAL APPLICATIONS OF STEROIDS IN OBSTETRICS AND GYNAECOLOGY

Prenatal Treatment of Mothers at Risk for Having An Affected Child Congenital Adrenal Hyperplasia (CAH)[46]

Prenatal maternal treatment with dexamethasone (up to 1.5 mg, daily in divided doses), can significantly reduce or eliminate fetal female genital virilization.[47]

Not metabolized by the placenta and efficiently crosses into fetal circulation.

For maximum effectiveness, treatment should begin between 4 and 5 weeks gestation.

After 9 weeks, prenatal maternal treatment poses some potential risks for the fetus, such as postnatal failure to thrive and psychomotor developmental delay, and can also have significant adverse effects on the mother, such as severe abdominal striae, hyperglycemia, hypertension, gastrointestinal symptoms, and emotional distress and lability.[48]

In light of the fact that only one in eight fetuses will benefit from maternal treatment (one in four will be affected, and half of those will be males), the optimal strategy involves early prenatal diagnosis by chorion villous sampling (CVS) with rapid sex determination and genotyping. Treatment will either be continued or initiated only in mothers who are carrying an affected female fetus. However, preoperative counselling, monitoring, and long-term follow-up are required and suggested. This is necessary due to the fact that even prenatal therapy with dexamethasone for a short period of time may damage postnatal physical, cognitive, and emotional development; provided within the context of academic research.[49,50]

Acute Emergencies
Cardiopulmonary Resuscitation

Inj. hydrocortisone is a highly effective treatment for acute emergencies resulting from atopy and other allergic reactions. Obstetric emergencies necessitate OT, Labour-ward administration, and injections. Intensivists administer 100 mg of sodium hydro-cortisone succinate intravenously as a life-saving drug.

Tubal Recanalisation Surgery

During tubal recanalisation surgery, gynecologists prefer continuous instillation of inj. hydrocortisone to keep local immunity lowered and avoid inflammations, to successfully achieve tubal recanalisation.

References

1. Nussey, S.; Whitehead, S. (2001). Endocrinology: An Integrated Approach. Oxford: BIOS Scientific Publishers.

2. Nussey, Stephen; Whitehead, Saffron (2001-01-01). The adrenal gland. BIOS Scientific Publishers.

3. Brook EM, Hu CH, Kingston KA, Matzkin EG (March 2017). "Corticosteroid Injections: A Review of Sex-Related Side Effects". Orthopedics. 40 (2): e211–e215. doi:10.3928/01477447-20161116-07. PMID 27874912.

4. Liu, Dora; Ahmet, Alexandra; Ward, Leanne; Krishnamoorthy, Preetha; Mandelcorn, Efrem D; Leigh, Richard; Brown, Jacques P; Cohen, Albert; Kim, Harold (2013-08-15). "A practical guide to the monitoring and management of the complications of systemic corticosteroid therapy". Allergy, Asthma, and Clinical Immunology. 9 (1): 30. doi:10.1186/1710-1492-9-30. ISSN 1710–1484. PMC 3765115. PMID 23947590.

5. Liggins GC (December 1969). "Premature delivery of foetal lambs infused with glucocorticoids". The Journal of Endocrinology. 45 (4): 515–523. doi:10.1677/joe.0.0450515. PMID 5366112.

6. Norwitz ER, Greenberg JA (2010). "Beyond antenatal corticosteroids: what did mont liggins teach us?". Reviews in Obstetrics & Gynecology. 3 (3): 79–80. PMC 3046760. PMID 21364857.

7. Liggins GC, Howie RN (October 1972). "A controlled trial of antepartum glucocorticoid treatment for prevention of the respiratory distress syndrome in premature infants". Pediatrics. 50 (4): 515–525. doi:10.1542/peds.50.4.515. PMID 4561295. S2CID 37818386.

8. Vyas J, Kotecha S (September 1997). "Effects of antenatal and postnatal corticosteroids on the preterm lung". Archives of Disease in Childhood. Fetal and Neonatal Edition. 77 (2): F147–F150. doi:10.1136/fn.77.2.f147. PMC 1720703. PMID 9377142.

9. Asztalos EV, Murphy KE, Matthews SG (October 2020). "A Growing Dilemma: Antenatal Corticosteroids and Long-Term Consequences". American Journal of Perinatology. 39 (6): s–0040–1718573. doi:10.1055/s-0040-1718573. PMID 33053595. S2CID 222421170.

10. Ninan K, Liyanage SK, Murphy KE, Asztalos EV, McDonald SD (April 2022). "Evaluation of Long-term Outcomes Associated With Preterm Exposure to Antenatal Corticosteroids: A Systematic Review and Meta-analysis". JAMA Pediatrics. 176 (6): e220483. doi:10.1001/jamapediatrics.2022.0483. PMC 9002717. PMID 35404395. S2CID 248083996.

11. Quinlivan JA, Beazley LD, Evans SF, Newnham JP, Dunlop SA (February 2000). "Retinal maturation is delayed by repeated, but not single, maternal injections of betamethasone in sheep". Eye. 14 (1): 93–98. doi:10.1038/eye.2000.20. PMID 10755109. S2CID 45299374.

12. Church MW, Adams BR, Anumba JI, Jackson DA, Kruger ML, Jen KL (2012-01-01). "Repeated antenatal corticosteroid treatments adversely affect neural transmission time and auditory thresholds in laboratory rats". Neurotoxicology and Teratology. 34 (1): 196–205. doi:10.1016/j.ntt.2011.09.004. PMC 3268869. PMID 21963399.

13. Asztalos E, Willan A, Murphy K, Matthews S, Ohlsson A, Saigal S, et al. (August 2014). "Association between gestational age at birth, antenatal corticosteroids, and outcomes at 5 years: multiple courses of antenatal corticosteroids for preterm birth study at 5 years of age (MACS-5)". BMC Pregnancy and Childbirth. 14 (1): 272. doi:10.1186/1471-2393-14-272. PMC 4261573. PMID 25123162.

14. Miracle X, Di Renzo GC, Stark A, Fanaroff A, Carbonell-Estrany X, Saling E (2008-01-01). "Guideline for the use of antenatal corticosteroids for fetal maturation". Journal of Perinatal Medicine. 36 (3): 191–196. doi:10.1515/JPM.2008.032. PMID 18576926.

15. Repeat Antenatal Steroids Trial - ClinicalTrials.gov [Internet]. [cited 2022 Nov 19]. Available from: https://clinicaltrials.gov/ct2/show/record/NCT00015002.

16. Murphy KE, Hannah ME, Willan AR, Hewson SA, Ohlsson A, Kelly EN, Matthews SG, Saigal S, Asztalos E, Ross S, Delisle MF. Multiple courses of antenatal corticosteroids for preterm birth (MACS): a randomised controlled trial. The Lancet. 2008 Dec 20;372(9656):2143–51.

17. Asztalos EV, Murphy KE, Willan AR, Matthews SG, Ohlsson A, Saigal S, Armson BA, Kelly EN, Delisle MF, Gafni A, Lee SK. Multiple courses of antenatal corticosteroids for preterm birth study: outcomes in children at 5 years of age (MACS-5). JAMA pediatrics. 2013 Dec 1;167(12):1102–10.

18. Antenatal Steroids [Internet]. [cited 2022 Nov 20]. Available from: http://www.perinatology.com/protocols/Steroids.htm. Archived from the original on 2012-09-03

19. McEvoy C, Schilling D, Spitale P, Peters D, O'Malley J, Durand M (May 2008). "Decreased respiratory compliance in infants less than or equal to 32 weeks' gestation, delivered more than 7 days after antenatal steroid therapy". Pediatrics. 121 (5): e1032–e1038. doi:10.1542/pe

20. "WHO. WHO recommendations on interventions to improve preterm birth outcomes". WHO. Retrieved 2020-12-01.

21. "Preterm labour and birth" (PDF). National Institute for Health and Care Excellence. 2015.

22. Antenatal Corticosteroid Therapy for Fetal Maturation | ACOG [Internet]. [cited 2022 Nov 20]. Available from: https://www.acog.org/en/Clinical/Clinical Guidance/Committee Opinion/Articles/2017/08/Antenatal Corticosteroid Therapy for Fetal Maturation.

23. "Antenatal corticosteroids given to women prior to birth to improve fetal, infant, child and adult health: Clinical Practice Guidelines" (PDF). Antenatal Corticosteroid Clinical Practice Guidelines Panel. 2015. Liggins Institute, The University of Auckland, Auckland. New Zealand.

24. Chow, SSW, Creighton, P, Chambers, GM, Lui, K. 2020. "Report of the Australian and New Zealand Neonatal Network" 2018. Sydney: ANZNN.

25. Skoll A, Boutin A, Bujold E, Burrows J, Crane J, Geary M, et al. (September 2018). "No. 364-Antenatal Corticosteroid Therapy for Improving Neonatal Outcomes". Journal of Obstetrics and Gynaecology Canada. 40 (9): 1219–1239. doi:10.1016/j.jogc.2018.04.018.

26. Operational_Guidelines-Use_of_Antenatal_Corticosteroids_in_Preterm_Labour, 2014 (PDF) https://nhm.gov.in/images/pdf/programmes/child-health/guidelines. Accessed: 2022-11-20

27. "Dexamethasone versus betamethasone as an antenatal corticosteroid (ACS)" (PDF). UN Commission / Born Too Soon Care Antenatal Corticosteroids Working Group. August 20, 2013.

28. Fanaroff AA, Hack M (October 1999). "Periventricular leukomalacia--prospects for prevention". The New England Journal of Medicine. 341 (16): 1229–1231. doi:10.1056/NEJM199910143411611. PMID 10519903.

29. Williams MJ, Ramson JA, Brownfoot FC. Different corticosteroids and regimens for accelerating fetal lung maturation for babies at risk of preterm birth. Cochrane Database Syst Rev. 2022 Aug 9;8(8):CD006764. doi: 10.1002/14651858.CD006764.pub4. PMID: 35943347; PMCID: PMC9362990.

30. Deshmukh M and Patole S. (2021). Antenatal corticosteroids for impending late preterm (34-36+6 weeks) deliveries—A systematic review and meta-analysis of RCTs. PLOS ONE, 16(3), e0248774. https://doi.org/10.1371/journal.pone.0248774

31. Sotiriadis, A., McGoldrick, E., Makrydimas, G., Papatheodorou, S., Ioannidis, J. P., Stewart, F., & Parker, R. (2021). Antenatal corticosteroids prior to planned caesarean at term for improving neonatal outcomes. The Cochrane database of systematic reviews, 12(12), CD006614. https://doi.org/10.1002/14651858.CD006614.pub4

32. Arsad N, Razak NA, Omar MH, Shafiee MN, Kalok A, Cheah FC, et al. Antenatal Corticosteroids to Asian Women Prior to Elective Cesarean Section at Early Term and Effects on Neonatal Respiratory Outcomes. Int J Environ Res Public Heal 2022, Vol 19, 5201.

33. What are the benefits and risks of giving corticosteroids to pregnant women at risk of premature birth? | Cochrane [Internet]. [cited 2022 Nov 20]. Available from: https://www.cochrane.org/podcasts/10.1002/14651858.CD004454.pub4

34. Ian Donald's Practical Obstetric Problems. 8th Edition. New Delhi, India: Wolters Kluwer (India); 2020. 13, Autoimmune Diseases; 268–283.

35. Park-Wyllie L, Mazzotta P, Pastuszak A, Moretti ME, Beique L, Hunnisett L, Friesen MH, Jacobson S, Kasapinovic S, Chang D, Diav Citrin O. Birth defects after maternal exposure to corticosteroids: prospective cohort study and meta-analysis of epidemiological studies. Teratology. 2000 Dec;62(6):385–92.

36. Neunert C, Lim W, Crowther M, Cohen A, Solberg Jr L, Crowther MA. The American Society of Hematology 2011 evidence-based practice guideline for immune thrombocytopenia. Blood, The Journal of the American Society of Hematology. 2011 Apr 21;117(16):4190–207.

37. Rodeghiero F, Stasi R, Gernsheimer T, Michel M, Provan D, Arnold DM, Bussel JB, Cines DB, Chong BH, Cooper N, Godeau B. Standardization of terminology, definitions and outcome criteria in immune thrombocytopenic purpura of adults and children: report from an international

working group. Blood, The Journal of the American Society of Hematology. 2009 Mar 12;113(11):2386–93.

38. Abdolmohammadi-Vahid S, Danaii S, Hamdi K, Jadidi-Niaragh F, Ahmadi M, Yousefi M. Novel immunotherapeutic approaches for treatment of infertility. Biomed Pharmacother. 2016;84:1449–59.

39. Robertson SA, Jin M, Yu D, Moldenhauer LM, Davies MJ, Hull ML, et al. Corticosteroid therapy in assisted reproduction - immune suppression is a faulty premise. Hum Reprod (Oxford, England). 2016;31:2164–73.

40. Benschop L, Seshadri S, Toulis KA, Vincent K, Child T, Granne IE, et al. Immune therapies for women with history of failed implantation undergoing IVF treatment. Cochrane Database Syst Rev. 2012.

41. Han AR, Ahn H, Vu P, Park JC, Gilman-Sachs A, Beaman K, et al. Obstetrical outcome of anti-inflammatory and anticoagulation therapy in women with recurrent pregnancy loss or unexplained infertility. Am J Reprod Immunol. 2012;68:418–27.

42. Addison RS, Maguire DJ, Mortimer RH, Roberts MS, Cannell GR. Pathway and kinetics of prednisolone metabolism in the human placenta. J Steroid Biochem Mol Biol. 1993;44:315–20.

43. Dan S, Wei W, Yichao S, Hongbo C, Shenmin Y, Jiaxiong W, et al. Effect of prednisolone administration on patients with unexplained recurrent miscarriage and in routine intracytoplasmic sperm injection: a meta-analysis. Am J Reprod Immunol. 2015;74:89–97.

44. Ryu RJ, Easterling TR, Caritis SN, Venkataramanan R, Umans JG, Ahmed MS, et al. Prednisone pharmacokinetics during pregnancy and lactation. J Clin Pharmacol. 2018.

45. Litwicka K, Arrivi C, Varricchio MT, Mencacci C, Greco E. In women with thyroid autoimmunity, does low-dose prednisolone administration, compared with no adjuvant therapy, improve in vitro fertilization clinical results?. Journal of Obstetrics and Gynaecology Research. 2015 May;41(5):722–8.

46. Speroff's Clinical Gynecologic Endocrinology and Infertility. 9th Edition. Wolters Kluwer; 2020. 8, Normal and Abnormal Sexual Development; 653–654.

47. Clayton PE, Miller WL, Oberfield SE, Ritzén EM, Sippell WG, Speiser PW; ESPE/LWPES CAH Working Group, Consensus statement on 21-hydroxylase deficiency from the Lawson Wilkins Pediatric Endocrine Society and the European Society for Paediatric Endocrinology, J Clin Endocrinol Metab 87:4048, 2002.

48. New MI, Carlson A, Obeid J, Marshall I, Cabrera MS, Goseco A, Lin-Su K, Putnam AS, Wei JQ, Wilson RC, Prenatal diagnosis for congenital adrenal hyperplasia in 532 pregnancies, J Clin Endocrinol Metab 86:5651, 2001.

49. Pang S, Clark AT, Freeman LC, Dolan LM, Immken L, Mueller OT, Stiff D, Shulman DI, Maternal side effects of prenatal dexamethasone therapy for fetal congenital adrenal hyperplasia, J Clin Endocrinol Metab 1992;75:249.

50. Nimkarn S, New MI, Prenatal diagnosis and treatment of congenital adrenal hyperplasia, Horm Res 2007;67:53.

Vaccination in Pregnancy

• Rashmi Jalvee • Reena Wani

Introduction

The development of vaccines against infectious disease is one of the greatest achievements of modern science. Vaccination is a method of primary prevention of diseases and therefore a cost-effective public health intervention. Over the decades, vaccination has made it possible to eradicate certain diseases (smallpox) and control of others (polio and pertussis).

Maternal immunisation refers to vaccinations administered during pregnancy. This offers dual benefit: Protection of pregnant women from disease (*viz.* influenza) and induction of an immune response that provides transplacental passive immunity to the infant after birth (*e.g.* whooping cough).

Principles of Immunology[1,2]

Immunity is the body's ability to protect and defend itself against disease causing pathogens by the action of specific antibodies or sensitized white blood cells. This immunity can be innate or adaptive.

- *Innate or native immunity:* An individual is born with components of native immunity. It is the body's first-line of defence with a rapid response; however, it is antigen non-specific and has poor specificity. It comprises of epithelial barriers and phagocytes—neutrophils, macrophages, and monocytes.

- Acquired or adaptive immunity is a type of immunity that develops over time due to exposure to a foreign antigen. It is acquired due to exposure to diseases or administration of vaccines. It is more powerful and specific although slower than innate immunity. T- and B-lymphocytes and antibodies and cytokines produced by them are components of adaptive immunity.

- *Active immunisation:* Here, an antigen is administered to stimulate production of antibodies. It can either be due to infection or immunisation.

- *Passive immunisation:* Here, antibodies are directly administered to confer rapid short-term immunity. It is used when the risk of infection is high and enough time is not available for the body to develop its own immune response.

The only naturally acquired passive immunity is the transplacental passive transfer of antibodies from the mother to the fetus and to the neonate through breastmilk. The antibodies acquired through the placenta are of the IgG type. Immunoglobulin (Ig) of the IgA type are primarily present in breastmilk and protects the neonatal intestinal mucosal surfaces.

IMMUNOLOGY OF PREGNANCY

In pregnancy, there is an adaptation of the maternal immune system to tolerate the semi-allogenic foetal conceptus. The innate immune system upgrades for maternal protection against infection and foetal protection against rejection; the acquired immune response toward foreign antigens (paternal/foetal antigens) is selectively down-regulated. These changes in the immune system of pregnant women are not known to affect the immunological response to vaccination.

Vaccination involves inducing an acquired immune response against microbes by administration of non-pathogenic variants or components of the organism. A vaccine is a biological preparation that induces immunity to a particular infectious disease. It serves not only to induce an active immunity but also provide immunological memory in the body.

The immune system can thus recognise and act rapidly against pathogens that have been encountered previously.

TYPES OF VACCINES[2,5]

Broadly, vaccines are divided as **(Table 26.1)**
- Live vaccines
- Killed/inactivated vaccines
- Purified macromolecules.

These include:
- Sub-unit vaccine
- Conjugate vaccine
- Toxoid vaccine
- Recombinant vaccine.

PRINCIPLES OF VACCINATION IN PREGNANCY[3,4]

- Ideally, women should be vaccinated against vaccine-preventable diseases before becoming pregnant.

Table 26.1: Types of vaccines

Type	Description	Examples
Live-attenuated vaccines	Contain attenuated form of the organism that is modified to abolish its virulence and yet retain their antigenicity. Contraindicated in pregnancy due to the potential risk of foetal infection. In exceptional cases where benefits may outweigh risks, the decision to administer a live vaccine to pregnant women should be made after consulting an infectious disease specialist.	MMR vaccine Rubella vaccine
Killed/Inactivated vaccines	The pathogen is destroyed during the process of vaccine manufacture through a physical or chemical process. Pathogen cannot replicate in the host. Often, multiple doses are necessary to build up and/or maintain immunity as the immunity conferred by killed vaccines is poorer than that by live vaccines.	Polio, hepatitis A, rabies vaccine.
Sub-unit vaccines	These contain only a part of the pathogen that is needed to produce a protective immune response.	*H. influenzae* vaccine, *S. pneumonia* vaccine.
Toxoid vaccines	These are made using inactivated bacterial toxins.	Tetanus toxoid, Diphtheria toxoid
Recombinant vaccines	Vaccines made using recombinant DNA technology.	Serogroup-B meningococcal vaccine

- Obstetric care providers should make a routine assessment of immunisation status of pregnant women.
- When given in pregnancy, the advantages and benefits of the vaccine should outweigh the risks.
- Generally, killed virus vaccines, immunoglobulins and toxoids are considered safe during pregnancy and evidence does not suggestany harmful effects on the fetus or pregnancy.
- During pregnancy, unless immediate vaccination is indicated, it is preferable to avoid immunisation in the first trimester to allow for completion of fetal organogenesis.

In the clinical context, vaccines can be broadly classified as shown in **Table 26.2.**

VACCINES INDICATED IN PREGNANCY

Tetanus Toxoid (TT)/Tetanus Diphtheria (Td)/ Reduced Diphtheria Toxoid, and Acellular Pertussis (Tdap) Vaccine

- In India, under the Ministry of Health and Family Welfare (MoHFW) guidelines,[6] as a

Table 26.2: Classification of vaccines

Vaccines contraindicated in pregnancy	• BCG vaccine • Measles vaccine • Mumps vaccine • Rubella vaccine • Varicella vaccine • Vaccinia vaccine • Human papillomavirus vaccine
Vaccines specially indicated in pregnancy	• Inactivated influenza vaccine • Pertussis (whooping cough) vaccine • Inactivated polio vaccine • Diphtheria toxoid • Tetanus toxoid
Vaccines recommended in pregnancy in certain situations	• Hepatitis A vaccine • Hepatitis B vaccine • Meningococcus vaccine • Pneumococcal vaccine • Rabies vaccine • Typhoid vaccine • Yellow fever vaccine

part of Universal Immunisation Program (UIP), all pregnant women were offered 2 doses of tetanus toxoid injection 4 weeks apart as a part of routine schedule.
- A single dose of TT booster was sufficient if the woman has received 2 doses of TT immunisation in a pregnancy within the last 3 years.
- Globally, although the policy recommendation to replace TT with Td has existed since 1998, the National Technical Advisory Group on Immunization (NTAGI), MoHFW has recommended the replacement of TT with Td vaccine in India's immunization programme for all age groups, including pregnant women in 2018.[7,8]
- Td vaccine is a combination of lower concentration of diphtheria antigen with tetanus. Td is now recommended instead of TT to protect mothers and babies tetanus and diphtheria.
- The American College of Obstetrics and Gynecology (ACOG)[10] and Centers for Disease Control (CDC)[9] recommend that all pregnant women should receive tetanus toxoid, reduced diphtheria toxoid, and acellular pertussis (Tdap) vaccine between 27–36 weeks.
- Tdap vaccine can be given immediately after delivery if the woman has never received any dose as an adolescent, adult or during a previous pregnancy.
- The rationale behind Tdap vaccination is the fact that pertussis infection in babies younger than 3 months is associated with a lot of morbidity and mortality. As infants receive the pertussis vaccine usually by 6 weeks of age, there is a window of vulnerability for the neonates which can be avoided as antepartum vaccination.

Influenza Vaccine[4,11–13]

- Although UIP in India does not recommend routine antenatal influenza immunisation, international guidelines recommend that pregnant women should receive antenatal seasonal influenza vaccination.

- Influenza infection in pregnancy is associated with more serious disease, increased risk of complications and need for hospitalisation in advanced pregnancy in addition to the adverse foetal effects like congenital malformations, spontaneous abortions, preterm births and low birth weight.
- ACOG recommends that all women who are or will be pregnant during influenza (flu) season should receive annual influenza vaccine.
- Influenza vaccination during pregnancy protects both the pregnant women and neonates from severe influenza disease.
- Influenza vaccine can be given at any period of gestation (first, second or third trimester).
- Maternal vaccination reduces both risk of transmission of infection to the neonate and provides passive immunity to infants in the first few months of life after birth.
- Pregnant women can receive both inactivated influenza vaccine (IIV) and recombinant influenza vaccine (RIV). However, live attenuated influenza virus vaccine should not be avoided in antenatal women.

USE OF SPECIFIC VACCINES IN PREGNANCY

Bacillus Calmette-Guérin (BCG)[3–5]

Although it has been seen that BCG vaccination is not associated with adverse effects to the baby, BCG is still avoided during pregnancy due to theoretical concerns associated with a live vaccine.

Measles, Mumps and Rubella (MMR)[3–5,14]

- MMR is a live-attenuated vaccine.
- Due to possible fetal teratogenic effects, MMR vaccine is contraindicated in pregnancy.
- Further, due to the theoretical risk of teratogenicity due to maternal immunisation with MMR, women should avoid becoming pregnant for 28 days after receiving MMR vaccine.

- However, guidelines do not recommend termination of pregnancy after inadvertent antenatal MMR vaccination as studies have not shown any link between rubella immunisation in early pregnancy and teratogenicity.

Rubella[3,4,5]

- Being a live-attenuated vaccine, rubella vaccination is contra-indicated in pregnancy.
- After rubella vaccination, women should avoid pregnancy for 28 days.
- Rubella vaccine can be safely given to breastfeeding women.

Varicella[3–5]

- Varicella zoster vaccine is a live-attenuated vaccine.
- Varicella vaccine is contraindicated in pregnancy due to known teratogenic fetal effects.[15,16]
- Non pregnant women vaccinated with varicella vaccine should avoid pregnancy for 28 days after taking the vaccine.

Human Papillomavirus (HPV)[4,16]

- HPV vaccine is not recommended due to limited data on its safety in pregnancy.
- However, if a woman accidentally gets pregnant after starting the vaccine series, she can be reassured that available evidence does not link HPV vaccines with any increase in adverse maternal or foetal effects.
- The second and/or third vaccine doses should be delayed and completed in the postpartum period.
- Being a sub-unit vaccine, women who are breastfeeding can receive the immunization safely.

Hepatitis A[3,5]

- The safety of hepatitis A vaccine in pregnancy is unknown.
- Being a formalin-inactivated vaccine, the risks to the foetus is likely to be low.

- Depending on the individual circumstances, the benefits and risks should be weighed and vaccination is decided.
- Hepatitis A vaccination is indicated in the presence of high-risk condition, *viz.* chronic liver disease, intravenous drug use, travel to an endemic area, clotting factor disorders, etc.

Hepatitis B[3,4,5]

- Infection with hepatitis B in pregnant women may cause severe maternal liver disease and chronic infection for the baby.
- Being an inactivated subunit vaccine, the risk to the fetus is negligible.
- Hence, pregnant women with high risk factors should receive hepatitis B vaccination.
- These high-risk conditions include:
  - Women with multiple sexual partners,
  - Women or partner with intravenous drug use,
  - Women who receive regular blood transfusion,
  - Women travelling to endemic area,
  - Female sex workers,
  - Those with chronic liver or kidney disease,
  - Sexual partners of patient with hepatitis B
  - Women who work in settings that increase exposure with body fluids, *viz.* medical and para-medical staff.

Meningococcal Vaccine[5,11,17]

- Both conjugated and quadrivalent vaccine MenACWY are not known to be associated with adverse maternal or foetal outcomes when administered in pregnancy.
- Vaccination is not recommended in pregnancy unless the mother is at increased risk of disease, *viz.*
  - Immunosuppressed women
  - Women with functional or anatomical asplenia
  - With complement deficiency

- Those travelling to endemic regions
- Women exposed to infected individuals
- Both vaccines can safely be given to lactating women.
- The safety of meningococcal B vaccine in pregnant and breastfeeding women has not been studied. Vaccination in pregnant and lactating women should be avoided, and should only be given if the benefits outweigh the potential risks.

Pneumococcal Conjugated Vaccine[3–5,11]

- It is preferable to give pneumococcal vaccine prior to conception in women with high-risk factors.
- The safety of both 13-valent polysaccharide vaccine and the 23-valent pneumococcal polysaccharide vaccine in pregnancy and lactating women has not been evaluated and should be deferred until after pregnancy.
- Vaccination is not recommended in pregnancy unless the pregnant woman is at risk of disease where the benefits may outweigh the potential risks, *viz.*
  - Heart disease
  - Chronic pulmonary disease
  - Sickle cell anaemia
  - Immunocompromised conditions, like HIV
  - Functional or anatomical aspenia

Typhoid Vaccine[3–5,18]

- The safety of both the typhoid vaccines has not been studied in pregnancy and should not be given to pregnant women.
- Oral live vaccine Ty21a is contraindicated in pregnancy.
- Pregnant women should avoid travel to endemic areas and if travel cannot be postponed, should receive inactive parenteral vaccine.

Rabies Vaccine[4,5,11]

- Rabies vaccine is an inactivated viral vaccine.
- After a potential exposure to rabies, rabies vaccine should be given during pregnancy

and lactation as the consequences of untreated rabies are potentially fatal.
- Pre-exposure prophylaxis for rabies may be considered in pregnancy, where the risk of exposure to rabies is significant.

Japanese Encephalitis (JE)[11]
- This is an inactivated vaccine.
- There is no data on the safety of vaccine in pregnancy.
- Women planning on travel to endemic areas should receive the vaccine.

Yellow Fever Vaccine[4,5,11]
- This is a live-attenuated vaccine.
- Pregnant women should defer travel endemic area.
- If travel cannot be postponed, immunisation with live attenuated viral vaccine may be given after discussion with an infectious disease specialist.

COVID-19 Vaccination in Pregnancy
- Since the beginning of Covid-19 pandemic in 2019, information about the SARS-CoV-2 virus and its treatment is constantly evolving.
- In majority of cases, Covid-19 infection in pregnant women is asymptomatic with mild disease.
- Compared with non-pregnant women, pregnant women are at increased risk of severe form of disease and complications *viz.*, intensive care unit (ICU) admission, need for assisted ventilation, sepsis and death.
- As per the National Technical Advisory Group on Immunization (NTAGI) recommendations, MoHFW has approved vaccinating pregnant women with Covid-19 vaccine after informing them about the risks of exposure to Covid-19 infection and the benefits and risks associated with the Covid-19 vaccines.[19]
- International guidelines also recommend that all pregnant and lactating women should receive Covid-19 vaccine.[20,21]

- Current evidence suggests that Covid-19 vaccination before and during pregnancy is safe, effective and beneficial to both the pregnant woman and baby.[22] The advantages of receiving the vaccine far outweigh any potential risk.
- Covid-19 vaccine can be taken in any trimester of pregnancy. However, it is preferable that the second dose be taken before 26 weeks of pregnancy. Evidence suggests that the production and subsequent transplacental transfer of antibodies was better following a second dose of vaccine.
- Interval between 2 doses of vaccine is the same as for non-pregnant adults.
- In India, currently, three vaccines have received approval for restricted use in emergency situation: An inactivated vaccine (Covaxin) and two based on non-replicating viral vector platform (Covishield and Sputnik V).[19]
- Other vaccines can be given simultaneously with Covid-19 vaccines but at different sites. For example, influenza, Td and Tdap.
- Contraindications to vaccination include:
  - Anaphylactic/allergic reaction to previous Covid-19 vaccine
  - Active Covid-19 infection
  - Confirmed Covid-19 infection in the pregnant women: Defer vaccination for 12 weeks from infection or 4 to 8 weeks from recovery
  - Covid-19 infection treated with convalescent plasma or anti-Covid-19 monoclonal antibodies.

Breastfeeding and Vaccination[5,23]
- Both live-virus vaccines (except smallpox and yellow fever) and inactivated can be safely given to lactating women without any adverse effects on women or their babies.
- Although there is a theoretical risk of viral replication with live vaccines, majority of live viruses in vaccines have not been isolated in human breast milk.

- It is advisable to defer yellow fever vaccine in breastfeeding women. However, if travel to an endemic area cannot be postponed, vaccination should not be withheld.[24]
- Toxoids, subunit, polysaccharide, inactivated, recombinant and conjugate vaccines pose no risk for mothers who are breastfeeding or for their infants.

CONCLUSION

- Obstetricians should routinely assess the vaccination status of their pregnant patients.
- Currently, Td/Tdap and influenza vaccine are recommended in pregnancy.
- Consider other vaccines in pregnancy in selective conditions where the benefits outweigh potential risks.
- Generally, live-attenuated vaccines are contraindicated in pregnancy because of theoretical risks to the foetus.
- Both live-virus vaccines (except smallpox and yellow fever virus) and inactivated vaccines can be safely administered to lactating women without any adverse effects to the women or their infants.
- It is important that healthcare professionals update themselves about the evolving guidelines and recent advances in vaccination in pregnancy. This will ensure better patient education and maximise vaccination uptake by pregnant women.

References

1. Coico S, Sunshine G, Benjamini E. Immunology: A short course. 5th ed. Hoboken: John Wiley and Sons; 2003.
2. https://www.cdc.gov/vaccines/pubs/pinkbook/downloads/prinvac.pdf
3. ACOG Committee Opinion No 741: Immunisation, Infectious disease and Public Health Preparedness Expert Work Group; June 2018.
4. Centers for Disease Control and Prevention. General recommendations on immunization: recommendations of the Advisory Committee on Immunization Practices (ACIP). MMWR Recomm Rep 2011;60:1–64.
5. PS Arunakumari, Sujatha Kalburgi, AmitaSahare. Vaccination in pregnancy. The Obstetrician and Gynecologist; 2015;17:257–63
6. https://main.mohfw.gov.in/sites/default/files/245453521061489663873.pdf
7. WHO/UNICEF Guidance Note: Ensuring Sustained Protection Against Diphtheria: Replacing TT with Td vaccine; Version 12 September 2018.
8. Td_vaccine_operational_guidelines.pdf (nhm.gov.in) 2018
9. CDC. Updated recommendations for use of tetanus toxoid, reduced diphtheria toxoid, and acellular pertussis vaccine (Tdap) in pregnant women – Advisory Committee on Immunization Practices (ACIP), 2012. MMWR. 2013; 62 (07): 131–5.
10. Update on Immunization and Pregnancy: Tetanus, Diphtheria, and Pertussis Vaccination: ACOG: Committee Opinion Number 718, September 2017.
11. Lin Kong K, Krishnaswamy S, Giles M. Maternal vaccinations. AJGP Vol. 49, No. 10, October 2020.
12. Royal Australian and New Zealand College of Obstetricians and Gynaecologists. Influenza vaccination during pregnancy (and in women planning pregnancy). East Melbourne, Vic: RANZCOG, 2017.
13. ACOG: Influenza Vaccination During Pregnancy. Committee Opinion No 732. April 2018.
14. CDC. Prevention of measles, rubella, congenital rubella syndrome, and mumps, 2013: summary recommendations of the Advisory Committee on Immunization Practices (ACIP). MMWR. 2013; 62 (No. RR-4): 13.
15. Royal College of Obstetricians & Gynaecologists. Chickenpox in pregnancy. RCOG Green-top guideline No.13. London: RCOG; 2015.
16. CDC. Use of 9-valent human papillomavirus (HPV) vaccine: updated HPV vaccination recommendations of the Advisory Committee on Immunization Practices (ACIP). MMWR. 2015; 64 (No. 11): 303.
17. Mbaeyi SA, Bozio CH, Duffy J, et al. Meningococcal Vaccination: Recommendations of the Advisory Committee on Immunization Practices, United States, 2020. MMWR Recom Rep 2020;69(No. RR-9):1–41.
18. CDC. Updated recommendations for the use of typhoid vaccine — Advisory Committee on Immunization Practices, United States, 2015. MMWR. 2015;64 (No. 11):307.

19. https://www.mohfw.gov.in/pdf/operational Guidance for COVID 19 vaccination on Pregnant Woman.pdf

20. COVID-19 Vaccination Considerations for Obstetric–Gynecologic Care: ACOG Practice Advisory; December 2020.

21. Royal College of Obstetricians and Gynecologists (RCOG). COVID -19 vaccines, pregnancy and breastfeeding. [Online] 16 April 2021. https://www.rcog.org.uk/en/guidelines-research-services/coronavirus-Covid-19-pregnancy-and-womens-health/Covid -19-vaccines-and pregnancy/Covid -19-vaccines-pregnancy-and-breastfeeding/

22. https://www.cdc.gov/coronavirus/2019-ncov/vaccines/recommendations/pregnancy.html

23. Kroger AT, Duchin J, Vázquez M. General Best Practice Guidelines for Immunization. Best Practices Guidance of the Advisory Committee on Immunization Practices (ACIP).

24. https://www.who.int/groups/global-advisory-committee-on-vaccine-safety/topics/yellow-fever-vaccines/breastfeeding

Combined Oral Contraceptive Medication

• Asha Dalal • Ashwin Shetty

Introduction

Combined oral contraceptive (COC) medication is a very popular contraceptive method globally.

Mechanisms of Action

The medication works by suppression of ovulation by inhibiting the release of gonadotrophin-releasing hormone (GnRh) from the hypothalamus and suppression of follicle-stimulating hormone (FSH) and luteinizing hormone (LH) from the pituitary. This disrupts the midcycle LH surge and prevents ovulation. Estrogen in the pill affects follicular development and progesterone helps in endometrial stabilization resulting in regular withdrawal periods and normal cycles.

Additionally, the estrogen component stabilizes sufficient endometrium production to maintain a regular bleeding pattern (cycle control). Additional progestin related mechanisms that contribute to the contraceptive effect include:

- Effects on the endometrium, rendering it less suitable for implantation. Long-term cyclic or daily progestin exposure leads to endometrial decidualization and eventual atrophy.
- Thickening of cervical mucus, which becomes less permeable to penetration by sperm.
- Impairment of normal tubal motility and peristalsis.

Ethinyl estradiol: Ethinyl estradiol, the most commonly used estrogen in combined oral contraceptive pills, is a potent synthetic estrogen.

Classification of Progestins Used in Combined Oral Contraceptive Pills

First generation
- Norethindrone acetate
- Ethynodiol diacetate
- Lynestrenol
- Norethynodrel.

Second generation
- DL-Norgestrel
- Levonorgestrel.

Third generation
- Desogestrel
- Gestodene
- Norgestimate.

Unclassified
- Drospirenone
- Cyproterone acetate.

Method of Administration

Cyclic use: Most pill preparations have 21 tablets for a 28-day cycle. This incorporates 7 days pill free interval or alternatively placebos taken for the 7 days, this is also known as a 21/7 regimen.

An alternative regimen is the 24/4 regimen where the pill is taken for 24 days followed by 4-day pill free break.[1]

Continuous or extended use: This allows the patient to choose, when she will have withdrawal bleeding. It is known that medical suppression of periods is safe and not having a withdrawal period is not detrimental. Popular use of extended cycles involves taking 2-pill packets or 3-pill packets back-to-back and withdrawal periods after 63 days.

Starting the Pill

When starting the pill for the first time, the pill is commonly started on the fifth day of the period. This does not provide immediate contraception and an additional contraceptive method is suggested for the first 7 days of the cycle.[2]

Alternatively, starting the pill on the first day of the menstrual cycle provides maximal contraceptive effect in the very first cycle.[2]

Postpartum: Immediately postpartum, there is increased risk of venous thromboembolism with COC use, hence use is delayed for at least 3 weeks post delivery. For breastfeeding mothers, there is a theoretical concern about reduction of lactation hence for them COC can be started 30 days after delivery.[2]

Missed Pills

If a single pill is missed, the patient is advised to take the pill soon as she remembers and then take the following pill as scheduled the next day.[2]

If two or more pills are missed then patient is advised to continue to take the remaining pills as schedule, however back-up barrier contraception will be needed.[2]

If this happens in the first week of the cycle and unprotected intercourse occurs, patient is advised to use emergency contraception.[2] If two or more pills are missed in the last week, *i.e.* from day 15 to day 21, patient is advised to finish the pills as scheduled but instead of stopping to have the 1 week break, she should go on to starting immediately a new pill packet the next day.[2]

Extra Pill

If patient has mistakenly taken 2 pills in one day, she should not skip a day but continue to take the pills as scheduled, she will finish her packet 1 day earlier.[2]

Duration of Use

Hormonal contraception can be continued until the age of menopause (average age 50 to 51 years) in healthy, nonsmoking and normal-weight women.[2]

Contraceptive Effectiveness

COC is highly user-dependent. If used perfectly, the risk of COC contraceptive failure is low.

With perfect use of COC (following directions for use) it has been estimated that 0.3% of users experience an unplanned pregnancy during the first year of use. In contrast, the first-year failure rate associated with typical use of COC (actual use including inconsistent or incorrect use) has been estimated to be around 9%.[3]

Most evidence suggests no association between weight/body-mass index (BMI) and effectiveness of COC.

A 2017 systematic review reported that 10 out of 14 studies of COC identified, did not report a difference in effectiveness by body weight or BMI.[4]

A systematic review concluded (on the basis of 10 small, biomedical studies) that missing one to four consecutive pills on days not adjacent to the hormone-free interval (HFI) resulted in little follicular activity and low risk of ovulation.[5]

Hepatic enzyme-inducing drugs increase the metabolism of estrogens and progestogens, which could reduce the contraceptive effectiveness of all COC methods. Women using enzyme-inducing drugs should be advised to switch to a contraceptive method (*e.g.* intrauterine methods or the progestogen-only injectable) that is unaffected by enzyme-inducers.[6]

It is an established practice that if, after advice to switch contraceptive method, a woman wishes to use COC concomitantly with an enzyme-inducing drug (with the exception of rifampicin or rifabutin which are potent enzyme-inducers) use of a minimum 50 µg (30 µg + 20 µg) ethinyl estradiol (EE) monophasic-combined pill may be considered during use of the enzyme-inducer and for a further 28 days after stopping. A continuous or tricycling regimen plus a shortened pill-free interval of 4 days should be used.

Women taking lamotrigine should be advised that COC may interact with lamotrigine; this could result in reduced seizure control or lamotrigine toxicity. The risks of using COC could outweigh the benefits.

Serum levels of lamotrigine can be reduced by COC. A case series reported increased seizure frequency in four women with reduced lamotrigine levels following the initiation of COC.[7]

Most broad-spectrum antibiotics are non-enzyme-inducing and patients on them need no additional contraception unless they have vomiting or severe diarrhea.[6]

Unacceptable Risk

Based upon the Centers of Disease Control and Prevention (CDC) Summary Chart of US Medical Eligibility Criteria (USMEC) and the WHO Medical Eligibility Criteria for Contraceptive Use 2015, Category 4 rating, some common medical conditions that represent an 'unacceptable health risk' for COC initiation include:[8,9]

- Age 35 years and smoking 15 cigarettes per day

- Multiple risk factors for arterial cardio-vascular disease (such as older age, smoking, diabetes, and hypertension)
- Hypertension (systolic ≥160 mmHg or diastolic ≥100 mmHg)
- Venous thromboembolism (VTE); unless on anticoagulation
- Known ischemic heart disease
- History of stroke
- Complicated valvular heart disease (pulmonary hypertension, risk for atrial fibrillation, history of subacute bacterial endocarditis)
- Current breast cancer
- Severe (decompensated) cirrhosis
- Hepatocellular adenoma or malignant hepatoma
- Migraine with aura
- Diabetes mellitus of >20 years duration or with nephropathy, retinopathy, or neuropathy.

Risks outweigh benefits—based upon the CDC's Summary Chart of US Medical Eligibility Criteria and the WHO Medical Eligibility Criteria for Contraceptive Use 2015, Category 3 rating, COC can still be used if alternatives are not acceptable to the patient. Patient should be counselled about the risks and a follow-up appointment be given to monitor safe use.[8,9] Some of these conditions include:[8,9]

- Age 35 years and smoking <15 cigarettes per day
- Hypertension (systolic 140 to 159 mmHg or diastolic 90 to 99 mmHg)
- Hypertension adequately controlled on medications
- Past breast cancer and no evidence of current disease for 5 years
- Current gallbladder disease
- Malabsorptive bariatric surgery
- Superficial venous thrombosis (acute or history)
- Inflammatory bowel disease with risk factors for VTE (active or extensive disease,

surgery, immobilization, corticosteroid use, vitamin deficiencies, or fluid depletion).

Assessment of Medical Eligibility for COC

Blood pressure: Women with severe hypertension (systolic pressure 160 mmHg or diastolic pressure 100 mmHg) should not use COC [United Kingdom Medical Eligibility Criteria 4 (UKMEC 4)].[6]

Women with less severe hypertension (systolic pressure 140–159 mmHg or diastolic pressure 90–99 mmHg), or with adequately controlled hypertension should not use COC (UKMEC 3). Blood pressure should therefore be evaluated before initiating COC.[6]

Weight (BMI): Women with BMI above 30 with other risk factors for cardiovascular disease, such as diabetes, hypertension, dyslipidemia, smoking should avoid COC, also patients with BMI greater than 35 should avoid COC (UKMEC 3).[6]

Clinical breast examination: Although women with current breast cancer should not use COC (UKMEC 4), screening asymptomatic women with a clinical breast examination before initiating COC is not necessary because of the low prevalence of breast cancer among women of reproductive age.[6]

For women using combined hormonal contraception, symptoms for which medical review is advised are:
- Calf pain, swelling and/or redness
- Chest pain and/or breathlessness and/or coughing-up blood
- Loss of motor or sensory function
- Breast lump, unilateral nipple discharge, new nipple inversion, change in breast skin
- New onset migraine
- New onset sensory or motor symptoms in the hour preceding onset of migraine
- Persistent unscheduled vaginal bleeding.

New Medical Diagnoses that should Prompt Women to Seek Advice from their Doctor

- High blood pressure
- Migraine or migraine with aura

- Deep vein thrombosis or pulmonary embolism
- Blood clotting abnormality
- Antiphospholipid antibodies
- Angina, heart attack, stroke or peripheral vascular disease
- Atrial fibrillation
- Cardiomyopathy
- Breast cancer or breast cancer gene mutation
- Liver tumor
- Symptomatic gallstones.

Non-contraceptive uses: COCs are also used widely to treat a variety of gynecologic disorders including:

Heavy Menstrual Bleeding

Use of COC can reduce heavy menstrual bleeding and menstrual pain.

Evidence from randomised controlled trials (RCTs) and non-randomized trials report a reduction in menstrual blood loss in women with heavy periods using COC.[26]

COC reduces menstrual pain, extended use of COC is effective for the treatment for primary dysmenorrhoea and may be superior to the traditional cyclic regimen, at least in the short-term.

Endometriosis

Use of COC (particularly extended-COC regimens), can reduce risk of recurrence of endometriosis after surgical management. Studies have shown that COC therapy is effective, safe and well-tolerated by women with endometriosis. A meta-analysis reported a significantly higher rate of remission from endometriosis symptoms and a lower rate of recurrence in women taking COC after surgery compared with surgery alone.[27]

Evidence suggests that a continuous rather than a cyclical COC regimen is advantageous in the management of endometriosis.

Acne

Evidence suggests that use of COC can improve acne vulgaris. A Cochrane review concluded that COCs are effective in reducing facial acne lesions.

COC-reduced acne lesion counts, severity grades and self-assessed acne compared to placebo.[28]

Premenstrual Syndrome (PMS)

Use of COC may be beneficial for women with PMS symptoms.

Premenstrual symptoms based on the limited available evidence symptoms of PMS/premenstrual dysphoric disorder (PMDD) could be improved in women who use COC for contraception. A continuous regimen may be considered. The 2016 Royal College of Obstetricians and Gynecologists (RCOG) Green-top Guideline Management of Premenstrual Syndrome[29] recommends that EE/drospirenone (DRSP), COC should be considered a first-line pharmaceutical intervention for management of PMS.

PMS symptoms improved significantly with the extended regimen compared to cyclical use.

Polycystic Ovary Syndrome

COC is recommended for first-line treatment of menstrual irregularity, acne and hirsutism in women with PCOS as per the Endocrine Society Clinical Practical Guideline Diagnosis and Treatment of Polycystic Ovary Syndrome.[30]

COC can be used for management of acne, hirsutism and menstrual irregularities associated with polycystic ovary syndrome (PCOS).

Cancer Reduction

COC use is associated with a significant reduction in risk of endometrial and ovarian cancer that increases with duration of COC use and persists for many years after stopping COC.

Endometrial Cancer

A meta-analysis of 36 international epidemiological studies found that every 5 years of COC use is associated with a relative risk of 0.76, resulting in a 50% reduction in risk of endometrial cancer with 10–15 years of use a persistent protective effect for as long as 30 years after cessation of COC exists.[31]

Ovarian Cancer

A systematic review of observational studies reported a reduction in risk of ovarian cancer in COC users compared to those who have never used COC. The meta-analysis found that the protective effect depends on the duration of use, those who have used COC for at least 10 years having a 50% reduction in incidence of ovarian cancer.[32]

BRCA Gene Mutation Carriers

On the basis of evidence from case-control studies that include small numbers of cases, systematic review with meta-analysis have concluded that amongst BRCA carriers, use of COC is associated with reduced risk of ovarian cancer with use, this is directly proportional to the duration of use.[33]

Colorectal Cancer

Use of COC is associated with a reduced risk of colorectal cancer. Evidence from meta-analyses of data from observational studies suggests that those who have used COC have a reduced risk of colorectal cancer compared to those who have never used COC.[34]

Menopause: Use of COC as an alternative to hormone replacement therapy (HRT) can be considered for use by medically eligible women until age of 50 as an alternative to HRT for relief of menopausal symptoms and prevention of loss of bone mineral density as well as for contraception.

Risks and side effects: The risks and side effects of COCs depend upon type and dose of estrogen and the progestin.

Early side effects: Nausea, breast tenderness, and headaches are usually minor complaints (<10% of women).

Amenorrhea: Amenorrhea occurs intentionally with continuous and extended COC regimens. However, amenorrhea may also occur unintentionally with 21/7 or 24/4 cyclic dosing schedules. Particularly with the lowest dose COC formulations, the low ethinyl estradiol level (relative to the much larger progestin doses) is inadequate to stimulate endometrial growth, which results in a lack of withdrawal bleeding.

Venous Thromboembolism

COC use has been associated with an increased risk of VTE. The risk of VTE depends on the estrogen dose and patient factors such as age, obesity, and smoking status. While the relative risk is increased, the absolute increase in risk is still low for most women and does not outweigh the numerous benefits of this contraceptive method, particularly when compared with the VTE risk during pregnancy and the postpartum period.[14]

Evidence from observational studies suggests that current use of COC is associated with a 3- to 3.5-fold increase in VTE risk compared with non-use of COC. It is important to note that despite this increased risk, the number of VTE events in women using COC remains very small.[14,15]

Risk of VTE is highest in the months immediately after initiation of COC or when restarting after a break of at least 1 month. The risk then reduces over the first year of use and remains stable thereafter.[14,15]

Women with inherited thrombophilias is an absolute contraindication to COC use (UKMEC 4).[6]

COC users with a mild thrombophilia and a family history of VTE have an 8- to 33-fold increase in VTE risk; for COC users with a severe thrombophilia and a positive family history, VTE risk is increased 70-fold.

Cardiovascular risk: COC use has been associated with increased risks of hypertension, myocardial infarction, and stroke in certain populations.

As per the Faculty of Sexual Health and Reproductive Healthcare (FSRH) UKMEC 2016[6] recommendations, the use of all COC is either strongly cautioned or avoided for women with hypertension, women over the age of 35 years who smoke, women with multiple risk factors for cardiovascular disease including smoking, hypertension, high BMI, dyslipidemias and diabetes, and for women with migraine with aura or migraine without aura that is of new onset during use of COC.

A Cochrane review of 24 observational studies found a significantly increased risk of myocardial infarction (MI) for current users of COC compared with non-users (RR 1.6; 95% CI 1.2–2.1).[16]

Cancer Risk

Breast cancer: Women should be advised that current use of COC is associated with a small increased risk of breast cancer which reduces with time after stopping COC.

A large Danish cohort study reported a relative risk of breast cancer of 1.19 (95% CI 1.13–1.26) for current or recent users of COC compared to those who had never used hormonal contraception. Risk appeared to increase with duration of use. No major differences in risk were observed with the different progestogens contained in the COC.[17]

More recent studies, including a meta-analysis of 44 observational studies, found no link between duration of COC use and breast cancer risk.[18]

Several studies do, however, suggest that women with a family history of breast cancer who have ever used COC are at no higher risk of breast cancer than women with a family history who have never used COC.[19]

Three meta-analyses based on observational studies conclude that carriers of BRCA mutations, who use COC have a reduced risk of ovarian cancer compared with never-users (RR 0.50, OR 0.57 and OR 0.58). This advantage would need to be weighed against the potential increased risk of breast cancer.[20]

Cervical cancer: Women should be advised that current use of COC for >5 years, is associated with a small increased risk of cervical cancer; risk reduces over time after stopping COC and is no longer increased by about 10 years after stopping.

Collaborative analysis of data from 24 worldwide observational studies, suggested that current use of COC for >5 years approximately doubled the risk of invasive cervical cancer (RR 190; 95% CI 169–213) compared with never-use of COC.[21]

Some women using COC report headaches, nausea, dizziness and breast tenderness.

Health Risks Associated with COC Use

Headache

A 2013 comprehensive literature review found no consistent association between COC use and headache, regardless of progestogen type and route of COC administration. Lower estrogen doses do not appear to be associated with fewer headaches.[22]

Unscheduled Bleeding

Unscheduled bleeding is a relatively common side effect of COC. The incidence is around 10–18% per cycle.

Unscheduled bleeding commonly occurs with COC use improves over the first 3–4 months of use. Formulations with higher doses of EE are probably associated with a lower risk of unscheduled bleeding when used in a traditional regimen, and pills containing second-generation progestogens could offer better cycle control than those containing norethisterone.[23]

Mood

There is no clear, consistent evidence that COC use causes depression; mood change is common and often related to external events. If a patient experiences low mood, a different formulation containing an alternative progestogen could be tried empirically. If the negative mood change is premenstrual, continuous use of COC may be of benefit.

Weight Gain

A 2014 Cochrane review of 49 RCTs identified only four trials that compared COC with placebo or with no intervention; the remainder compared different COC formulations. The limited evidence does not support a causal association between the use of COC and weight gain, and there is no consistent evidence that different COC formulations affect weight differently.[24]

Libido

Despite the fact that active testosterone levels (where measured) were reduced during COC use, COC users reported an increase in sexual desire in 15 studies and no impact on sexual desire in 12 studies.[25]

VAGINAL COMBINED CONTRACEPTIVE DEVICES

Etonogestrel and ethinyl estradiol ring: The etonogestrel/ethinyl estradiol (ENG/EE, commercial names NuvaRing, EluRyng) ring is a flexible device measuring 54 mm in diameter and 4 mm in cross-section that is worn vaginally for 3 weeks and then removed (and discarded) for 1 week.

There is an immediate increase in serum hormonal concentration after insertion with a slow decrease over the cycle. The concentration of EE is lower with the ENG/EE vaginal ring compared with other combined hormonal contraceptives.[35]

Segesterone and ethinyl estradiol ring: The one-year reusable segesterone acetate/ethinyl estradiol (SA/EE, commercial name Annovera) ring is 56 mm in overall diameter and 8.4 mm in cross-sectional diameter. The ring is worn for 3 weeks and removed for 1 week, and that pattern is repeated for a total of 13 cycles. This pattern of use results in regular withdrawal bleeding and an overall pooled unintended pregnancy rate (Pearl index) of 2.98 per 100 woman-years.

Other product advantages include that it does not require refrigeration for storage.[36]

The combined hormonal rings provide the same benefits of combined oral contraceptive (COC) pills, including contraception, regulation of bleeding, endometrial protection, and, in some, reduction of dysmenorrhea and endometriosis-related pain. In addition, the ring is a good option for people who want the benefits of combined oral contraceptives (OCs), but prefer to avoid a method that requires daily user compliance.

Local: Ring users report more vaginitis, vaginal wetness, and leukorrhea compared with COC users. In a meta-analysis of trials comparing the ENG/EE vaginal ring with various estrogen-progestin contraceptive pills, the odds of vaginitis were approximately 2.5 times greater [odds ratios (OR) 2.48 to 2.84] and the odds of leukorrhea were three to six times greater (OR 3.21 to 6.42) for those using the contraceptive ring.

References

1. Vandever MA, Kuehl TJ, Sulak PJ, et al. Evaluation of pituitary-ovarian axis suppression with three oral contraceptive regimens. Contraception 2008; 77:162.

2. Curtis KM, Jatlaoui TC, Tepper NK, et al. U.S. Selected Practice Recommendations for Contraceptive Use, 2016. MMWR Recomm Rep 2016; 65:1.

3. Trussell J. Contraceptive failure in the United States. Contraception 2011;83:397–404.

4. Dragoman MV, Simmons KB, Paulen ME, et al. Combined hormonal contraceptive (CHC) use among obese women and contraceptive effectiveness: a systematic review. Contraception 2017;95:117–29.

5. Zapata LB, Steenland MW, Brahmi D, et al. Effect of missed combined hormonal contraceptives on contraceptive effectiveness: a systematic review. Contraception 2013;87:685–700.

6. Faculty of Sexual & Reproductive Healthcare (FSRH). Drug interactions with Hormonal Contraception (November 2017). 2017. https://www.fsrh.org/standards-and-guidance/currentclinical-guidance/drug-interactions.

7. Sabers A, Buchholt JM, Uldall P, et al. Lamotrigine plasma levels reduced by oral contraceptives. Epilepsy Res 2001;47:151–4.

8. Curtis KM, Tepper NK, Jatlaoui TC, et al. U.S. Medical Eligibility Criteria for Contraceptive Use, 2016. MMWR Recomm Rep 2016; 65:1.

9. Department of Reproductive Health, World Health Organization. Medical eligibility criteria for contraceptive use, 5th ed, World Health Organization, Geneva 2015.

10. Iversen L, Sivasubramaniam S, Lee AJ, et al. Lifetime cancer risk and combined oral contraceptives: the Royal College of General Practitioners' Oral Contraception Study. Am J Obstet Gynecol 2017; 216:580.e1.

11. Moorman PG, Havrilesky LJ, Gierisch JM, et al. Oral contraceptives and risk of ovarian cancer and breast cancer among high-risk women: a systematic review and meta-analysis. J Clin Oncol 2013; 31:4188.

12. Gambacciani M, Cappagli B, Lazzarini V, et al. Longitudinal evaluation of perimenopausal bone loss: effects of different low dose oral contraceptive preparations on bone mineral density. Maturitas 2006; 54:176.

13. Allen RH, Cwiak CA, Kaunitz AM. Contraception in women over 40 years of age. CMAJ 2013; 185:565.

14. Lidegaard Ø, Løkkegaard E, Svendsen AL, et al. Hormonal contraception and risk of venous thromboembolism: national follow-up study. BMJ 2009;339:b2890.

15. Suissa S, Blais L, Spitzer WO, et al. First-time use of newer oral contraceptives and the risk of venous thromboembolism. Contraception 1997;56:141–6.

16. Roach REJ, Helmerhorst FM, Lijfering WM, et al. Combined oral contraceptives: the risk of myocardial infarction and ischemic stroke. Cochrane Database Syst Rev 2015;CD011054.

17. Mørch LS, Skovlund CW, Hannaford PC, et al. Contemporary Hormonal Contraception and the Risk of Breast Cancer. N Engl J Med 2017;377:2228–39.

18. Vessey M, Painter R. Oral contraceptive use and cancer. Findings in a large cohort study, 1968-2004. Br J Cancer 2006;95:385–9.

19. Gaffield ME, Culwell KR, Ravi A. Oral contraceptives and family history of breast cancer. Contraception 2009;80:372–80.

20. Moorman PG, Havrilesky LJ, Gierisch JM, et al. Oral contraceptives and risk of ovarian cancer and breast cancer among high-risk women: a systematic review and meta-analysis. J Clin Oncol 2013;31:4188–98.

21. International Collaboration of Epidemiological Studies of Cervical Cancer, Appleby P, Beral V, et al. Cervical cancer and hormonal contraceptives: collaborative reanalysis of individual data Copyright ©Faculty of Sexual & Reproductive Healthcare 2019 77 FSRH guideline: CHC for 16,573 women with cervical cancer and 35,509 women without cervical cancer from 24 epidemiological studies. Lancet 2007;370:1609–21.

22. MacGregor EA. Contraception and headache. Headache 2013;53:247–76.

23. Ahrendt H-J, Makalová D, Parke S, et al. Bleeding pattern and cycle control with an estradiolbased oral contraceptive: a seven-cycle, randomized comparative trial of estradiol valerate/ dienogest and ethinyl estradiol/ levonorgestrel. Contraception 2009;80:436–44.

24. Gallo MF, Lopez LM, Grimes DA, et al. Combination contraceptives: effects on weight. Cochrane Database Syst Rev 2014;CD003987.

25. Pastor Z, Holla K, Chmel R. The influence of combined oral contraceptives on female sexual desire: a systematic review. Eur J Contracept Reprod Health Care 2013;18:27–43.

26. Bitzer J, Heikinheimo O, Nelson AL, et al. Medical management of heavy menstrual bleeding: a comprehensive review of the literature. Obstet Gynecol Surv 2015;70:115–30.

27. National Institute for Health and Care Excellence (NICE). Endometriosis: diagnosis and management. NICE guideline [NG73]. 2017. https://www.nice.org.uk/guidance/cg30.

28. Arowojolu AO, Gallo MF, Lopez LM, et al. Combined oral contraceptive pills for treatment of acne. Cochrane Database Syst Rev 2012;CD004425

29. The 2016 Royal College of Obstetricians and Gynaecologists (RCOG) Green-top Guideline Management of Premenstrual Syndrome.

30. The Endocrine Society Clinical Practical Guideline Diagnosis and Treatment of Polycystic Ovary Syndrome.

31. Collaborative Group on Epidemiological Studies on Endometrial Cancer. Endometrial cancer and oral contraceptives: an individual participant meta-analysis of 27 276 women with endometrial cancer from 36 epidemiological studies. Lancet Oncol 2015;16:1061–70.

32. Havrilesky LJ, Moorman PG, Lowery WJ, et al. Oral contraceptive pills as primary prevention for ovarian cancer: a systematic review and meta-analysis. Obstet Gynecol 2013;122:139–47

33. Iodice S, Barile M, Rotmensz N, et al. Oral contraceptive use and breast or ovarian cancer risk in BRCA1/2 carriers: a meta-analysis. Eur J Cancer 2010;46:2275–84.

34. Gierisch JM, Coeytaux RR, Urrutia RP, et al. Oral contraceptive use and risk of breast, cervical, colorectal, and endometrial cancers: a systematic review. Cancer Epidemiol Biomarkers Prev 2013;22:1931–43

35. Van den Heuvel MW, van Bragt AJ, Alnabawy AK, Kaptein MC. Comparison of ethinylestradiol pharmacokinetics in three hormonal contra-ceptive formulations: the vaginal ring, the transdermal patch and an oral contraceptive. Contraception 2005;72:168.

36. Annovera [package insert]. New York, NY. Manufactured for Population Council. August 2018. www.accessdata.fda.gov/drugsatfda_docs/label/2018/209627s000lbl.pdf (Accessed on August 13, 2018).

Progesterone Only Pills and Depot-Medroxyprogesterone Acetate

• Isha Wadhawan • Avir Sarkar • Anjaly Raj • Mala Arora

PROGESTERONE ONLY PILL

Introduction

Progesterone-only pills (POPs) are contraceptive pills containing synthetic steroids with progestogenic properties. Every obstetrician should be able to guide and support women to make informed decisions about their contraceptive of choice, after explaining the effectiveness, method of use and side effects.

There are 4 different POPs currently available:

1. Levonorgestrel (LNG), 30 μg ⎫ Traditional
2. Norethisterone (NET), 350 μg ⎬ POPs
3. Desogestrel (DSG), 75 μg
4. Drosperinone (DRSP), 4 μg

MECHANISM OF ACTION

1. Makes the cervical mucus 'hostile'-reduced volume, increased viscosity and cellularity of cervical mucus hampers sperm penetration
2. Endometrial thinning-making it unfavorable for implantation
3. Reduced tubal motility
4. DSG and DRSP, in addition, also have anti-gonadotropic effects, thus inhibiting ovulation. The traditional POPs do not reliably inhibit ovulation.[1]

Effectiveness

- Contraceptive effectiveness of these pills depends on their correct use and compliance to timing of pill intake. Ideally the pill should be taken at the same time every day. Risk of pregnancy in first year of typical use of POP is 9%. However, if used perfectly, they are >99% effective.
- It is hypothesized that DSG and DRSP are more effective than traditional POPs, since they suppress ovulation and have longer pill-free interval. But currently, there is no research evidence to suggest difference in the contraceptive efficacy between various POPs.

Contraceptive effectiveness is affected by:

1. Vomiting soon after pill intake will not allow adequate absorption of pill resulting in failure of contraception. The recommended time after pill intake until unaffected by vomiting varies, being 2 hours for the traditional POPs and 3–4 hours for DSG POP and DRSP POP. In such situations, take a pill of the same type as soon as possible. If replacement pill is not taken within
   - 3 hours of intake of traditional POPs
   - 12 hours of intake of DSG POP
   - 24 hours of intake of DRSP POP

Then follow steps for missed pill management.

2. Diarrhea soon after taking POP may also affect the absorption and women should be advised to take a pill of the same type as soon as possible after an episode of severe watery diarrhea. At present, there are no recommendations or any evidence regarding the time period after pill intake when diarrhea would affect absorption.

3. Drug interactions

- Contraceptive effectiveness of POPs could be affected when used along with enzyme inducing drugs, even up to 28 days after stopping the drug. Enzyme inducers can increase the metabolism of progestogens and contraceptive efficacy is thus reduced.

- Women on enzyme-inducing drugs should be made aware of the possibility of failure of contraception with POP and must be offered other options of contraception that are unaffected by enzyme-inducing drugs, such as depot-medroxyprogesterone acetate (DMPA) or intrauterine contraceptive devices.

- The effectiveness of POP may also be reduced by regular concomitant use of ulipristal acetate (UPA) for non-emergency contraception indications.

Contraceptive efficacy of POPs is not affected by body weight, body-mass index (BMI) or bariatric surgery.

How to start: POPs can be prescribed to all medically eligible women between menarche to 55 years of age **(Table 28.1)**.

The following minimum criteria should be checked before initiating POPs:

1. Medical eligibility assessment which includes comprehensive assessment of medical conditions and drug history

2. Any concomitant use of interacting drugs or herbal medications

3. No known allergy to POP content (some DSG POP contain soya which may cause cross reaction in those with allergy to peanuts)

4. Rule out risk of existing pregnancy and assess need for emergency contraception, additional contraceptive precautions and follow-up pregnancy testing

5. Advise about
   - Contraceptive effectiveness with perfect and typical use
   - How to take pills and importance of compliance to timing
   - Management of late/missed pills
   - Potential bleeding patterns and side effects
   - Any requirement of additional contraceptives
   - Interactions with other medications
   - Alternate options, like long-acting reversible contraception (LARC)

6. Also consider assessment of sexually transmitted infection (STI) risk assessment and cervical screening
   - Clinical examination and laboratory investigations are not routinely needed prior to initiating traditional POPs or DSG POP.

Table 28.1: Starting procedures for traditional POP, DSG POP and DRSP POP

Traditional POP and DSG POP	DRSP POP
Standard start • On day 1–5 of menses • By day 5 after abortion • By day 21 after childbirth	Standard start • On day 1 of menses • On day 1 after abortion • By day 21 after childbirth
Quick start (after day 5 of menses) When started at any time other than above mentioned, use **additional contraceptive methods for 2 days** and take a follow-up pregnancy test if indicated.	**Quick start (after day 1 of menses)** When started at any time other than above mentioned, use **additional contraceptive methods for 7 days** and take a follow-up pregnancy test if indicated.

- Prior to prescription of DRSP, consider checking urea and electrolytes and blood pressure in those individuals with mild-to-moderate renal function impairment or significant risk factors for chronic kidney disease (CKD), particularly if age >50 years.

Traditional POPs and DSG POP are taken as daily pills with no hormone-free interval (HFI), while DRSP POP is available as 24 active pills with 4 days of HFI.

- In women, undergoing medical termination of pregnancy, POP can be started along with mifepristone without affecting effectiveness of medical abortion.

Starting POP after emergency contraceptive (EC) use:

- POP can be initiated immediately after levonorgestrel-EC. Additional contraception (condoms), should be used for 2 days in case of traditional/DSG POPs and for 7 days when using DSRP POP. Pregnancy test should be done 21 days after last unprotected sexual intercourse (UPSI).
- However, if a woman who has used UPA-EC, delay POP for 5 days after taking UPA-EC as the effectiveness of UPA-EC to delay ovulation may be inhibited by POP. Additional contraceptive precautions should be followed as mentioned above and pregnancy test should be done 21 days after UPSI.

Missed Pill (Table 28.2)

Management

- Take missed pill as soon as possible.
- Take the next pill at usual time (this may mean taking 2 pills in a day).
- Use additional contraception for 48 hours after starting correct pill intake.
- EC must be considered if UPSI occurred at any time between first missed pill to 48 hours after starting correct pill intake.
- Pregnancy test should be considered 21 days after occurrence of UPSI.

Table 28.2: Definition of missed pill

POP	Missed pill
Traditional	Delay of pill intake by >3 hours (>27 hours since last pill)
DSG	Delay of pill intake by >12 hours (>36 hours since last pill)
DRSP	Delay of pill intake by >24 hours (>48 hours since last pill) Or > 24 hours after a new pack should have been started after HFI

Management

- Take missed pill as soon as possible.
- Take the next pill at usual time (this may mean taking 2 pills in a day).
- Use additional contraception for 7 days after starting correct pill taking.
- EC must be considered.
- If any active pill(s) was missed and UPSI occurred between first missed pill to 7 days after starting correct pill intake.
- If any active pill(s) was missed in first 7 days of a packet and UPSI happened during HFI or first week.
- If any of the last 7 active pills were missed, HFI must be omitted.
- Pregnancy test should be considered 21 days after occurrence of UPSI.

Contraindications

Medical Eligibility Criteria for Contraceptive Use by WHO (WHO MEC) classifies the use of various contraceptive methods for different conditions in 4 classes as noted in the Table 28.3. The classification is given both for initiation and continuation of a particular method in a specific medical condition.

MEC 4 (use has unacceptable risks): Current breast cancer

MEC 3 (risks of use more than the benefits)
1. Current and history of ischemia heart disease—for POP continuation (UKMEC 2 for initiation)
2. History of stroke—for POP continuation (UKMEC 2 for initiation)
3. Past breast cancer

Table 28.3: MEC categories for contraceptive eligibility[26]

1	A condition for which there is no restriction for the use of the contraceptive method.
2	A condition where the advantages of using the method generally outweigh the theoretical or proven risks.
3	A condition where the theoretical or proven risks usually outweigh the advantages of using the method.
4	A condition which represents an unacceptable health risk if the contraceptive method is used.

4. Severe decompensated cirrhosis/hepato-cellular adenoma or carcinoma

- In women with breast cancer, before initiating any hormonal contraception consultation with their oncology team may be considered.
- POPs can be used safely in women with history of ectopic pregnancy. POP reduce incidence of all pregnancies including ectopic pregnancies. Traditional and DSG POP are effective when initiated within 5 days of ectopic pregnancy and DRSP POP when initiated within day 1 without need for additional contraceptive precautions.

Special Considerations for DRSP

DRSP POP has additional aldosterone antagonistic actions resulting in increased sodium and water excretion and potassium reabsorption. As a result of these effects, additional precautions following must be followed when DRSP is used:

- Should not be used in severe renal insufficiency and acute renal failure.
- Avoid in hyperkalemia, untreated hypo-aldosteronism (Addison's disease), individuals on concomitant therapy with potassium sparing diuretics, aldosterone antagonists and potassium supplements
- Use with caution in those with mild-to-moderate renal impairment and treated hypoaldosteronism.

Side Effects

Most common side effect is unpredictable/unscheduled bleeding pattern and is often the reason for discontinuation of POPs.[2] Bleeding patterns vary depending on the type of POP. Before prescribing POP, women should be made aware of this side effect and that with regular use, the incidence of unpredictable bleeding decreases and amenorrhea increases.[3,4]

Problematic bleeding must be assessed for underlying causes. Change of POP maybe beneficial in some women. In cases of problematic bleeding with DSG POP, often a double dose (150 µg) daily is prescribed in clinical practice. However, there is no published evidence for effectiveness of double dose in such situations. Short-term strategies like estrogen supplementation, use of non-steroidal anti-inflammatory drugs (NSAIDs) or tranexamic acid may also be useful.

Health Risks

- There are no adverse effects on lactation or on infant.[5]
- No evidence currently exists to suggest that POP use is associated with depression or mood changes, headache, acne, significant weight gain, clinically significant effect on bone mineral density or formation of ovarian cysts.
- There is no evidence to suggest an increase in venous thromboembolic events (VTE), thrombotic stroke or myocardial infarction. POPs are safe in thrombophilia, those with history of VTE, obese and overweight and dose need not be changed.
- *Cancers:* No increase in risk of breast cancer and no association with endometrial cancer/ovarian cancer/cervical cancer.

Non-contraceptive Benefits

- POPs, specifically DSG and DSRP have proved to be beneficial in controlling heavy menstrual bleeding and dysmenorrhea.

- Owing to its anti-androgenic and diuretic properties, DSRP may be useful in acne, hirsutism and for weight reduction. But these effects have not been specifically studied as yet.

Follow-up

Women on POP should be advised to follow-up annually and at any time they face problematic side effects, wish to discontinue or switch to other methods.

How to Stop

On discontinuing POP, return of fertility is immediate. If woman does not wish pregnancy, she should be offered alternate methods of contraception.

Contraception is not required after 55 years of age and POP can be discontinued.

Switching from Other Methods of Contraception to POP
(Flowcharts 28.1–28.4)

Combined Oral Contraceptives

- Women on combined oral contraceptives (COCs) can be offered POP on day 1 or 2 of hormone-free interval (HFI) or in week 2 or 3 of COC schedule without any alternate contraceptive precautions.

If on day 1 to day 5 of cycle, traditional/DSG-based POP can be started. DRSP POP can be started only on day 1 of cycle.

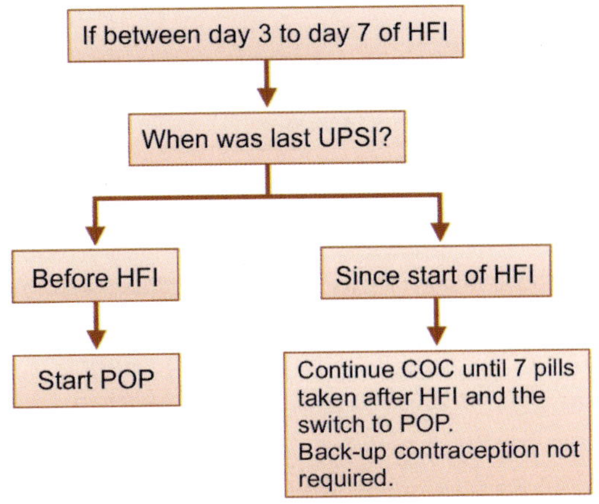

Flowchart 28.1: Transitioning from COCS to POPs in the HFI

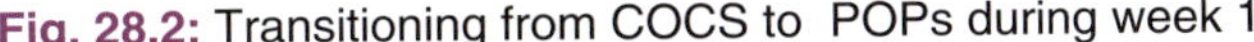

CONCLUSION

POPs are safe option for contraception, particularly useful in postpartum period since it does not affect lactation or growth and development of the infant. These pills have a very low failure rate when used perfectly, however the need for compliance to timing of pill intake and unpredictable bleeding episodes discourage women to select POPs. There is scope for further research into the side effects and health risks associated with POP use as currently there is limited evidence available.

Fig. 28.2: Transitioning from COCS to POPs during week 1

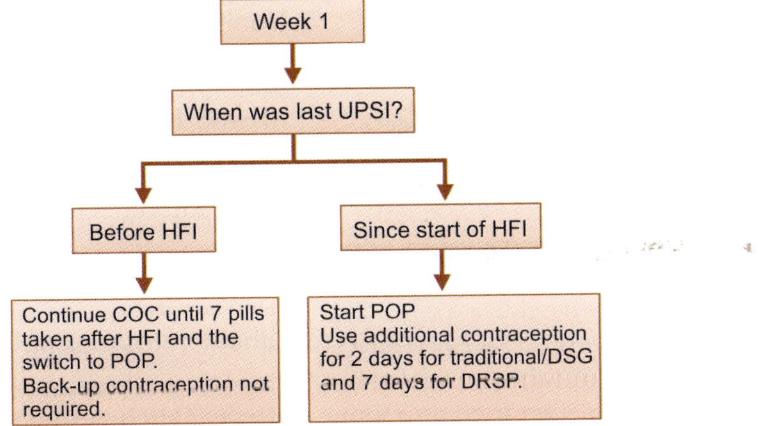

Flowchart 28.3: Transitioning from DMPA to POPs

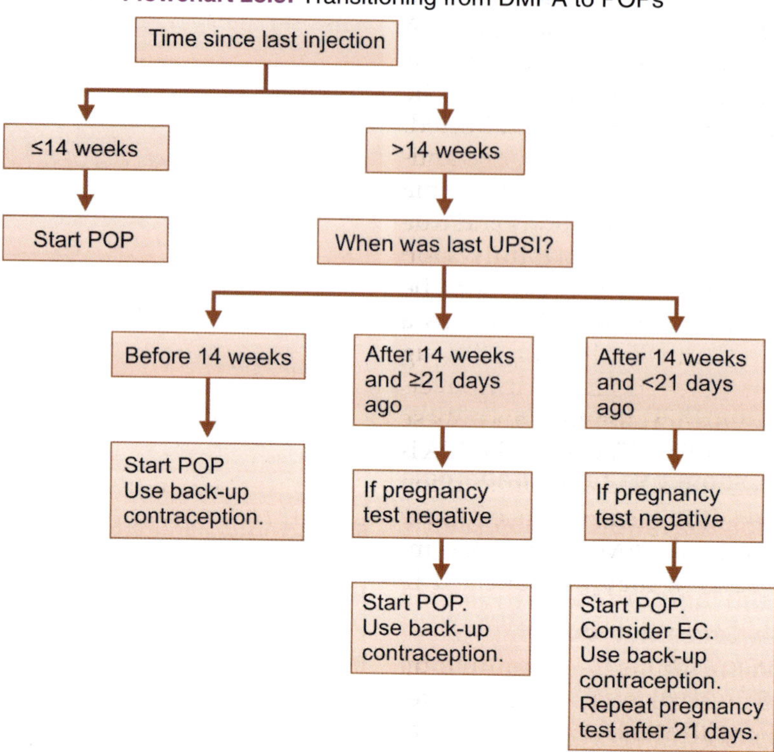

Flowchart 28.4: Transitioning from Copper IUCD to POPs

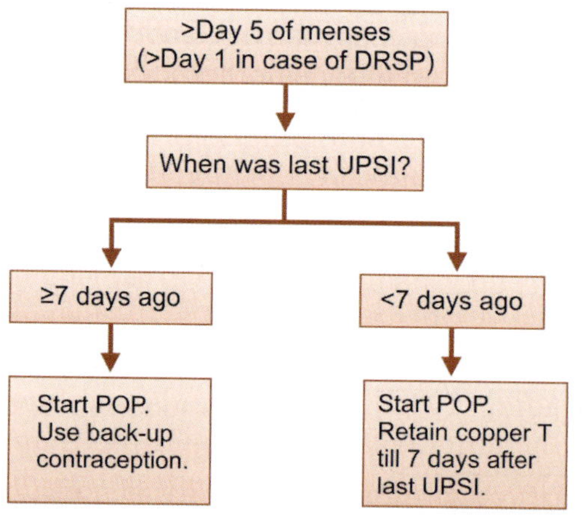

Introduction

Depot medroxyprogesterone acetate (DMPA) is a progesterone containing injectable medication. It is more often used as a long- acting reversible contraceptive method. A number of times it is also utilized for its non-contraceptive benefits in the treatment of abnormal uterine bleeding, endometriosis, premenstrual syndrome and others.

MECHANISM OF ACTION AND PHARMACOKINETICS

The primary mechanism of action of DMPA is inhibition of ovulation.[6,7] Additionally, it thickens cervical mucus and makes endo- metrium unfavourable for implantation.[8] As a result, it provides effective contraception.

By inhibiting ovulation, DMPA also decreases pain associated with endometriosis and adenomyosis. Similarly, symptoms of premenstrual dysphoric syndrome and abnormal uterine bleeding are also suppressed.

Other Pharmacokinetic Considerations

Hepatic enzymes-inducing drugs do not affect DMPA serum levels. Therefore, it can be easily used for HIV patients taking antiretroviral medications. Similarly, DMPA is an effective means of contraception for women with epilepsy and on antiepileptic treatment as its serum levels are unaffected. However, patients on anti-retrovirals and anti-epiletics may be at higher risk for osteopenia due to the effect of the medications and due to prolonged periods of immobilization and hospitalizations, and this needs to be considered while considering DMPA as a contraceptive option.[6] Evaluation of drug levels and BMI have noted similar drug levels and return to ovulation for thin and obese women in initial studies.[9] Therefore, DMPA is considered effective method of contraception for obese women. However, serum levels are lower in women with a BMI over 40 kg/m^2 and therefore caution may be exercised in such cases.[9]

Return to fertility: Though, it may take up to a year for ovulatory cycles[8] to start after discontinuation of DMPA, it can be sooner and therefore if DMPA is discontinued for those not desiring fertility, an alternate method must be initiated at the time the next injection would be due.

CONTRACEPTIVE USE AND CONSIDERATIONS

- In India, it is available as an intra muscular preparation by the name Depo-Provera®, that contains 150 mg of medroxyprogesterone acetate in 1 ml.[6] There are other formulations used overseas.

- It comes in a prefilled syringe as a water based suspension. The syringe must be shaken vigorously before use. BMI evaluation may be performed at each visit. Standard sites of administration are the gluteus maximus muscle (upper outer quadrant) or lateral thigh. The deltoid may be preferred in obese individuals to ensure intramuscular drug delivery. Manufacturer instructions should be reviewed and appropriate training must be conducted.

- It is administered every 12 weeks and offers an effective long-acting reversible contraceptive (LCRC) method. The failure rate is 0.2% with perfect use[10] and up to 6% with typical use.[11]

- At each visit, users should be screened for general wellbeing, side effects if any, and medical eligibility reassessed. They should be notified of their next injection date. Though, ideal administration interval in 12 weeks, DMPA may be administered as early as 10 weeks and as late as 14 weeks [even 16 weeks as per the World Health Organization (WHO)] from the last injection with good efficacy. Documentation and record-keeping are essential. There is no limit for age till it may be used or length of use as long as criteria is met **(Flowchart 28.3)**.

- Cervical mucus thickening occurs effectively at up to 7 days after administration of DMPA. It is advisable to use a second agent until one week after administration.[8]

- DMPA is more cost effective than COCs after 1 year of use.[6,12] However, it is less cost-effective than other LARCs [copper intrauterine device (Cu-IUD), LNG-IUS] since the failure rate is higher with typical use. This is likely due to the requirement for multiple injections and therefore higher chance of default.[6,12]

- Ideal time to start DMPA is up to cycle day 5. It may be administered for the first

Box 28.1: To rule out pregnancy either of the following criteria should be met.

- No intercourse since last menstrual period (LMP) (or birth or abortion or ectopic pregnancy)
- Consistent use of a reliable method of contraception.
- A negative urine pregnancy test (that detects ~20 mIU/ml) and no intercourse in >21 days.
- Within first 5 days of normal cycle [or abortion, ectopic pregnancy, evacuation of gestational trophoblastic neoplasia (GTN)]
- Within 21 days postpartum
- Exclusively breastfeeding, amenorrheic and <6 months postpartum.

time on later day in the cycle as long as it is fairly clear that the user is not pregnant.

Quick Starting DMPA

Consider oral contraceptive pills (OCPs) for bridging for a week.[13] It may be taken immediately after emergency contraception (EC) with levonorgestrel 1.5 mg.[13] In such cases, a pregnancy test may be taken 3 weeks after unprotected intercourse.

In the event that ulipristal acetate, 30 mg, is used for EC, the DMPA injection is to be taken after 5 days for EC to be effective.[13] This is because ulipristral acetate is a progesterone receptor modulator, with primarily inhibitory effects on the progesterone receptor, and therefore its effectiveness as EC may be reduced with DMPA administration. Similarly, DMPA as a method contraception may not be as effective in women using ulipristal acetate, 5 mg, for treatment of uterine fibroids.

Switching from Another Method

1. *Combined hormonal contraceptives (CHC):* No back-up method is needed with DMPA is administered on day 1–2 of cycle or within week 2 or 3 of taking a CHC provided, it was being used correctly until initiation of DMPA. If started with days 3–7 of a CHC cycle a bridging method for a week is required as ovulation may still occur prior to establishment of DMPA effectiveness if CHC is stopped.

2. *POPs:* When switching from traditional POPs, a bridging period of a week is always required. However, with desogestrel no bridging period is needed if it was being used correcting.

3. *Copper IUD:* When switching on day 1–5 of cycle, no need for additional contraception. However, at any other time in the cycle, additional 7 days of contraception is needed while DMPA takes effect. One may retain the IUD for bridging.

4. *LNG-IUS:* Switching on any day of the cycle, requires bridging for 7 days. Again, the user may retain the LNG-IUS for an additional week.

5. *Progesterone implant:* If bridging is done prior to completion of 3 years since implant placement, it will still be effective and no second method is required.

- There is no evidence to demonstrate any harmful effects on a pregnancy conceived by user just before or while on DMPA. A small Thai suggests possibility of growth restriction, low birth weight and neonatal demise,[14] however confounding variables were not well adjusted. Other long term observational data are reassuring.[14]

Non-contraceptive Benefits

DMPA is also recommended for management of heavy menstrual bleeding[7] since most users experience decreased menstrual flow with its use and majority become amenorrhoeic.[7] Likewise, it may also help reduce symptoms of endometriosis and dysmenorrhea.[6] DMPA use also reduces rates of ovarian and endometrial cancers.[21] There is limited evidence supporting its benefit in reducing pain during sickle cell crisis.[6]

It is important to counsel women regarding these changes in menstrual patterns so that they do not view these as side effects. Knowledge regarding additional advantages may improve acceptance and compliance.

Side Effects

- As noted previously altered bleeding patterns may be viewed as side effects by some women. Many women have decreased flow to amenorrhea, and at times spotting to prolonged flow, especially when on DMPA long term.[15] However, it is essential to evaluate any unscheduled bleeding for other pathologies including cervical dysplasia, polyps, hyperplasia or any endocrinopathy before chalking it up to DMPA.

- Another common reason for discontinuation is weight gain. Weight gain noted is higher than other non-hormonal methods and COCs.[16] Among the adolescent population, this weight gain is noted more often in new users and those with her a higher BMI.[17]

- An important health concern of DMPA is the effect on bone mineral density (BMD) due to decrease in oestrogen levels. Therefore, caution is advised during prescription to teenagers who may not have achieved peak bone mass and to older patient nearing menopause. There is definitive evidence for decrease in BMD with DMPA use, that in young women is reversible with discontinuation.[18] Furthermore, it has been shown that the greatest decline in BMD occurs in the first year of use, and though it tapers it continues with each passing year.[18] However, there is not any conclusive data to prove increase in clinical risk.[19] The studies reporting a modest increased rate of fracture risk are noted to have not adjusted for baseline fracture risk or confounding factors and are not adequately powered.[19] Therefore, DMPA may still be chosen as first-line treatment for the younger patients if no other method seems acceptable and also in older women if osteoporosis risk is otherwise not elevated. Such patients should be reviewed periodically. Routine screening for osteoporosis with dual X-ray absorptiometry (DEXA) scan is not recommended, but may be performed as deemed clinically appropriate.

- There have been occasional reports of injection site reactions. Also, though not conclusive, there are a few reports of increased acne, decreased libido, mood swings, depressive symptoms, vaginal dryness, headache, alopecia with DMPA.[20]

- Risk of ovarian and endometrial cancer is likely to reduce with DMPA use.[21]

- There is a weak association between cervical cancer rates and long-term DMPA use, however, this may be due to confounding factors.[22] It is important to screen all women, including those seeking DMPA as contraception for cervical cancer. Additionally, sexually shared infection prevention counselling should also be provided including discussion on use of barrier methods with all other contraceptives and testing done as deemed fit.

- DMPA use and breast cancer risk is not well-studied, however a meta-analysis of 54 studies noted a small increase in risk without statistical significance.[23] Another data reported small increase in risk with recent use which may be reduced after stopping DMPA.[23]

Table 28.4: Selective summary of MEC by WHO for POPs and DMPA (5th edition, released in 2015)[26]

Condition	POPs	DMPA	Comments
Age Menarche to <18 yrs 18 to 45 yrs >45 yrs	 1 1 1	 2 1 2	Some evidence support loss of bone mineral density with DMPA use. Whether this loss is clinically significance, needs to assessed.
Breastfeeding <6 weeks post-delivery >6 weeks post-delivery	 2 1	 3 1	Potential exposure to DMPA or POP in the neonate in first 6 weeks is a matter of concern.
Postabortal	1	1	Both methods may be initiated immediately after the abortion (e.g. in the same sitting that a D&E is performed).
Smoking	1	1	

Contd...

Table 28.4: Selective summary of MEC by WHO for POPs and DMPA (5th edition, released in 2015) (*Contd...*)

Condition	POPs	DMPA	Comments
Obesity			There is evidence for differential weight gain among normal weight and obese adolescents who use DMPA.
>30 kg/m² BMI	1	1	
Menarche to <18 yrs and BMI >30 kg/m²	1	2	
Hypertension			
Well-controlled	1	2	
Poorly controlled/with vascular disease	2	3	
Multiple risk factors for arterial cardiovascular disease	2	3	Risk may increase significantly with use of progesterone containing contraceptives.
Diabetes	2	2 (except 3 for diabetes complicated with vascular disease)	
DVT/PE			Though there is poor quality evidence, WHO is stricter with progesterone-containing methods with respect to VTE risk.
• History/or stable on treatment/known case of condition predisposing to VTE (antiphospholipid, mutations)	2	2	
• Acute event	3	3	
STIs (for both increased risk for STIs, active STIs including vaginitis, cervicitis, hepatitis B)	1	1	
HIV (high risk for HIV, mild HIV not on treatment)	1	1	
HIV on antiretrovirals	1 or 2 (for NNRTIs)	1	NNRTIs may interact with POPs thereby reducing their effectiveness.
Anticonvulsant therapy			Effectiveness of POPs is likely to be reduced on enzyme-inducing medications.
• Enzyme inducers	3	1	
• Lamotrigine	1	1	
Headaches			
• Migraines with aura	Initiation = 3, continuation = 2	Initiation = 3, continuation = 2	
• Others	1	1	
Depressive disorders	1	1	
Cervical neoplasia			Evidence suggests possible increased risk of developing cancer in women with CIN.
• CIN	1	2	
• Cervical cancer	1	2	
Breast diseases			
• Benign	1	1	
• Current breast cancer	4	4	
• Past breast cancer	3	3	
Ovarian cancer	1	1	
Endometrial cancer	1	1	

- No conclusive evidence exists for increased incidence of venous thromboembolism with DMPA use. Therefore, the WHO Medical eligibility criteria labels it as a MEC-2 for users with previous thromboembolism, systemic lupus erythematosus (SLE) anti-phospholipid syndrome, etc.
- DMPA does not increase risk of cardio-vascular disease or cerebrovascular accident.[24] Its effect on lipid profile and cardio-metabolic parameters is not well studied.
- There is insufficient evidence to support association between DMPA use and acquisition with HIV.[25] However, all users must be educated on safe sex practices and use of barrier methods to protect against sexual shared infections.

CONCLUSION

DMPA is an effective method of long active reversible contraceptive measure that is simple, easy to use and safe. It is also utilized in number of gynecological conditions like abnormal uterine bleeding and endometriosis. Certain factors may need to be considered during its prescription including patient age, BMI, desire for return to fertility, risk of osteoporosis, risk of breast cancer and venous thromboembolism.

References

1. Teal S, Edelman A. Contraception Selection, Effectiveness, and Adverse Effects: A Review. JAMA. 2021;326(24):2507–2518.
2. de Melo NR. Estrogen-Free Oral Hormonal Contraception: Benefits of the Progestin-Only Pill. Women's Health. 2010;6(5):721–735.
3. Apter D, Colli E, Gemzell-Danielsson K, et al. Multicenter, open-label trial to assess the safety and tolerability of drospirenone 4.0 mg over 6 cycles in female adolescents, with a 7-cycle extension phase. Contraception. 2020 Jun;101(6):412–419.
4. Archer DF, Ahrendt H-J, Drouin D. Drospirenone-only oral contraceptive: results from a multicenter noncomparative trial of efficacy, safety and tolerability. Contraception 2015; 92: 439–44.
5. Philips SJ, Tepper KN, Kapp N, et al. Progestogen-only contraceptive use among breastfeeding women: a systematic review. Contraception. 2016; 94(3): 226–252.
6. National Institute for Health and Care Excellence (NICE). Long-acting Reversible Contraception (Update). 2014.
7. Mishell DR Jr. Pharmacokinetics of depot medroxyprogesterone acetate as contraception. J Repod Med 1996; 41: 381–390.
8. Petta CA, Faundes A, Dunson TR, et al. Timing of the onset of contraceptive effectiveness in Depo-Provera users. II Effects on ovarian function. Fertil Steril 1998; 70: 817–820.
9. Segall-Gutierrez P, Taylor D, et al. Follicular development and ovulation in extremely obese women receiving depo-medroxyprogesterone acetate subcutaneously. Contraception 2010; 81: 487–495.
10. Sekadde-Kigondu C, Mwathe EG, Ruminjo JK, et al. Acceptability and discontinuation of Depo-Provera, IUCD and combined pill in Kenya. East Afr Med J 1996; 73: 786–794.
11. Winner B, Peipert JF, Zhao Q, et al. Effectiveness of long-acting reversible contraception. N Engl J Med 2012; 366: 1998–2007.
12. Mavranezouli I. The cost-effectiveness of long-acting reversible contraceptive methods in the UK: analysis based on a decision-analytic model developed for a NICE clinical practice guideline. Hum Reprod 2008; 23: 1338–1345.
13. Faculty of Sexual & Reproductive Healthcare. Quick Starting Contraception. 2010. http: // www.fsrh.org / pdfs / CEUGuidance Quick StartingContraception.pdf [Accessed 27 November 2014].
14. Pardthaisong T, Yenchit C, Gray R. The long-term growth and development of children exposed to Depo-Provera during pregnancy or lactation. Contraception 1992; 45: 313–324.
15. Said S, Omar K, Koetsawang S, et al. A multi-centred phase III comparative clinical trial of depot-medroxyprogesterone acetate given three-monthly at doses of 100 mg or 150 mg: II. The comparison of bleeding patterns. World Health Organization Task Force on Long-Acting Systemic Agents for Fertility Regulation Special Programme of Research, Development and Research Training in Human Reproduction. Contraception 1987; 35: 591–610.
16. Curtis KM, Ravi A, Gaffield ML. Progestogen-only contraceptive use in obese women. Contraception 2009; 80: 346–354.

17. Beksinska ME, Smit JA, Kleinschmidt I, et al. Prospective study of weight change in new adolescent users of DMPA, NET-EN, COCs, nonusers and discontinuers of hormonal contraception. Contraception 2010; 81: 30–34.

18. Gai L, Zhang J, Zhang H, et al. The effect of depot medroxyprogesterone acetate (DMPA) on bone mineral density (BMD) and evaluating changes in BMD after discontinuation of DMPA in Chinese women of reproductive age. Contraception 2011; 83: 218–222.

19. Lopez LM, Chen M, et al. Steroidal contraceptives and bone fractures in women: Evidence from observational studies. Cochrane Database Syst Rev 2012; 8: CD009849.

20. Ott MA, Shew ML, Ofner S et al. The influence of hormonal contraception on mood and sexual interest among adolescents. Arch Sex Behav 2008; 37: 605–613.

21. Wilailak S, Vipupinyo C, Suraseranivong V, et al. Depot medroxyprogesterone acetate and epithelial ovarian cancer: a multicentre case-control study. BJOG 2012; 119: 672–677.

22. Harris TG, Miller L, Kulasingam SL et al. Depot-medroxyprogesterone acetate and combined oral contraceptive use and cervical neoplasia among women with oncogenic human papillomavirus infection. Am J Obstet Gynecol 2009; 200: 489.e1–e8.

23. Li CI, Beaber EF, Tang MT et al. Effect of depo-medroxyprogesterone acetate on breast cancer risk among women 20 to 44 years of age. Cancer Res 2012; 72: 2028–2035.

24. World Health Organization. Cardiovascular disease and use of oral and injectable progestogen only contraceptives and combined injectable contraceptives. Results of an international, multicentre, case control study. Contraception 1998; 57: 315–324.

25. World Health Organization. Hormonal Contraception and HIV: Technical Statement. 2012. http://whqlibdoc.who.int/hq/2012/WHO_RHR_12.08_eng.pdf [Accessed 27 November 2014].

26. Medical Eligibility Criteria for Contraceptive Use. 5th ed. Geneva: World Health Organization; 2015. PMID: 26447268.

Emergency Contraception

• Vijaya Babre • Vandana Walvekar

Introduction

Global and Indian scenario—worldwide approximately 42 million abortions performed each year, out of these unsafe abortions are 20 million. Worldwide nearly 1 in 10 pregnancy ends in unsafe abortion. India has the highest number of unsafe abortions in the world, with one woman dying every 2 hours due to unsafe abortions.

Emergency contraception (EC) is a birth control technique, used after unprotected sexual intercourse to prevent pregnancy. Emergency contraceptive pills (ECPs) are also sometimes called the morning-after pill or postcoital contraception. Medicines act by prevention or delay ovulation or fertilization, which is necessary for pregnancy.

History

In 1966, gynecologist John McLean Morris and biologist Gertrude Van Wagenen at the Yale School of Medicine, introduced the use of oral estrogen to produce beneficial effects for women.

- The first widely used methods were 5-day treatments with high-dose of estrogens, using diethylstilbestrol (DES) in the United States and ethinyl estradiol (EE) in the Netherlands by Haspels.
- Early 1970s, the Yuzpe regimen was developed by A. Albert Yuzpe in 1974; progestin-only postcoital contraception was invented.
- In 1975, study on use of copper IUD as emergency contraception (EC)
- Danazol was tried in the early 1980s, but was found to be ineffective as EC.
- 1980: Yuzpe regimen became the standard option for EC
- 1998: After large WHO trial, levonorgestrel widely used as EC.
- 2002: In China, first time mifepristone was registered for use as EC.

Definition

Emergency contraception is a birth-control method used to reduce the risk of pregnancy following unprotected sexual intercourse or when other regular contraceptive measures have not worked properly or have not been used correctly.

Indications

1. After voluntary sexual act without contraceptive protection.
2. Incorrect or inconsistent use of regular contraceptive methods: Failure to take oral contraceptives for >3 days, being late for contraceptive injection, being late for POPs consumption.
3. In case of contraceptive failure or mishaps, miscalculation of infertile period, failed

coitus interruptus, expulsion of an intra-uterine device and, or in case of slippage/leakage/breakage of condom.

4. In cases of sexual assault.

EMERGENCY CONTRACEPTION METHODS: HORMONAL AND MECHANICAL

Hormonal Emergency Contraception

Combined estrogen and progesterone pills—Yuzpe regimen.

1. Progesterone-only pills—levonorgestrel (LNG)
   a. Canadian Prof. Albert Yuzpe, who created the Yuzpe regimen in early 1970s, has a combination of ehinyl estradiol and levonorgestrel. In 1980s, Yuzpe regimen became the standard treatment for EC. Oral doses of 0.1 mg (100 µg) ethinyl estradiol (EE) and 0.5 mg (500 µg) levonorgestrel 12 hours apart. Failure rate is 0–2%.
   b. Ovral 2 tablets 12 hours apart or Mala-D, Mala-N, Ovral-L low dose OC pills 4 tablets 12 hours apart.

2. Progestin only (levonorgestrel)
   National Reproductive and Child Health Program, Drug Controller of India, has approved levonorgestrel, 0.75 mg, tablets for use as ECP. Levonorgestrel-only pills 2 doses of 0.75 mg, to be taken by mouth 12 hours apart within 72 hours of un-protected sexual intercourse (UPSI). Take a single dose 1.5 mg LNG within 72 hours of UPSI. Failure rate of this method is 0–1%.

3. Antiprogesterone (mifepristone) low dose 10 mg up to 72–120 hours of UPSI. Mechanism of action is anti-implantation agent if used after intercourse, abortifacients in early pregnancy. Failure rate of this method is 0.06%.

4. Ulipristal acetate is selective progesterone receptor modulator given once, single, 30 mg, within 120 hours of UPSI. It is approved by European Medicines Agency 2009 and United States Food and Drug Administration (US FDA) 2010.

Mechanical Emergency Contraception

Intrauterine device-Cu T 200, multiload Cu 250, multiload 375, Cu T 380 A. Intrauterine devices (IUDs) can be inserted up to 5 days of UPSI. IUDs are a choice for women who want to use IUD as an ongoing method of contraception. Failure rate of this method is 0–0.1%.

Contraindications are acute pelvic inflammatory disease (PID), abnormal uter-ine bleeding (AUB), suspected pregnancy and uterine anomaly. Side effects are irregular vaginal bleeding, pain, expulsion and pelvic infection.

MEDICAL ELIGIBILITY CRITERIA FOR CLIENTS FOR ECPS

Condition	Category	Clarifications/evidence
Pregnancy	NA	Clarification: Although this method is not indicated for a woman with a known or suspected pregnancy, there is no known harm to the woman, the course of her pregnancy, or the fetus if ECPs are accidently used
Breastfeeding	1	
History of ectopic pregnancy	1	
History of severe CVS complications* (ischemic heart disease, cerebrovascular attack, or other thromboembolic conditions)		
Angina pectoris*	2	
Migraine*	2	

Contd..

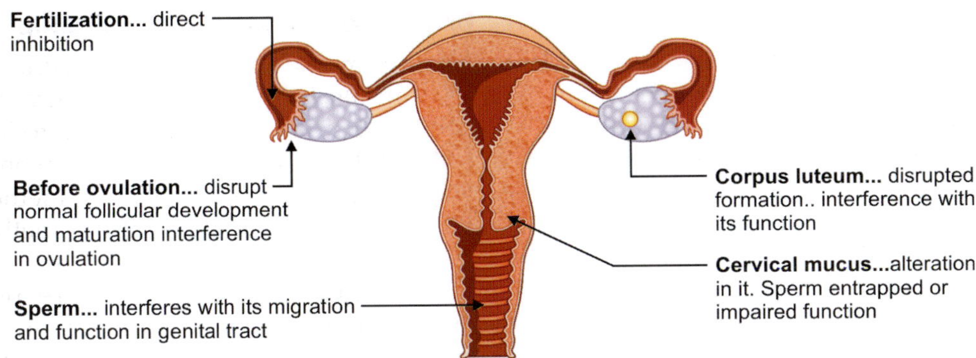

Fig. 29.1: Mechanism of action

Contd..

Condition	Category	Clarifications/ evidence
Severe liver disease (including jaundice)*	2	
Repeated ECP use	1	Clarification: Recurrent ECP use is an indication that the woman requires further counselling on other contraceptive options. Frequently repeated ECP use may be harmful for women with conditions classified as 2, 3 or 4 for COC, CIC or POC use.
Rape*	1	

Reference: WHO Medical Eligibility Criteria 2004
Here Category means:
1. A condition for which there is no restriction for use of a contraceptive method
2. A condition where the advantages of using the method generally outweigh the theoretical or proven risk
Guidelines for administration of ECPs by Health care providers, Family Planning Division Ministry of health and family Welfare of India, Nov 2008.

MECHANISM OF ACTION (Fig. 29.1)

1. LNG and ulipristal acetate (UPA) mechanism of action is to interfere with the process of ovulation, if taken before in pre-ovulatory phase of cycle.
2. If luteinizing hormone (LH) surge started, then LNG can inhibit the surge and the follicular growth and development and maturation or the release of the egg itself.
3. It has been shown that UPA prevents ovulation both before and after the surge has started, delaying follicular rupture for at least 5 days of ovulation if not prevented, either LNG or UPA is administered on the day of the luteinizing hormone peak.
4. Various studies have shown that LNG does not prevent implantation of a fertilized egg into the uterus. Previous UPA research have shown mild endometrial changes in some aspects of endometrial function and receptivity.
5. A higher percentage of pregnancies were prevented when LNG and UPA were given pre-ovulatory compared with post-ovulatory administration.
6. It has been postulated that mechanisms include interference with corpus luteum function, thickening of the cervical mucus resulting in trapping of sperm, alterations in the tubal transport of sperm or egg, or inhibition of sperm function.
7. If LNG and UPA are administered after implantation have no effect on an existing pregnancy and do not increase rates of miscarriage.

Side Effects

Emergency contraceptive pills are safe. Most side effects are mild and self-limiting.

Altered Vaginal Bleeding Patterns

Most women who have used ECPs get their next menstrual period within 7 days of the expected time. On an average, menses are reported to be 1 day earlier after use of the LNG regimen and 2 days later than expected after use of the UPA regimen.

Nausea and Vomiting

Nausea occurs in <20% of women taking the LNG regimen and approximately 12% of women taking the UPA regimen. If vomiting occurs within 2 hours after taking a dose of the LNG regimen or the combined hormonal regimen, another dose should be taken as soon as possible. If vomiting occurs within 3 hours after taking a dose of UPA ECPs, the dose should be repeated as soon as possible.

Other Symptoms

Other symptoms that may occur in users of ECPs include headache, abdominal pain, breast tenderness, dizziness, or fatigue. These side effects generally resolve within 24 hours.

Effects on Pregnancy

Studies have shown that pregnancy occurs despite using the LNG regimen or who used it inadvertently after becoming pregnant. This regimen does not harm either a pregnant woman or her fetus. It does not increase the rates of miscarriage, ectopic pregnancy, low birth weight, congenital malformations, or pregnancy complications.

SPECIAL CONSIDERATIONS OF USE OF EMERGENCY CONTRACEPTION

1. Use in Adolescents

Use of emergency contraception by adolescents should not be limited by clinical or programmatic concerns. ECPs are safe for all women regardless of age. EC should be included in routine family planning guidelines for adolescents, females, and families of adolescents with disabilities, regardless of current intentions of sexual behavior.

WHO recommends offering EC to girls who have been raped involving penovaginal penetration and who present within 5 days of the incident. This includes girls who have attained menarche as well as those who are in the beginning stages of puberty (as they may be ovulating even prior to the onset of menstruation). UPA and LNG are recommended as first-line treatment. If these are not available, the combined hormonal regimen may be offered.

2. Breastfeeding

A woman who is <6 months postpartum and is exclusively breastfeeding, and has not had menstrual period since delivery is unlikely to be ovulating and requirement of ECPs is unlikely. However, a woman who does not meet all three criteria may be at risk for pregnancy.

According to WHO's medical eligibility criteria, the LNG regimen of ECPs is indicated during lactation and that the UPA regimen can generally be used by breastfeeding women, but as a precaution breast milk should not be given for 1 week and should be expressed and discarded.

3. Use of ECPs before Sexual Intercourse

The systematic review of pericoital use of hormonal contraception containing LNG suggested that it is safe and moderately effective. Pericoital use means that the method is taken immediately before or after every episode of coitus during one or more menstrual cycles. A more recent study evaluated the efficacy, safety, and acceptability.

4. Use After more than One Episode of Unprotected Intercourse

After multiple unprotected sexual intercourse, women should try to use ECPs as soon as possible. Waiting until a series of episodes is not recommended. Similarly, a woman should not refrain from taking ECPs simply because she has had multiple episodes of unprotected intercourse. She should be aware that the efficacy of the ECPs may be limited if the latest episode of unprotected intercourse was >4 or 5 days prior. She should use only one ECP treatment at a time in spite of the number of prior unprotected acts. If all episodes of unprotected intercourse were within the last 120 hours, using UPA ECPs is suggested. If all episodes took place within the last 72 hours, she can either use LNG or UPA ECPs.

5. Repeated Use

ECPs are not intended for deliberate repeated use or use as a regular routine contraceptive method, repeated use of ECPs is safe compared to the potential health risks of pregnancy or unsafe abortion, women should be able to access and use ECPs as many times as they need. However, ongoing methods of contraception are more effective than ECPs, and only barrier methods, such as condoms, protect against human immunodeficiency virus (HIV) and sexually transmitted infections (STIs).

6. Drug Interactions

Over the past few years, there has been more information about potential interactions of ECPs with other drugs. No drug interaction poses any health or safety risk but some may impact the effectiveness of LNG and UPA ECPs.

LNG regimen: Inducers of hepatic CYP450 enzymes may reduce the effectiveness of LNG ECPs. These include the HIV medicines efavirenz and ritonavir, some drugs for tuberculosis and epilepsy, and

herbal medicines containing St. John's wort. A woman using these drugs and in need of EC, should be offered the Cu-IUD or a double dose of LNG (3 mg).

UPA regimen
- Inducers of hepatic CYP450 enzymes may also reduce the effectiveness of UPA ECPs. Cu-T should be given as an option of EC to women using these drugs. A double dose of UPA is not recommended.
- UPA may not be effective, if progestogen is taken 7 days prior to taking UPA or within 5 days after UPA.
- Use of UPA as EC in women with severe asthma treated by oral glucocorticoid is not recommended.
- ECP recommends that not to use UPA in women with severe hepatic impairment.
- Drugs that increase gastric pH (such as esomeprazole) may interfere with UPA, but the clinical significance of this interaction for UPA ECPs is unclear.

8. Ectopic Pregnancy

All birth control methods reduce the absolute risk of ectopic pregnancy by preventing pregnancy overall. A systematic review of world literature found that neither regimen increases the risk that a pregnancy will be ectopic.

9. Obesity

Research conducted in the past few years seems to suggest that the effectiveness of LNG and UPA ECPs could be reduced in overweight women and/or high BMI. According to WHO ECPs may be less effective among women with BMI ≥ 30 kg/m^2 than among women with BMI <25 kg/m^2. Recent pharmacokinetic studies show that clinical obesity reduces the bioavailability of LNG but not UPA. Given that the negative effect of obesity is greater on LNG's effectiveness than it is on UPAs, Cu-IUD and UPA regimen should be recommended as the first-line treatment for obese-BMI women. A double dose of LNG can also be considered if the Cu-IUD or UPA is not an option. Women should never be denied access to EC due to higher weight.

Recommendations of Family Planning Division, Ministry of Health and Family Welfare, Government of India

1. ECPs with LNG taken as single dose of 1.5 mg, or alternatively, LNG taken in 2 doses of 0.75 mg each, 12 hours apart within 72 hours of UPSI.
2. Combined oral contraceptives (COCs) taken as a split dose—one dose of 100 µg of EE plus 500 µg of LNG followed by second dose of 100 µg of EE plus 500 µg of LNG, 12 hours later (Yuzpe method) within 72 hours of UPSI.
3. IUD insertion up to 5 days of UPSI.

WHO Recommendations

1. ECPs with UPA, taken as single dose of 30 mg up to 120 hours of UPSI.
2. ECPs with LNG taken as single dose of 1.5 mg, or alternatively, LNG taken in 2 doses of 0.75 mg each, 12 hours apart within 72 hours of UPSI.
3. COCs taken as a split dose one dose of 100 µg of EE plus 500 µg of LNG followed by second dose of 100 µg of EE plus 500 µg of LNG, 12 hours later (Yuzpe method) within 72 hours of UPSI.
4. IUD insertion up to 5 days of UPSI.

Suggested Reading

1. 'Emergency Contraception'. www.acog.org. Retrieved 2020-06-18.
2. FSRH Faculty of Sexual and Reproductive Healthcare Guideline, Contraception after Pregnancy, January 2012.
3. Guidelines for administration of ECPs by Health care providers, Family Planning Division Ministry of health and family Welfare of India, Nov 2008.
4. Guidelines for Administration of Emergency Contraceptive Pills by Healthcare providers Family Planning Division Ministry of Health and Family welfare Government of India, November 2008.
5. Leung, Vivian WY; Levine, Marc; Soon, Judith A. (February 2010). 'Mechanisms of action of hormonal emergency contraceptives'; Pharmacotherapy. 30 (2): 158–168. doi:10.1592/phco.30.2.158. PMID 20099990. S2CID 41337748.
6. Medical eligibility criteria (2015).
7. Reference Manual for Oral Contraceptive Pills March 2016, Family Planning Division Ministry of Health and Family welfare Government of India.
8. Responding to children and adolescents who have been sexually abused: WHO clinical guidelines. Geneva: World Health Organization; 2017.
9. Trussell, James; Schwarz, Eleanor Bimla (2011). 'Emergency contraception'. In Hatcher, Robert A; Trussell, James; Nelson, Anita L; Cates, Willard, Jr.; Kowal, Deborah; Policar, Michael S. (eds.). Contraceptive technology (20th revised ed.). New York: Ardent Media. pp. 113–145. ISBN 978-1-59708-004-0. ISSN 0091-9721. OCLC 781956734. p. 121:
10. Van der Wijden C, Manion C. Lactational amenorrhoea method for family planning. Cochrane Database of Systematic Reviews 2015, Issue 10. Art. No.: CD001329. DOI:10.1002/14651858.CD001329.pub2.

Contraceptive Vaginal Ring

• Ruchika Garg • Malavika JC

Introduction

Contraceptive vaginal ring is a form of combined hormonal contraceptive method. Combined (estrogen-progestin) hormonal contraception is available in various forms such as an oral pill, transdermal patch or a vaginal ring. All these methods are user-controlled. When used consistently and correctly, they are safe and highly effective.

What is a Vaginal Ring?

Contraceptive vaginal ring is a small flexible soft plastic ring that is placed inside the vagina. It releases both estrogen and progesterone continuously into the bloodstream, thereby preventing pregnancy. The main advantage of vaginal ring over other combined methods is the longer duration of action and avoids the difficulty with daily or weekly use and hence ensures better compliance.

What are the Types of Vaginal Ring Available in the Market?

Combined hormonal contraceptive vaginal rings are available under the following brand names:

NuvaRing: It is a one-month ring . It is flexible latex-free device measuring around 2 inches in diameter. It contains ethinyl estradiol (EE) and etonogestrel (ENG). It needs to be worn in the vagina for 3 weeks and removed and discarded for 1 week. It releases 120 µg of EE and 15 µg of ENG continuously into the bloodstream over 21 days.[1] The dose of EE released by the vaginal ring is much lower than that released by other combined hormonal contraceptive methods.

Annovera: It is a one-year ring. It can be rinsed and reinserted every month. Overall it can be used for 13 cycles. It contains EE and segesterone acetate (SA). The ring has to be placed in the vagina for 3 weeks and removed for 1 week. Annovera comes with a case to safely store the ring during the ring-free week.[2]

MECHANISM OF ACTION

Both estrogen and progesterone are continuously released into the bloodstream.

Estrogen acts by preventing ovulation and progesterone acts by thickening the cervical mucus making it difficult for the sperm to enter the cervix and even the endometrium is rendered hostile for implantation.

Time to Insert the Vaginal Ring

Vaginal ring can be inserted at any time of the menstrual cycle provided pregnancy is ruled out.

If the vaginal ring is inserted in the vagina within first 5 days of menstrual cycle, then the chances of pregnancy are very less.

If the vaginal ring is inserted in any other time of the menstrual cycle, then additional contraception needs to be used for first 7 days after insertion to avoid pregnancy.

Ideally, ring should be left in the vagina for 21 days and removed for 7 days. There is protection against pregnancy in the ring-free period. There is also a choice for the woman to have a shorter ring-free break or no break at all. This is known to be as safe and effective as the standard use (7-day break).

The partner may feel the vaginal ring while having sex, but it is not harmful.

Postpartum insertion: Vaginal ring can be used safely by breastfeeding woman after 42 days of giving birth, a back-up contraception should be used for 7 days in such situations.

If the woman is not breastfeeding and vaginal ring is inserted on day 21 after giving birth, then no back-up contraception is needed. If it is >21 of days of giving birth, then additional contraception should be used for first 7 days of the ring insertion.

Post-abortion insertion: Vaginal ring can be inserted immediately after abortion without the need of back-up contraception.

If 5 days has elapsed since abortion, then a back-up contraception needs to be used for 7 days after the insertion of the ring.

How to Insert the Vaginal Ring?

After cleaning the hands, the ring needs to be squeezed between the thumb and the finger and should be gently inserted into the vagina and the ring should be pushed up till it feels comfortable. It is not required for the ring to completely cover the cervix as with diaphragm and cervical cap.

After the ring is inside the vagina for 21 days (3 weeks), then it should be removed. After a ring-free period of 7 days, a new ring should be inserted.

The ring should be inserted on the same day of the week when it was removed, *e.g.* if the ring was removed on Monday, then a new ring should be inserted the next Monday and the ring should be removed after 3 weeks on Monday itself.

Delayed Insertion

- Woman who forget to insert a new ring on time and if it is <48 hours due for insertion of a new ring , then the woman can insert the ring immediately without the need for additional contraception.[3]
- If the woman has forgotten to insert the new ring for >48 hours, then a new ring should be inserted immediately and an additional contraception is needed for 7 days.

How to Remove the Vaginal Ring?

With clean hands, insert a finger into the vagina, hook around its edge and gently pull out the ring. After removing the ring, it should be placed in a bag provided and thrown into the bin. There should not be any pain while removing the ring. In case of Annovera, the ring should be rinsed, cleaned and placed in a case.

In the ring-free interval, there can be a period type bleed.

After 7 days ring-free period, insert a new vaginal ring. The new ring can be placed irrespective of the menstrual bleed.

DELAYED REMOVAL

If the Nuvaring is *in situ* for >3 weeks but <5 weeks, then remove the ring and insert a new ring after 1-week ring free period. If the woman desires, she can insert a new ring immediately after removing the old one foregoing the 1-week ring free interval, although the woman may experience break-through bleeding.

If the NuvaRing is *in situ* for >5 weeks, then the ring should be removed and replaced with a new ring immediately. But an additional contraception, like condoms is necessary for the first 7 days following insertion of the new vaginal ring.

Rationale behind this is the fact that sufficient amount of estrogen and progesterone is released by the vaginal ring to prevent pregnancy (by inhibition of ovulation) for 5 weeks. Hence, even if the woman forgets removing the vaginal ring after 3 weeks , the efficacy is maintained up to 5 weeks.[4]

What if the Vaginal Ring Falls Out?

For NuvaRing: If the ring falls out, then the ring should be cleaned and placed in the vagina immediately.

If the ring has been out of the vagina for >3 hours, then a back-up contraception should be used.

For Annovera: If the ring falls out or it is out of the vagina for up to 2 hours , then the ring is washed with a mild soap and water and dried and inserted into the vagina and no back-up contraception is needed.[2]

If the ring is out of the vagina for >2 hours, then re-insert the ring after washing it, and an additional contraception (*e.g.* condoms) is needed for 7 days.

How to Take Care of the Vaginal Ring?

Place NuvaRing at room temperature. It should be kept away from direct sunlight. In such conditions, it can be stored up to 4 months.

If the NuvaRing is not used within 4 months, then it has to be stored in the refrigerator.

Annovera, once removed out of the vagina, should be washed with a mild soap and lukewarm water, dried with a clean cloth or a paper towel and stored in a case. Avoid extreme temperatures.

Annovera, when placed inside the vagina, concurrent use of oil or silicone based products like suppositories, creams, gels, lubricants should be avoided. Water-based lubricants can be used.

Administration and Use

Before prescribing vaginal ring:
- Pregnancy should be excluded

- Measure blood pressure: Ideally, blood pressure should be measured before starting any form of combined hormonal contraceptives.
- Physical examination and Laboratory tests: are not mandatory.[3]

Who can Use the Vaginal Ring?

Woman without the following conditions may use the vaginal ring.

Vaginal ring is not suitable for women with:
- History of arterial or venous thrombosis
- Hypertensive and cardiac problems
- Age >35 years
- Overweight
- Smoking or stopped smoking recently in the past 1 year
- History of migraine with aura (warning symptoms)
- Suffering from breast cancer or had breast cancer in the past 5 years.
- Diabetic with complications
- Taking medicines which interact with the ring
- Can't hold the ring in the vagina.

If the woman does not smoke and is not suffering from any medical comorbidities, then the vaginal ring can be used in woman up to 50 years of age.

BENEFITS AND RISKS OF VAGINAL RING

Benefits

It does not interfere with sex.
- Improved compliance as the woman does not have to think about it every day .
- It is easy to insert and remove.
- Action of vaginal ring is unaffected by conditions like vomiting and diarrthoea.
- Provides better cycle control and reduces bleeding and dysmenorrhea.
- It helps woman with pre-menstrual symptoms.

Risks

- At the beginning, woman may not feel comfortable inserting and removing the vaginal ring.
- Vaginal ring does not protect against sexually transmitted infections.
- Interaction with some drugs may render it less effective.
- Woman needs to remember the day on which vaginal ring needs to be removed and when the new one needs to be inserted.
- Sometimes, the ring can get expelled during the act of sex or following a bowel movement.
- Some woman may experience spotting and bleeding in the first few months following insertion.
- It may cause increased vaginal discharge.
- Headaches, nausea, breast tenderness and mood changes can occur just as with other combined hormonal methods.

Serious Risks

Vaginal rings carry same serious risk as with any other combined hormonal methods.

Cardiovascular and thromboembolic events—combined hormonal contraceptives are known to increase the risk of thrombo-embolic events compared to the non-users.[1,2] Although the risk of venous thromboembolism (VTE) is lower in ring users compared to other combined methods.[5]

Hence, woman with a history of previous VTE should not choose a vaginal ring.

Risk of Cancer

Women using vaginal ring have a very small increased risk of being diagnosed with breast cancer but this risk reduces once the woman stops using the ring.

There is also a small increased risk of developing cervical cancer with long-term use of any combined hormonal contraception.

Follow-Up

- A routine follow-up examination is not needed.
- Blood pressure should be checked yearly.

Return of fertility: Majority of woman resume ovulation and regular menses within a month of removal of vaginal rings.[1] In a study conducted on 45 participants using Nuvaring, ovulation was reported to be as early as 13 days after removal of ring and the median time to ovulate was 19 days after removal of vaginal ring.[6] Similarly with Annovera initial trials reported return of regular menses within 6 months of discontinuation.[2]

Use with other vaginal devices and products: Vaginal rings are known to interfere with other female barrier contraceptive methods, such as diaphragm, cervical cap or the female condoms. Hence, female barrier contraceptives cannot be used as back-up contraception along with vaginal rings.[7]

Concomitant use of tampons during menses does not affect the hormone absorption from the vaginal ring.[1]

Vaginal rings are compatible with water-based vaginal lubricants and spermicides, but oil-based products including silicone-based lubricants are not compatible with vaginal rings.[1,2]

INTERACTIONS WITH OTHER MEDICATIONS

Interactions of vaginal ring is similar to combined oral contraceptives (COCs) and most of the information is based on it.

Vaginal rings interact with other systemic medications and consequently increase or decrease each-others levels.

- Decrease in estrogen/progestin levels—drugs which increase the activity of liver microsomal enzymes decrease systemic exposure to the estrogen and progestins in contraceptive vaginal rings, and thus contraceptive efficacy is reduced.

Some such medications are

- Antiepileptics, such as barbiturate, phenytoin, carbamazepine, oxcarbazepine and topiramate
- Antifungal like griseofulvin
- Antitubercular drugs, like rifampicin, rifabutin

- Anti-HIV medications, like efavirenz, nelfinavir, ritonavir, darunavir, lopinavir, Nevirapine.[1,2]
- Individuals using the above medications should use an additional form of contraception, such as condoms or choose an alternative form of contraceptions.

Altered levels of certain medications: Plasma levels of lamotrigine is known to decrease when used along with combined hormonal methods. Hence, seizure control may not be optimal and a higher dose of lamotrigine may be needed to attain good seizure control.[8,9]

Combined hormonal methods are avoided in those women on antiviral medications for hepatitis C (ritonavir, paritaprevir) since alanine transaminase (ALT) levels are significantly elevated.

Use with other vaginal medications: Water-based vaginal drugs used in treatment of vaginal candidiasis or bacterial vaginosis can be used along with vaginal rings.[1,2]

Oil-based suppositories, such as miconazole suppositories are associated with increased hormonal levels and hence avoided along with vaginal rings.[1,2]

SPECIAL SITUATIONS

1. If the vaginal ring is out for unknown duration of time, then pregnancy has to be ruled out before inserting a new ring.[7]
2. Continuous use of ring for menstrual suppression—some women desire fewer days of withdrawl bleed and may prefer using vaginal ring for extended period. Vaginal ring may be used without ring-free period, wherein a new ring is inserted immediately after the removal of old ring. This omits hormone-free interval. Extended use of ring is effective, but the woman may suffer from unscheduled bleeding and spotting.[10,11]
3. Data supporting continuous use of the Annovera are not yet available, but continuous use may be associated with increase in unscheduled bleeding.

4. *Broken ring:* Very rarely, the contraceptive ring may break at the weld joint.[1] The break does not affect the contraceptive effectiveness, but it is more likely that the ring slips out. Hence, in the event of broken ring, the ring needs to be removed and replaced with a new one.

NON-CONTRACEPTIVE BENEFITS OF VAGINAL RING

Cycle control: Cycle control is a major benefit provided by all combined hormonal contraceptive methods. In this regard, vaginal ring is equivalent or possibly superior to other combined hormonal contraceptives.[12–14]

Vaginal ring users less frequently experience breakthrough bleeding unlike with other combined methods.[12,14–16]

Endometriosis: Vaginal ring appears to reduce endometriosis-related pain. A cohort study was conducted comparing Nuva-Ring with a transdermal patch for relief of persistent endometriosis-related pain and it was reported that both treatments reduced dysmenorrhea[13] but ring users were more satisfied compared to the patch users (72% versus 48%).

Diabetic or pre-diabetic woman: Woman who are diagnosed with insulin resistance or those who are at risk of insulin resistance may benefit from the contraceptive ring as compared to COCs, because the vaginal ring had no impact on insulin resistance while COCs were known to increase insulin levels.[17]

Improved psychosexual function: Vaginal ring users have been studied to have improved psychosexual function.[18–20]

What is correct use?

Correct and consistent use of the contraceptive vaginal ring is very similar to other combined hormonal methods. NuvaRing should be ideally placed, used as 3 weeks in and 1 week out. Some women prefer to extend the use for up to 5 weeks to regulate their cycles.[15,21,22]

When used correctly, the ring is almost 99% effective in preventing pregnancy.

CDC reports a 7% pregnancy rate with typical use.

ACCEPTABILITY OF VAGINAL RINGS

Vaginal rings are highly acceptable as it is easy to use, once a month administration, remains effective even if removal or reinsertion of the ring is not done precisely on time.

A low level of systemic hormone is maintained enough to prevent ovulation(vaginal delivery of hormones improve its bioavailability).

Even, the effect is rapidly reversible. Users of NuvaRing report a satisfaction rates of 84 to 96% and are more likely to recommend the method to other women.[21,23,24]

Minor complaints like feeling of the ring, coital problems and expulsion of the ring is complained by <3% of the women.[25,26]

Compared to COCs, vaginal ring users are more satisfied.[25,26]

Vaginal ring users are less likely to discontinue as compared to COC users (11% versus 16%).

SUMMARY: FACTS ABOUT THE VAGINAL RING

When used correctly and consistently.

- Vaginal ring is >99% effective.
- Compliance is better since each ring provides contraception for a month
- Does not interfere with sex, when the ring is in place.
- Vaginal rings do not protect against sexually transmitted infections (STIs), and hence condoms may be used concomitantly.
- Unlike COCs, vaginal ring works even when the woman has vomiting or diarrhea.
- Regular menses is lighter, less painful and also prevents premenstrual symptoms.

- Minimal side effects, like white discharge may be there.
- Complications, like VTE are rare but a possibility.
- When the ring comes out accidentally, it should be washed with mild soap and water and dried and reinserted in the vagina.
- To improve the effectiveness, a new ring should be inserted on the same day of the week when it was removed.
- When the ring is out of the vagina for >3 hours, then an additional back-up contraception should be used.
- When medications interacting with the vaginal ring is taken, an additional back-up contraception is advised.

RECENT DEVELOPMENTS IN VAGINAL RINGS

- *Progering:* A new progesterone-releasing vaginal ring widely available in South America and Africa, commonly advised for lactating woman.[27,28] Each ring releases 10 mg progesterone daily. It is approved for 3 months use. It acts to thicken the cervical mucus and also inhibits ovulation and affects endometrial receptivity. Unscheduled bleeding is a common complaint.[29] A ring that releases a synthetic progestin (Nesterone®) is under development.
- A newer combined hormonal ring containing estrogen in the form of EE and progesterone in the form of Nestrone, a 19-nor-testosterone derivative is under trial. Nestrone does not bind to either estrogen or androgen receptors and hence side effects like acne are reduced. This novel method was created with the goal to reduce the thrombogenic risk.[30,31]

A comparison of vaginal ring with other birth-control methods is given in **Table 30.1**.

Table 30.1: Comparison of vaginal ring with other birth-control methods

Criteria	Ring	Patch	Pill	Shot	IUD	Implant
Effectiveness (typical use)	93%	93%	93%	96%	99.2% (Copper) 99.6% (hormonal)	99.9%
Schedule	Replace monthly	Replace weekly	Take daily	Get every 3 months	Lasts up to 12 years	Lasts up to 5 years
Risks	Rare, but include: • Blood clots • Stroke • Heart attack	Rare, but include: • Blood clots • Stroke • Heart attack	Rare, but include: • Heart attack • Blood clots • Stroke • Liver tumors	Temporary osteoporosis	• Loss of the IUD or IUD moving out of place • Ectopic pregnancy • Infection	• Scarring • Infection
Side effects	• Sore breasts • Spotting • Headaches • Nausea	• Sore breasts • Spotting • Headaches	• Sore breasts • Nausea • Spotting • Headaches	• Changes to your period • Nausea • Weight gain • Headaches • Depression • Sore breasts • Bruising at the injection site	• Pain during insertion and days afterward • Irregular periods and spotting for hormonal IUD • More bleeding and cramping during periods for copper IUD	• Arm pain • Heavier, longer periods in some people • Headaches • Weight gain • Ovarian cysts • Nausea • Breast pain

IUD: Intrauterine device

References

1. Nuvaring [package insert]. Whitehouse Station, NJ. Merck and Co, Inc. 2001–2018. http://www.merck.com/product/usa/pi_circulars/n/nuvaring/nuvaring_pi.pdf.
2. Annovera [package insert]. New York, NY. Manufactured for Population Council. August 2018. www.accessdata.fda.gov/drugsatfda_docs/label/2018/209627s000lbl.pdf
3. Curtis KM, Jatlaoui TC, Tepper NK, et al. US Selected Practice Recommendations for Contraceptive Use, 2016. MMWR Recomm Rep 2016;65:1.
4. Mulders TM, Dieben TO. Use of the novel combined contraceptive vaginal ring NuvaRing for ovulation inhibition. Fertil Steril 2001;75:865.
5. Han L, Jensen JT. Does the Progestogen Used in Combined Hormonal Contraception Affect Venous Thrombosis Risk? Obstet Gynecol Clin North Am 2015;42:683.
6. Mulders TM, Dieben TO, Bennink HJ. Ovarian function with a novel combined contraceptive vaginal ring. Hum Reprod 2002;17:2594.
7. Nuvaring- etonogestrel and ethinyl estradiol insert, extended release. US Food and Drug Administration (FDA) approved product information. Revised May 30, 2017.
8. Curtis KM, Tepper NK, Jatlaoui TC, et al. U.S. Medical Eligibility Criteria for Contraceptive Use, 2016. MMWR Recomm Rep 2016;65:1.
9. Dragoman M, Curtis KM, Gaffield ME. Combined hormonal contraceptive use among women with known dyslipidemias: a systematic

review of critical safety outcomes. Contraception 2016;94:280.

10. Miller L, Verhoeven CH, Hout Ji. Extended regimens of the contraceptive vaginal ring: a randomized trial. Obstet Gynecol 2005;106:473.

11. Barreiros FA, Guazzelli CA, Barbosa R, et al. Extended regimens of the contraceptive vaginal ring: evaluation of clinical aspects. Contraception 2010;81:223.

12. Bjarnadóttir RI, Tuppurainen M, Killick SR. Comparison of cycle control with a combined contraceptive vaginal ring and oral levonorgestrel/ethinyl estradiol. Am J Obstet Gynecol 2002;186:389.

13. Vercellini P, Barbara G, Somigliana E, et al. Comparison of contraceptive ring and patch for the treatment of symptomatic endometriosis. Fertil Steril 2010;93:2150.

14. Westhoff C, Osborne LM, Schafer JE, Morroni C. Bleeding patterns after immediate initiation of an oral compared with a vaginal hormonal contraceptive. Obstet Gynecol 2005;106:89.

15. Oddsson K, Leifels-Fischer B, de Melo NR, et al. Efficacy and safety of a contraceptive vaginal ring (NuvaRing) compared with a combined oral contraceptive: a 1-year randomized trial. Contraception 2005;71:176.

16. Oddsson K, Leifels-Fischer B, Wiel-Masson D, et al. Superior cycle control with a contraceptive vaginal ring compared with an oral contraceptive containing 30 microg ethinylestradiol and 150 microg levonorgestrel: a randomized trial. Hum Reprod 2005;20:557.

17. Cagnacci A, Ferrari S, Tirelli A, et al. Route of administration of contraceptives containing desogestrel/etonorgestrel and insulin sensitivity: a prospective randomized study. Contraception 2009;80:34.

18. Guida M, Di Spiezio Sardo A, Bramante S, et al. Effects of two types of hormonal contraception--oral versus intravaginal--on the sexual life of women and their partners. Hum Reprod 2005; 20:1100.

19. Morotti E, Casadio P, Guasina F, et al. Weight gain, body image and sexual function in young patients treated with contraceptive vaginal ring. A prospective pilot study. Gynecol Endocrinol 2017;33:660.

20. Guida M, Cibarelli F, Troisi J, et al. Sexual life impact evaluation of different hormonal contraceptives on the basis of their methods

of administration. Arch Gynecol Obstet 2014; 290:1239.

21. Roumen FJ, Apter D, Mulders TM, Dieben TO. Efficacy, tolerability and acceptability of a novel contraceptive vaginal ring releasing etonogestrel and ethinyl oestradiol. Hum Reprod 2001; 16:469.

22. Roumen FJ, op ten Berg MM, Hoomans EH. The combined contraceptive vaginal ring (NuvaRing): first experience in daily clinical practice in The Netherlands. Eur J Contracept Reprod Health Care 2006;11:14.

23. Dieben TO, Roumen FJ, Apter D. Efficacy, cycle control, and user acceptability of a novel combined contraceptive vaginal ring. Obstet Gynecol 2002;100:585.

24. Merki-Feld GS, Hund M. Clinical experience with NuvaRing in daily practice in Switzerland: cycle control and acceptability among women of all reproductive ages. Eur J Contracept Reprod Health Care 2007;12:240.

25. Ahrendt HJ, Nisand I, Bastianelli C, et al. Efficacy, acceptability and tolerability of the combined contraceptive ring, NuvaRing, compared with an oral contraceptive containing 30 microg of ethinyl estradiol and 3 mg of drospirenone. Contraception 2006;74:451.

26. Schafer JE, Osborne LM, Davis AR, Westhoff C. Acceptability and satisfaction using Quick Start with the contraceptive vaginal ring versus an oral contraceptive. Contraception 2006;73:488.

27. RamaRao S, Obare F, Ishaku S, et al. Do Women Find the Progesterone Vaginal Ring Acceptable? Findings from Kenya, Nigeria, and Senegal. Stud Fam Plann 2018;49:71.

28. Massai R, Quinteros E, Reyes MV, et al. Extended use of a progesterone-releasing vaginal ring in nursing women: a phase II clinical trial. Contraception 2005;72:352.

29. Nath A, Sitruk-Ware R. Progesterone vaginal ring for contraceptive use during lactation. Contraception 2010;82:428.

30. Jensen JT, Edelman AB, Chen BA, et al. Continuous dosing of a novel contraceptive vaginal ring releasing Nestorone® and estradiol: pharmacokinetics from a dose-finding study. Contraception 2018;97:422.

31. Archer DF, Thomas MA, Conard J, et al. Impact on hepatic estrogen-sensitive proteins by a 1-year contraceptive vaginal ring delivering Nestorone® and ethinyl estradiol. Contraception 2016;93:58.

Gestational Trophoblastic Neoplasia

• Danny Laliwala • Shalini Bathija

MODIFIED WHO CLASSIFICATION OF GESTATIONAL TROPHOBLASTIC DISEASE (GTD)

Molar pregnancies

1. Hyaditiform mole
   - Complete
   - Partial
2. Invasive mole

Trophoblastic tumors

1. Choriocarcinoma
2. Placental site trophoblastic tumors
3. Epitheloid tumors

Incidence: 1/1000 to 1/1500 pregnancies

Risk factors[1]

1. Extremes of maternal age
2. Old paternal age
3. Previous spontaneous abortion
4. Previous GTD (10 times risk)
5. Oral contraceptive pills (OCPs) use (2 times risk)
6. Vitamin A deficiency
7. Smoking, irregular menses

Investigations: Complete blood count (CBC), pelvic ultrasonography (USG), X-ray chest, thyroid-stimulating hormone (TSH).

Treatment of Molar Pregnancies[2]

1. *Surgical evacuation,* preferably under sonographic guidance along with escalating doses of oxytocin. Can also add methylergonovine or carboprost in case of heavy bleeding. Rh-negative women to be given anti-D 300 µg, IM, after procedure.
2. *Hysterectomy:* Rarely needed
3. *Theca lutein cysts:* Regress post-evacuation. If persist, aspiration can be done.
4. *Chemotherapeutic agents:* Whether to add a chemotherapeutic agent prophylactically to prevent risk of future gestational trophoblastic neoplasia (GTN) is controversial. There is a 20% risk of these patients developing a persistent tumour; but due to the side effects of these medications, it is to be evaluated whether these should be given to all or it should be given when hormonal follow-up is not possible. The single-agent chemotherapy drugs given as the first line for GTN are (when WHO progostic score is <6).
   a. Methotrexate
   b. Actinomycin-D

Indications for chemotherapy following the diagnosis of GTDs, include:

1. Evidence of metastasis to brain, liver or gastrointestinal (GI) tract or on X-ray >2 cm radio-opacities.
2. Histopathological diagnosis of choriocarcinoma
3. Heavy vaginal bleeding or evidence of GI or intraperitoneal hemorrhage

Table 31.1: Management of complete and partial moles (WHO Classification)

	Complete mole	*Partial mole*	
Clinical features	*Common:* ↑ vaginal bleeding (97%) *Uncommon:* Anemia Increase uterine size Hyperemesis gravidarum Pre-eclampsia (27%) Theca lutein cysts	Features similar to missed abortion/incomplete abortion	
Karyotype	46XX, 46XY (diploid) 23X-bearing haploid sperm penetrates 23X egg (inactivated)—only paternal chromosome duplication	69XXX, 69XXY (triploid) 23X- or 23Y bearing haploid 2 sperms penetrated 23X egg (activated)	
Diagnosis 1. USG Color doppler	'Snowstorm appearance'—chorionic villi form cluster of vesicles which fill uterine cavity. Change in uterine artery waveform, large vascular channels due to AV shunting. Uterine artery PI may predict response to chemotherapy. Chorionic villi clusters (no amnion)	Fetal tissue with abnormal thick placenta + anechoic cyts	
2. Pathology Fetal tissue Trophoblastic proliferation Placenta	$--$ ++++ Villi completely fill endometrial cavity.	Fetal tissue and amnion ++ Focal/minimal Lesser extent of villous edema and trophoblastic proliferation	
Other investigations	CBC, TSH, X-ray chest		
Risk of post-molar GTN	15–20%	4–6%	
Frequency of hCG testing	After 48 hours of suction and evacuation → fortnightly (2 weekly) → monthly UPT depending on normalisation of β-hCG.	After 48 hours of suction evacuation → 2 samples if normal 4 weeks apart, stop testing.	
Follow-up post-treatment	If β-hCG reverted to normal within 56 days of pregnancy event, follow-up will be for 6 months from suction curettage	If β-hCG not reverted to normal within 56 days of pregnancy event → follow-up will be for 6 months from normalisation of β-hCG level.	Follow-up is concluded when β-hCG has returned to normal on 2 samples 4 weeks apart.

4. Pulmonary, vulval or vaginal metastasis
5. Rising β-hCG levels after evacuation
6. Serum β-hCG >20000 IU/L, after 4 weeks of evacuation
7. Increased serum β-hCG, 6 months after evacuation.

METHOTREXATE

This novel drug was found by an Indian biochemist, Yellapragada Subba Rao.

Mechanism of Action (Flowchart 31.1)

This is a folic acid analogue that competitively inhibits dihydrofolate reductase (DHFR) and thymidylate synthetase (TS). It inhibits the folate-dependent enzymes of *de novo* purine and thymidylate synthesis.

It is partially selective for tumour cells and kills rapidly dividing normal cells, especially the intestinal epithelium and bone marrow.

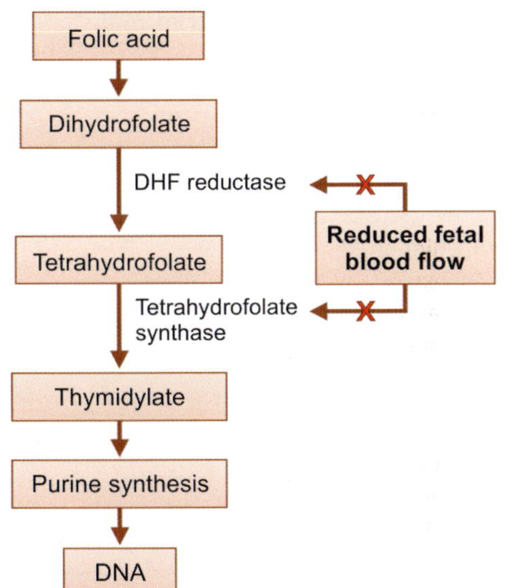

Flowchart 31.1: Mechanism of action

Dose of MTX for GTN with Modified WHO Prognostic Scoring ≤6

1. MTX—1 mg/kg or 50 mg/m², intramuscular single dose followed by inj. folinic acid 0.1 mg/kg, IM.

2. 8-day alternate regimen: MTX—1 mg/m², IM, given on days 1, 3, 5 and 7 (better response rate) with leucovorin (folinic acid)—leucoverin rescue therapy.
   It is folic acid in its reduced form which allows nucleic acid synthesis to proceed even in presence of MTX. It prevents excessive toxic side effects of MTX.
   Dose—0.1 mg/kg, IV, on days 2, 4, 6, 8.

3. Daily (5-day regimen)—IM or IV, 0.4 mg/kg/day.

Investigations: Before starting MTX therapy—complete blood count, blood group, liver function tests, serum creatinine.

Side effects: These are usually seen on the gastrointestinal tract and the bone marrow, which usually correct within 10 to 14 days.

These include stomatitis, alopecia, dermatitis, allergic interstitial pneumonitis, pericarditis nephrotoxicity, diarrhea, myelosuppression (neutropenia, thrombocytopenia), defective oogenesis and abortion.

Methotrexate teratogenicity—craniofacial abnormalities.

Side effects higher with 8-day regimen compared with weekly regimen.

Contraindications to MTX therapy
- Lactating women
- Peptic ulcer
- Acute pulmonary disease
- Anemia, leucopenia, thrombocytopenia
- Immunodeficiency

Drug interactions: Renal clearance of MTX is decreased by non-steroidal anti-inflammatory drugs (NSAIDs), probenicid, penicillin. Thus, can give lower dose of MTX.

Tetracyclines, salicylates, sulfonamide, multivitamins, folic acid, decrease action of MTX. Thus, higher dose needed in their presence.

ACTINOMYCIN D

Origin: Drug comes from bacteria *Streptomyces parvulus*.

Mechanism of action: Intercalation of DNA and stabalisation of cleavable complexes of topoisomerase I and II with DNA.

Dose: Single dose 1.25 mg every 2 weeks or biweekly pulse therapy.

Side effects: Alopecia, grade-4 toxicity.

CHEMOTHERAPY FOR HIGH-RISK GTN (WHO PROGNOSTIC SCORING >7)[3]

Etoposide, methotrexate, actinomycin-D, cyclophosphamide, vincristine (oncovin)— EMACO Regimen.

EMA—day 1
EA—day 2
CO—day 8

Course repeated in 14–21 days, till hCG normalizes and 6 weeks after that.

Cases refractory to EMACO regimen or relapse with EMACO:

1. Etoposide, methotrexate, actinomycin-D, etoposide, cisplatin (EMA-EP)
2. Etoposide, methotrexate, actinomycin-D, paclitaxel, cisplatin (EMA-TP)
3. Etoposide, methotrexate, actinomycin-D, paclitaxel, etoposide (EMA-TE)
4. Bleomycin, etoposide, cisplatin (BEP).

References

1. Hoffman Bl, Schorge JO, Halvorson LM, Hamid CA, Corton MM, Schaffer JI, Gestational trophoblastic diseases, Williams Textbook of Gynecology, McGraw Hill, 2021;4th ed.: 774–790.
2. Chu E, Cancer Chemotherapy. In: Katzung BG, Vanderah TW editors. Basic and Clinical Pharmacology, 15thed, McGraw Hill Lange, 2021;948–977.
3. Management of Gestational Trophoblastic Disease, RCOG Green-top guideline no. 38, Sept 2020.

Index